Goat Medicine and Surgery

Goat Medicine and Surgery

DAVID HARWOOD BVETMED FRCVS

Chairman Goat Veterinary Society
Honorary Veterinary Surgeon, British Goat Society
Visiting Reader in Veterinary Field Pathology, Department of Pathology and Infectious Diseases
School of Veterinary Medicine, University of Surrey
Guildford, UK
Formerly Veterinary Investigation Officer, Animal and Plant Health Agency, UK

KARIN MUELLER MVSC DCHP DIPECBHM MRCVS

RCVS and European Diplomate & Specialist in Cattle/Bovine Health
Senior Lecturer Animal Husbandry & Reproduction
Institute of Veterinary Science, University of Liverpool
Liverpool, UK

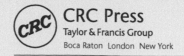

CRC Press
Taylor & Francis Group
Boca Raton London New York

CRC Press is an imprint of the
Taylor & Francis Group, an **informa** business

CRC Press
Taylor & Francis Group
6000 Broken Sound Parkway NW, Suite 300
Boca Raton, FL 33487-2742

First issued in paperback 2020

ISBN-13: 978-1-4987-4863-6 (hbk)
ISBN-13: 978-0-367-89342-2 (pbk)

Library of Congress Cataloging-in-Publication Data

Names: Harwood, David, BVM, author. | Mueller, Karin, author.
Title: Goat medicine and surgery / David Harwood and Karin Mueller.
Description: Boca Raton : CRC Press, [2018]
Identifiers: LCCN 2017034019 (print) | LCCN 2017035549 (ebook) | ISBN 9781315152233 (Master eBook) | ISBN 9781498748636 (hardback : alk. paper)
Subjects: LCSH: Goats--Diseases. | MESH: Goat Diseases
Classification: LCC SF968 (ebook) | LCC SF968 .H27 2018 (print) | NLM SF 968 | DDC 636.3/90896--dc23
LC record available at https://lccn.loc.gov/2017034019

Visit the Taylor & Francis Web site at
http://www.taylorandfrancis.com

and the CRC Press Web site at
http://www.crcpress.com

CONTENTS

Preface		xix
Abbreviations		xxi

CHAPTER **1**	**INTRODUCTION**	**1**
	EVOLUTION	1
	GOAT BREEDS AND THEIR PURPOSES	3
	GENOMICS	3
	BEHAVIOUR	4
	NUTRITION	7
	ENVIRONMENT	11
	Housing	11
	Fencing	12
	Tethering	12
	HANDLING	12
	PHYSIOLOGY AND BODY FEATURES	13
	Lactation	13
	Horns	13
	Coat	13
	Wattles	14
	Weight	14
	Longevity	14
	HISTORY TAKING AND CLINICAL EXAMINATION	14
	Farm related history of interest	14
	For the individual animal, history of interest	14
	Basic clinical examination	14
	ADMINISTERING MEDICATION	15
	Oral administration	15
	Subcutaneous injection	16
	Intramuscular injection	16
	Intravenous injection and catheterisation	17
	Intraperitoneal injection	18
	Subconjunctival injection	18
	ROUTINE PROCEDURES AND HEALTH PLANNING	18
	BIOSECURITY	18
	LEGISLATION	20

CHAPTER 2	**REPRODUCTIVE SYSTEM**	**21**
	THE DOE	**21**
	NORMAL STRUCTURE AND FUNCTION	21
	FERTILITY	21
	FECUNDITY	22
	OESTROUS CYCLE AND SIGNS OF OESTRUS	22
	CONTROL OF OESTRUS	23
	Out-of-season breeding	23
	Synchronisation during the breeding season	23
	OVARIAN DISORDERS	24
	Anoestrus	24
	Cystic ovarian disease	25
	BREEDING	25
	Natural service	25
	Artificial insemination	26
	Embryo transfer	27
	Pregnancy diagnosis	28
	Misalliance	28
	UTERINE DISORDERS	28
	Anatomical abnormalities – congenital	28
	Anatomical abnormalities – acquired	29
	Endometritis	30
	Uterine neoplasia	31
	HERD INFERTILITY PROBLEM	32
	INFECTIOUS DISEASES	32
	Caprine herpesvirus 1	32
	EMBRYONIC LOSS AND ABORTION	33
	ABORTION	34
	Common infectious causes of abortion	**35**
	Toxoplasmosis	35
	Chlamydiosis (syns. enzootic abortion, ovine enzootic abortion)	36
	Q fever	38
	Brucellosis	39
	Listeriosis	40
	Less common infectious causes of abortion	**41**
	Salmonellosis	41
	Neosporosis	42
	Tick-borne fever	42
	Arbovirus infections	42
	Campylobacter infection	42
	Leptospirosis	43
	Border disease virus/bovine viral diarrhoea virus (BDV/BVDV)	43
	Caprine herpesvirus	43
	Rift Valley fever	43
	Maceration – non-specific	43

Non-infectious causes of abortion   **43**
Pharmacological products   43
Toxicity   44
Vitamin/mineral deficiencies   44
Malnutrition/pregnancy toxaemia   44
Habitual abortion in Angora goats   44
Mummification – non-specific   44
THE BUCK   **45**
NORMAL STRUCTURE AND FUNCTION   45
OUT-OF-SEASON BREEDING   45
Indications   45
Technique   45
EXAMINATION FOR BREEDING SOUNDNESS   45
Indications   45
Aetiology   46
History   47
Physical examination   47
Genital tract examination   47
Semen evaluation   47
TESTICULAR AND EPIDIDYMAL ABNORMALITIES   49
Testicular hypoplasia   49
Testicular degeneration or atrophy   49
Orchitis and epididymitis   50
Cryptorchism (syn. retained gonad)   51
ACCESSORY SEX GLAND DISORDERS   52
PENIS AND PREPUCE ABNORMALITIES   52
Penile deviation   52
Penile trauma   53
Phimosis and paraphimosis   54
Balanoposthitis   54
Neoplasia of the male reproductive tract   55
CASTRATION   56
VASECTOMY   57
TEMPORARY SUPPRESSION OF FERTILITY   59
OTHER MALE DISORDERS   59
Gynaecomastia   59
Venereal disease   59

CHAPTER **3**   **PREGNANCY AND PARTURITION**   **61**

PREGNANCY   61
Pregnancy diagnosis   61
PREPARTUM PROBLEMS   63
Hypocalcaemia and pregnancy toxaemia   63
Mummification, maceration and fetal maldevelopment   63
Pseudopregnancy (syns. cloudburst, hydrometra)   63

Hydrops uteri   64
Vaginal and cervical prolapse   65
Rupture or herniation of the uterus   66
Induction of parturition   67
Ante-natal preparation   67
PARTURITION   67
   Normal parturition   67
   Dystocia   68
   Failure of cervical dilation (syn. ringwomb)   70
   Uterine torsion   71
   Caesarean section   72
   Fetotomy   75
POST-PARTURIENT PROBLEMS   77
   Haemorrhage   77
   Laceration of the cervix   77
   Laceration of the vagina   78
   Recto-vaginal fistula   78
   Vaginal prolapse – post-parturient   79
   Uterine rupture   79
   Uterine prolapse   79
   Retained fetal membranes   81
   Metritis   82
   Necrotic vaginitis   84
   Bladder eversion or herniation   84

CHAPTER 4   **NEONATOLOGY**   **85**

INTRODUCTION   85
WEAK NEWBORN KIDS   85
   Congenital abnormalities   85
   Genetic abnormalities   85
   Developmental insult abnormalities   85
   Mineral shortfall abnormalities   86
   Known heritable abnormalities   86
RESPIRATION   86
   Normal adaptation   86
   Asphyxia   86
CARDIAC FUNCTION AND CIRCULATION   88
   Normal adaptation   88
   Absent heartbeat   88
   Cardiovascular defects   88
THERMOREGULATION   89
   Normal adaptation   89
   Hypothermia   89

IMMUNE SYSTEM   90
   Normal adaptation   90
   Failure of passive transfer   91
   Neonatal septicaemia (syn. sepsis)   93
GASTROINTESTINAL TRACT   95
   Normal adaptation   95
   Hypoglycaemia   95
   Meconium retention   96
   Atresia ani, recti or coli   96
   Cleft palate (syn. palatoschisis)   97
URINARY FUNCTION   97
   Normal adaptation   97
   Urine retention   97
MUSCULOSKELETAL FUNCTION   98
   Normal adaptation   98
   Contracted tendons   98
   Flexor tendon laxity   99
   Arthrogryposis   99
   White muscle disease   100
METABOLIC DISORDERS   100
   Neonatal acidosis   100
   Floppy-kid syndrome   100
   Beta-mannosidosis   101
   Iodine deficiency (congenital hyperplastic goitre)   101
NEUROLOGICAL FUNCTION   101
   Normal adaptation   101
   Congenital central nervous system abnormalities   102
   Congenital swayback   102
MISCELLANEOUS   102
   Neonatal maladjustment syndrome   102
   Prematurity   103
   Low birth weights   103
   Sticky kid disease   104
ARTIFICIAL REARING   104
   Fostering   104
   Supplementing   104
   Routine artificial rearing   105

CHAPTER 5   **DIGESTIVE TRACT AND ABDOMEN**   **109**

CLINICAL EXAMINATION OF THE DIGESTIVE SYSTEM   109
   Oral and dental examination   109
   Abdominal examination   109
   Ancillary diagnostics   111

NON-INFECTIOUS DISEASES OF THE DIGESTIVE TRACT AND ABDOMEN   114

Dental problems   **114**
    Normal structure and function   114
    Mandibular brachygnathia and prognathia (syns. underbite/overbite)   115
    Dental disease   115

Oral problems (excluding dental)   **118**
    Normal structure and function   118
    Neoplasia   118
    Drenching/bolus gun injury   119
    Tongue lesions   120

Oesophageal problems   **120**
    Megaoesophagus   120
    Obstruction (syn. choke)   121

Forestomach problems   **121**
    Normal structure and function   121
    Rumen tympany (syn. bloat)   121
    Rumen acidosis (syn. carbohydrate overload)   122
    Traumatic reticuloperitonitis   124

Surgery of the rumen   **124**
    Trocarisation   124
    Rumen fistula   124
    Rumenotomy   124

Abomasal problems   **125**
    Normal structure and function   125
    Abomasal emptying defect (syns. pyloric stenosis,
      abomasal impaction, distal vagal indigestion)   125
    Abomasal displacement   126
    Abomasal ulceration   127
    Abomasitis (syn. abomasal bloat)   128

Intestinal problems   **130**
    Normal structure and function   130
    Intussusception   130
    Torsion of the mesentery or mesenteric root   131
    Intestinal obstruction   132
    Rectal prolapse   132
    Exploratory laparotomy   134

Liver and pancreas problems   **136**
    Normal structure and function   136
    Liver abscessation   136
    Hepatic lipidosis (syn. fatty liver necrosis)   136
    Ovine white liver disease   136
    Metastatic tumours   136

Pancreatic disorders   **136**

Umbilical disorders   **137**
    Normal structure and function   137
    Umbilical hernia   137

Umbilical infections 138
Patent urachus 139
Umbilical surgery 139
INFECTIOUS DISEASES OF THE DIGESTIVE SYSTEM AND ABDOMEN 142
Rotavirus 142
Cryptosporidiosis 142
Coccidiosis 144
Escherichia coli 146
Salmonellosis 147
Yersiniosis 148
Clostridium perfringens (syn. enterotoxaemia) 149
Johne's disease (syn. paratuberculosis) 151
Parasitic gastroenteritis 153
Liver fluke (syns. fascioliasis, fasciolosis) 159
Small liver fluke (syn. lancet fluke) 160
Tapeworms (cestodes) 160
Metacestode disease 161
Peste des petits ruminants (syn. goat plague) 161
Bluetongue 163
Miscellaneous conditions 163

CHAPTER 6   RESPIRATORY SYSTEM 165

NORMAL STRUCTURE AND FUNCTION 165
CLINICAL EXAMINATION OF THE RESPIRATORY SYSTEM 165
General aspects 165
Specific observations 165
Ancillary diagnostics 167
TREATMENT PRINCIPLES 167
Tracheotomy 167
NON-INFECTIOUS DISEASES OF THE RESPIRATORY SYSTEM 169
Conditions affecting the nasal passages and sinuses 169
Laryngeal problems 169
Aspiration pneumonia 170
Pleural effusion 170
Pneumothorax 171
Toxicities 171
Neoplasia 172
INFECTIOUS DISEASES OF THE RESPIRATORY SYSTEM 172
Contagious caprine pleuropneumonia 172
Pasteurellosis 173
Parasitic pneumonia 174
MISCELLANEOUS CONDITIONS 176
Other Mycoplasma organisms 176
Peste des petits ruminants (syn. goat plague) 176
Caprine arthritis encephalitis 176

	Caseous lymphadenitis	176
	Tuberculosis	176
	Fungal pneumonia/allergic pneumonitis	176
	Vena cava thrombosis	177

CHAPTER 7 — CARDIOVASCULAR DISEASE AND DISORDERS OF THE HAEMATOPOIETIC SYSTEM — 179

	NORMAL STRUCTURE AND FUNCTION	179
	CLINICAL EXAMINATION OF THE CARDIOVASCULAR SYSTEM	179
	Clinical assessment	179
	Ancillary diagnosis	180
	Blood sampling and basic in-house analysis	180
	CARDIOVASCULAR DISEASE	181
	Septal defects	181
	Endocarditis	182
	Pericarditis	183
	Cardiomyopathies	184
	Other conditions	185
	DISORDERS OF BLOOD VESSELS	185
	Venous thrombosis	185
	Caudal vena cava thrombosis	186
	Other vascular abnormalities	187
	DISORDERS OF THE HAEMATOPOIETIC SYSTEM	187
	Normal structure and function	187
	Anaemia	187
	Milk goitre/thymic enlargement	189
	Neoplasia of lymph nodes or thymus	190
	Swelling disease	191
	Caseous lymphadenitis	191
	Babesiosis	193

CHAPTER 8 — NERVOUS SYSTEM DISORDERS — 195

	CLINICAL EXAMINATION OF THE NERVOUS SYSTEM	195
	Consciousness, alertness and behaviour	195
	Reflexes, upper motor neurons and lower motor neurons	195
	Vestibular syndrome	197
	Spinal lesions	197
	Peripheral nerves	197
	Specific assessment considerations	198
	Cerebrospinal fluid collection and analysis	199
	Imaging and further diagnostics	201
	NON-INFECTIOUS DISEASES	201
	Central nervous system	**201**
	Disbudding injury	201
	Acquired storage disease	201

Inherited central nervous system disorders 202
Swayback (syn. enzootic ataxia) 202
Polioencephalomalacia (syn. cerebrocortical necrosis) 202
Floppy kid syndrome 204
Peripheral nervous system **204**
Peripheral nerve paralysis 204
INFECTIOUS DISEASES 206
Listerial encephalitis 206
Bacterial meningitis/encephalitis 208
Tetanus 209
Enterotoxaemia 210
Scrapie and bovine spongiform encephalopathy 210
Rabies 212
Aujeszky's disease (syn. pseudorabies) 212
Caprine arthritis encephalitis 213
Louping ill 213
Coenurosis (syn. gid) 213
Cerebrospinal nematodiasis (syn. meningeal worm) 214

CHAPTER **9** **MUSCULOSKELETAL DISEASE INCLUDING FOOT DISORDERS** 215

CLINICAL EXAMINATION OF THE MUSCULOSKELETAL SYSTEM 215
Clinical assessment 215
Ancillary diagnosis 216
NON-INFECTIOUS DISEASES 217
Nutritional muscular dystrophy/white muscle disease 217
Rickets 217
Osteodystrophy of mature bone 218
Fractures 219
Bone sequestrum 221
Joint dislocation 223
Tendon injuries 223
Cartilage disorders 224
INFECTIOUS DISEASES 225
Caprine arthritis encephalitis 225
Bacterial arthritis (syn. joint ill) 227
Mycoplasma arthritis 228
Clostridial myositis 229
Arbovirus infection (Akabane, Schmallenberg) 229
FOOT DISORDERS 229
Laminitis 229
Scald and footrot 230
Treponeme-associated foot disease 232
Overgrown claws 233
Routine foot trimming 233
White line disease 234

Pedal joint abscess 235
Foreign bodies and foot lameness 235
Foot and mouth disease 235

| CHAPTER 10 | **URINARY TRACT DISEASE** | **237** |

NORMAL STRUCTURE AND FUNCTION 237
CLINICAL EXAMINATION OF THE URINARY TRACT 237
    Clinical assessment 237
    Ancillary diagnostics 237
NON-INFECTIOUS DISEASES 240
    Urethral obstruction caused by urolithiasis 240
    Urethrotomy and urethrostomy 242
    Tube cystotomy 243
    Renal insufficiency and failure 244
    Toxic nephrosis 245
    Neoplasia 245
INFECTIOUS DISEASES 245
    Cystitis and pyelonephritis 245

| CHAPTER 11 | **SKIN DISEASES** | **249** |

CLINICAL EXAMINATION OF THE SKIN AND INTEGUMENT 249
    Clinical assessment 249
    Ancillary diagnostics 249
NON-INFECTIOUS SKIN DISEASES 250
    Pemphigus foliaceus 250
    Zinc deficiency (zinc-responsive dermatosis) 250
    Pygmy goat syndrome (syn. seborrhoeic dermatitis) 251
    Photosensitisation 252
    Physical and toxic causes 253
    Fibre break or loss 253
    Hypotrichosis 253
INFECTIOUS SKIN DISEASES (PARASITIC) 253
    Chorioptic mange 253
    Sarcoptic mange 255
    Demodectic mange 256
    Psoroptic mange 257
    Lice 257
    Ticks 258
    Flies 258
    Insect bite reactions 260
    Besnoitiosis 260
INFECTIOUS SKIN DISEASES (VIRAL/BACTERIAL/FUNGAL) 260
    Contagious pustular dermatitis (syns. orf, contagious ecthyma) 260
    Goat pox 262

Bluetongue   263
Peste des petitis ruminants   263
Foot and mouth disease   263
Aujeszky's disease (syn. pseudorabies)   263
Staphylococcal dermatitis/folliculitis   263
Malassezia   264
Mycotic dermatitis (syns. dermatophilosis, streptothricosis)   264
Ringworm (syn. dermatophytosis)   265
CUTANEOUS SWELLINGS   265
Caseous lymphadenitis   265
Morel's disease   265
Lymphoma   265
Neoplasia   265
Thymus enlargement   266
Haematoma   266
Injection site abscesses   266
SURGERY OF SKIN ADNEXA   267
Disbudding   267
Dehorning   267

CHAPTER 12   **MAMMARY GLAND DISORDERS**   271

NORMAL STRUCTURE AND FUNCTION   271
CLINICAL EXAMINATION OF THE UDDER   271
Sampling for culture   272
Ultrasonography   272
NON-INFECTIOUS DISEASES   272
Trauma   272
Neoplasia   272
Enlarged pendulous udder   272
Maiden milkers   272
Post-partum agalactia   273
Induction of lactation   273
INFECTIOUS DISEASES   274
Contagious agalactia   274
Mastitis   275
Udder impetigo (syn. staphylococcal folliculitis of the udder)   281
SURGERY OF THE MAMMARY GLAND   281
Supernumerary teat removal   281
Teat surgery   282
Mastectomy   283

CHAPTER 13   **SENSORY ORGAN DISEASE**   285

THE EYE   **285**
NORMAL STRUCTURE AND FUNCTION   285

CLINICAL EXAMINATION OF THE EYE   285
  Further diagnostics   286
FIRST AID FOR OCULAR TRAUMA   287
NON-INFECTIOUS DISEASE   287
  Entropion   287
  Foreign bodies   288
  Corneal ulceration and stromal abscessation   289
  Neoplasia   290
INFECTIOUS DISEASE   291
  Infectious keratoconjunctivitis (syn. pink eye)   291
  Uveitis and iritis   293
OCULAR SURGERY   293
  Tarsorrhaphy   293
  Third eyelid flap   293
  Conjunctival pedicle flap   294
  Enucleation   294
SYSTEMIC DISEASES AFFECTING THE EYE   295
THE EAR   **295**
CLINICAL EXAMINATION OF THE EAR   295
NON-INFECTIOUS DISEASE   295
  Ear lacerations   295
  Tagging injuries   296
  Aural haematoma   296
INFECTIOUS DISEASE   297
  Otitis   297
  Ear tip necrosis   298

CHAPTER **14**   **METABOLIC DISORDERS**   **299**

  Hypocalcaemia (syns. milk fever, eclampsia, parturient paresis)   299
  Hypomagnesaemia (syns. grass tetany, grass staggers)   300
  Pregnancy toxaemia   301
  Lactational ketosis (syn. acetonaemia) and fatty liver complex   303
  Metabolic acidosis   304
  Floppy kid syndrome   304
  Swelling disease in Angora goats   304

CHAPTER **15**   **TRACE ELEMENT AND VITAMIN DISORDERS**   **305**

TRACE ELEMENTS   305
  Copper deficiency   306
  Selenium/tocopherol (vitamin E) deficiency
    (syns. nutritional muscular dystrophy, white muscle disease)   308
  Cobalt deficiency   309
  Iodine deficiency   310
  Zinc deficiency   311

VITAMINS   311
    Retinol (vitamin A) deficiency   311
    Thiamine (vitamin B1) deficiency   311
    Cyanocobalamin (vitamin B12) deficiency   312
    Calciferol (vitamin D) deficiency   312
    Tocopherol (vitamin E) deficiency   312

CHAPTER 16   POISONING AND TOXICITIES   313

INTRODUCTION   313
GENERAL APPROACH   313
COMMON POISONS AND TOXINS   314
    Genus *Rhododendron*   314
    Yew   315
    Other plants, trees and shrubs potentially toxic to goats   316
    Oxalate poisoning   316
    Nitrate poisoning   317
    Copper poisoning   318
    Urea poisoning   319
    Mycotoxins   319
    Water source poisons   321

CHAPTER 17   EXOTIC AND EMERGING DISEASES   323

INTRODUCTION   323
    Foot and mouth disease (aphthous fever)   323
    Bluetongue   326
    Tuberculosis   328
    Anthrax   329
    New and emerging diseases   330

CHAPTER 18   ANAESTHESIA, FLUID THERAPY, EUTHANASIA   333

SEDATION   333
    General principles   333
    Sedatives   333
    Reversal   334
GENERAL ANAESTHESIA   334
    General principles   334
    Preoperative starvation   334
    Preoperative assessment   334
    Intraoperative support   334
    Hypothermia   334
    Induction   335
    Inhalation anaesthesia   335
    Injection anaesthesia   335

Monitoring	336
Recovery	336
LOCAL AND REGIONAL BLOCKS	336
General principles	336
Drugs	337
Specific blocks	337
ANALGESIA	341
General principles	341
Opioids	341
Non-steroidal anti-inflammatory drugs	342
Corticosteroids	342
NMDA receptor antagonists	342
FLUID THERAPY	342
Assessing hydration status	342
Fluid rates	343
Route of administration	343
Choice of fluids	343
EUTHANASIA	344
Lethal injection	344
Free-bullet firearms	344
Captive bolt	345
Conditionally acceptable methods	345
Emergency on-farm slaughter of neonatal kids	345
Unacceptable methods	346
CHAPTER 19 **POST-MORTEM EXAMINATION AND SAMPLING**	**347**
INTRODUCTION	347
HISTORY	347
HEALTH AND SAFETY	348
PREPARATION	348
POST-MORTEM EXAMINATION APPROACH	348
SAMPLING PROTOCOLS	351
Bacteriology	351
Histopathology	351
Aborted goat kids	352
APPENDICES	**353**
1 LABORATORY REFERENCE INTERVALS	353
2 CONVERSION FACTORS	355
3 FURTHER READING	356
INDEX	**357**

One of the main objectives in writing *Goat Medicine and Surgery* was to bring together in a single text all the medical and surgical considerations when faced with a goat health or welfare problem, be it a single emergency procedure or a long-standing herd problem. The book begins by providing the reader with some background information on goat evolution, behaviour, nutrition and basic physiology, and is then divided into a series of chapters dealing with individual conditions based on body systems including reproduction.

Each chapter highlights relevant aspects of the specific clinical examination, giving guidance on baseline clinical and physiological parameters and the ancillary diagnostic tools that may be available, such as relevant laboratory tests and ultrasonography or radiography. Each condition is then described in a consistent format, covering its aetiology, pathophysiology, presenting signs, diagnosis, differential diagnosis, treatment, management and control.

The book is richly illustrated with over 450 images. Expansions for abbreviations used in the text are listed on page xxi.

Anaesthetic procedures and surgical and other interventions are dealt with in a structured format and, where possible, within the relevant chapter. Miscellaneous procedures such as fluid therapy, euthanasia and post-mortem examination are also covered.

Although written by two UK based authors, the book provides a comprehensive overview of goat health and welfare and the diseases and conditions to which they are susceptible around the world. It will be a useful addition to the library of veterinarians, undergraduate students and anyone interested in understanding and improving goat health.

David Harwood
Karin Mueller

ACDP	Advisory Committee on Dangerous Pathogens	CT	computed tomography
		CV	cardiovascular
AI	artificial insemination	DJD	degenerative joint disease
ALD	angular limb deformity	DGGE	denaturing gradient gel electrophoresis
ALP	alkaline phosphatase	DM	dry matter (diet)
AST	aspartate transaminase/aspartate aminotransferase	EAE	enzootic abortion of ewes (see OEA)
		EBV	estimated breeding value
BAER	brainstem auditory evoked response	ECF	extracellular fluid
BD	border disease	eCG	equine chorionic gonadotropin
BDV	border disease virus	ECG	electrocardiography
BHB	beta-hydroxybutyrate	EDTA	ethylenediamine tetra-acetic acid
BCS	body condition score	EEJ	electroejaculation
BPD	biparietal diameter	EHEC	enterohaemorrhagic *E. coli*
bpm	beats per minute (heart); breaths per minute (lungs)	ELISA	enzyme-linked immunosorbent assay
		EMG	electromyography
BSE	bovine spongiform encephalopathy	EPEC	enteropathogenic *E. coli*
BTV	bluetongue virus	epg	eggs per gram
BVD	bovine viral diarrhoea	ET	embryo transfer; endotracheal (tube).
BVDV	bovine viral diarrhoea virus	ETEC	enterotoxigenic *E. coli*
CAE	caprine arthritis encephalitis	EU	European Union
CAEV	caprine arthritis encephalitis virus	FB	foreign body
CCN	cerebrocortical necrosis (see PEM)	FEC	faecal egg count
CCPP	contagious caprine pleuropneumonia	FMD	foot and mouth disease
CIDR	controlled internal drug release (intravaginal progesterone releasing device)	FSH	follicle stimulating hormone
		GA	general anaesthesia
		gGT	gamma-glutamyl transferase (liver function test)
CK	creatinine kinase (measure of muscle pathology)	GI	gastrointestinal
		GLDH	glutamate dehydrogenase (liver function test)
CL	corpus luteum		
CLA	caseous lymphadenitis	GnRH	gonadotropin-releasing hormone
CMT	California mastitis test	GSH-Px	glutathione peroxidase (a selenium dependent enzyme)
CNS	central nervous system		
COD	cystic ovarian disease		
CODD	contagious ovine digital dermatitis	Hb	haemoglobin
CP	crude protein	hCG	human chorionic gonadotropin
CPD	contagious pustular dermatitis (orf)	HCl	hydrochloride
CpHV-1	caprine herpesvirus 1	Hct	haematocrit
CRI	constant rate infusion	IFAT	indirect fluorescent antibody test
CRT	capillary refill time	Ig	immunoglobulin (IgA, IgE, IgG, IgM)
CSF	cerebrospinal fluid	IKC	infectious keratoconjunctivitis

i/m	intramuscular
IOP	intraocular pressure
i/p	intraperitoneal
i/v	intravenous
ISR	injection site reaction
IU	International unit
IVRA	intravenous regional anaesthesia
KOH	potassium hydroxide
L1	first-stage larvae – also L2, L3 (nematode life cycle)
LDH	lactate dehydrogenase
LH	luteinising hormone
LMN	lower motor neurone
MAP	*Mycobacterium paratuberculosis* subsp. *paratuberculosis*
MCH	mean corpuscular haemoglobin
MCHC	mean corpuscular haemoglobin concentration
MCV	mean corpuscular volume
mEq	milliequivalent
MGA	megestrol acetate
MHz	megahertz
MJ ME	megajoules of metabolisable energy
ML	macrocyclic lactone (includes the avermectins and the milbemycins)
MRI	magnetic resonance imaging
MTB	*Mycobacterium tuberculosis*
MV	maedi visna (sheep)
MZN	modified Ziehl–Neelsen
NaCl	sodium chloride
NaHCO$_3$	sodium bicarbonate
NDF	neutral detergent fibre (in diet)
NEB	negative energy balance
NO$_2$	nitrogen dioxide
NSAID	non-steroidal anti-inflammatory drug
NTEC	necrotoxigenic *E. coli*
OC	osteochondrosis
OD	outer diameter (tubing); optical density (laboratory test results)
OEA	ovine enzootic abortion (see EAE)
Off-cascade	Relating to use of drugs. The UK veterinary prescription cascade can not be applied to such drugs
Off-licence	Relating to use of drugs. Such drugs are licensed in food producing animals, but for any of: a different species, another indication, another route of administration, another dose rate

OIE	World Organisation for Animal Health (formerly Office International des Epizooties)
OWLD	ovine white liver disease
PAGE	polyacrilamide gel electrophoresis
PCR	polymerase chain reaction
PCV	packed cell volume
PDA	patent ductus arteriosus
PDS	polydioxanone
PEM	polioencephalomalacia (see CCN)
PGE	parasitic gastroenteritis
PGF$_{2\alpha}$	prostaglandin-F 2 alpha
PME	post-mortem examination
PMI	point of maximum intensity
PO$_2$	partial pressure of oxygen
PPR	Peste des petits ruminants
PPV	positive pressure ventilation
PrP	prion protein
PSP	phenolsulphonphthalein
RAMALT	rectoanal mucosa-associated lymphoid tissue
RFM	retained fetal membranes
SAP	serum alkaline phosphatase
SARA	subacute ruminal acidosis
s/c	subcutaneous
SCC	somatic cell count; squamous cell carcinoma
SDH	sorbitol dehydrogenase (liver enzyme)
SICCT	single intradermal comparative cervical test
SRLV	small ruminant lentivirus
T3	triiodothyronine
T4	thyroxine
TB	tuberculosis
TBC	total bacterial count
TLC	'tender loving care'
TMR	total mixed ration
TP	total protein
TSE	transmissible spongiform encephalopathy.
WBCC	white blood cell count
UHT	ultra-high temperature (usually referring to high temperature processing of e.g. milk)
UK	United Kingdom
UMN	upper motor neurone
US/USA	United States of America
UV	ultraviolet
ZN	Ziehl–Neelsen

CHAPTER 1

INTRODUCTION

EVOLUTION

Goats are one of the earliest examples of a domesticated animal. Around 12,000 to 14,000 years ago, our Neolithic ancestors began the process of domestication of the arable crops and livestock resources available to them at that time. It is this process that underpins what we recognise today as our modern agricultural and farming practices. Approximately 40 distinct livestock species have been domesticated, but only six species are currently found on all continents, namely goats, cattle, sheep, pigs, horses and donkeys.

Archaeological records can give us some indication of timescales, with the goat exhibiting the earliest signs of domestication around 10,000 years BP. BP is the abbreviation for the archaeological term 'before present', which is based on the year 1950 when carbon dating first became widely available. For comparison, these same records show sheep domestication at 8,500 years BP and cattle at 7,000 years BP. All figures refer to the earliest archaeological evidence of domestication based on the circumstances in which such evidence was found. The oldest goat remains indicative of domestication were found in Iran, but the process appears to have fanned out from there to the near and middle east and the northern Indian subcontinent.

Records suggest that modern goats have all evolved from the wild Bezoar goat (or Bezoar Ibex) of the Zagros Mountains in Iran and Iraq, a species still found in the region today.

The key elements to domestication include:

- Breeding in captivity with control of the breeding cycle.
- Modification to make them more useful/productive.
- Provision of shelter from predators and the environment.
- Provision of food.

From a domestication perspective, goats are without doubt the best example of a multipurpose species, providing the following benefits for those who have domesticated them:

- Milk.
- Meat.
- Skins to keep warm, for carrying water (and wine), as flotation devices for crossing water.
- Fibre for clothing.
- Dried faeces for fuel.
- Transport through pulling small carts.
- Goat kid skin used as parchment.

As a result of domestication and a much closer contact between our ancestors and the species they began to 'keep', it is hardly surprising that goats began to feature in many other aspects of their lives, and goats have regularly been referred to in the arts, mythology, the bible and common folklore.

Following this early domestication, goats today are one of the most widely kept domestic animals worldwide, mainly as a result of the relative ease with which they can be kept and the obvious benefits provided to those who keep them. In 2011, it was estimated that there were more than 924 million live goats around the globe, according to the UN Food and Agriculture Organization. The largest population is in China, with an estimated 149 million goats making up around 16% of the total world goat population. India follows with approximately 125.7 million and Pakistan with 56.7 million, followed by Bangladesh, Nigeria, Sudan, Ethiopia, Iran, Mongolia and Indonesia. According to 2012 data there are just over 2.6 million goats in the USA, heavily concentrated in the south west, particularly in Texas. Australia reports between 3 and 4 million goats, of which only around 0.4 million are farmed, the remainder being referred to as range or 'free living' goats. Within Europe, Greece has the largest population of around 5 million, followed by Spain (3 million) and France (1 million). The UK has a relatively small population of around 100,000.

The evolution of goat keeping will vary from country to country. In the UK, for example, many families kept one or more 'house goats', to produce

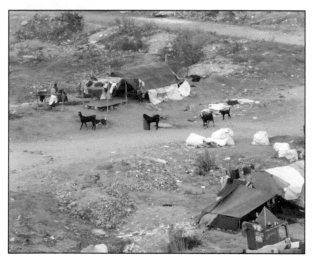

Fig. 1.1 **Nomadic goats in India.**

milk for their own consumption. This practice began to decline towards the end of the 18th century with the Enclosure Movement, which effectively began to place what was formerly common land into private ownership. The availability of common land then declined as it was fenced off and farmed. From the late 19th century through to around 1940, goat keeping was mainly confined to rural families and those with poorly paid jobs such as miners and railwaymen. Due to the need for food and the effects of food rationing during the Second World War, goat keeping did enter a period of growth, but there was then a gradual decline after the war ended. The British Goat Society (holding the pedigree goat herd books) was founded in 1879, and with the exception of the Hereford cattle herd book is the oldest such record in the UK.

Modern goat keeping gives us a full spectrum of activity from nomadic tribes moving from location to location with their animals, to the range keeping activities in Australia, to units fattening goat kids for meat and to intensive goat dairy production systems in which several thousand goats are housed and milked through highly automated parlours. Alongside these production systems are those in which goats are kept in small numbers as a hobby, as pets and at public attractions where their docile and inquisitive behaviour make them popular with all ages (**Figs. 1.1–1.3**).

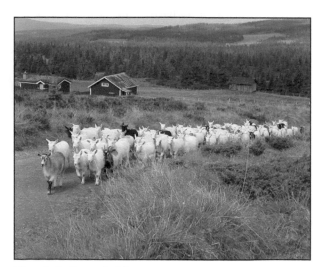

Fig. 1.2 **Goats in Norway.**

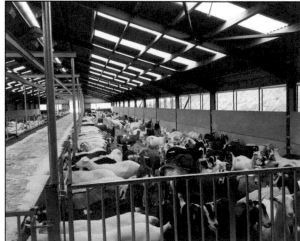

Fig. 1.3 **Intensive dairy goat farming in the UK. Note the high stocking rate and raised feeding table.**

This background information gives the reader an insight into the wide range of environmental, management and socio-economic factors that have an influence on goat health and welfare worldwide, each of which needs to be considered when arriving at a diagnosis and formulating therapeutic and prophylactic regimes.

GOAT BREEDS AND THEIR PURPOSES

The goat is a member of the family Bovidae and is closely related to the sheep, as both are in the goat-antelope subfamily Caprinae. Goats (genus *Capra*) have 60 chromosomes and sheep (genus *Ovis*) have 54. Goats and sheep can very rarely breed with each other, and although most offspring will be stillborn, there are a number of reports of offspring surviving with a chromosome count of 57. Such offspring are often referred to colloquially as a 'geep'.

It is estimated that there are now over 300 distinct breeds of goat kept worldwide, many having been bred selectively to enhance a particular trait to increase productivity, quality or survivability. As an example, the Saanen and its derivatives comprise the most popular dairy breed. Other dairy breeds include the Toggenburg (**Fig. 1.4**) and its derivatives, the British Alpine and the Anglo-Nubian. The most popular fibre breed is the Angora, which produces mohair. Cashmere is not a breed of goat but describes the soft underhair that grows as an insulating layer, and goats are farmed commercially for this. One of the most popular meat breeds is the Boer goat, originating from South Africa and bred specifically for carcass conformation and meat yield. Pygmy goats are commonly kept as pets in the UK because of their small size. The breed originates from West Africa and they are more accurately described as West African Dwarf goats.

There will be local variation in terminology used, but in broad terms, female goats are referred to as 'does' or 'nannies', entire males as 'bucks' or 'billies', and their offspring are 'kids'. Castrated males are 'wethers'. Meat for human consumption from younger animals is called kid or cabrito (Spanish), and from older animals is simply known as goat meat or, sometimes, is called chevon.

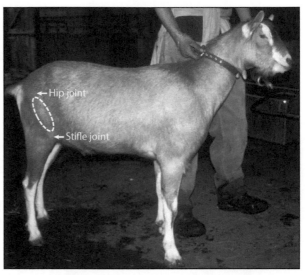

Fig. 1.4 **The distinct face marking of Toggenburgs is similar to that of the British Alpine, but their base colour is grey to grey–brown. This image also shows restraint by a neck collar. The dotted line outlines the quadriceps muscle (suitable for intramuscular injections).**

Goat meat is consumed by around 75% of the world's population. In countries such as the UK and USA, the majority of goat meat has traditionally been eaten by some ethnic communities only, but there is increasing evidence of a wider developing demand for goat meat. Gourmet wholesale and retail markets (many of which are internet based) and local restaurants are beginning to stock goat meat, leading to new goat meat units, both specialist and those rearing male kids surplus to the dairy sector (**Fig. 1.5**).

Part of this increasing popularity is the goat's reputation as a healthy meat alternative in comparison with other red meats. It is low in fat, cholesterol, calorific energy and saturated fat (50% lower in calories than beef and around 30% lower in saturated fat than chicken; *Table 1.1*).

GENOMICS

The goat genome was the first reference genome for small ruminant animals to be defined. This has led to an increased interest in harnessing these techniques to improve goat health and productivity, focussing on identifying desirable and undesirable traits.

Table 1.1 **Composition of meat of various species (per 85 g [3 oz] roasted meat).**					
	CALORIES	**FAT (G)**	**SATURATED FAT (G)**	**PROTEIN (G)**	**IRON (G)**
Goat	122	2.58	0.79	23	3.2
Beef	245	16.0	6.8	23	2.0
Pork	310	24.0	8.7	21	2.7
Lamb	235	16.0	7.3	22	1.4
Chicken	120	3.5	1.1	21	1.5

Source: United States Department of Agriculture.

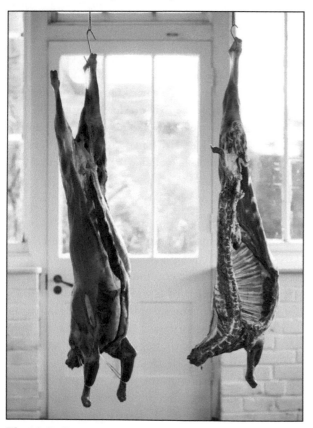

Fig. 1.5 Goat carcases recently slaughtered and dressed.

Using commercial milk production as an example, it is recognised that there are considerable differences between the performances of daughters from different sires in their milk yield, milk quality, conformation, disease resistance, live weight, feed intake and other traits. By selecting goats that are genetically more productive by using, for example, estimated breeding values (EBVs) as an aid to selection, cumulative benefits can be realised.

It is important to ensure that top performing goats have high functional fitness. By using conformation assessment and scoring of relevant physical attributes (such as legs, feet, udders and teat conformation), EBVs can be developed. Combining these with production trait EBVs should ensure that high productivity is achieved without compromising overall robustness.

Accelerating the rates of response to selection can be achieved by improving the accuracy of selection, reducing the generation interval (keeping younger, more productive animals with a higher genetic merit than the previous generation) and only selecting the very best animals for breeding.

This is an evolving process, and it will become more widely available and technologically advanced.

BEHAVIOUR

Goat behaviour can be interesting, unusual and at times frustrating. Domestication has had an impact on what could be described as a goat's natural behaviour when running wild, although the constant objective for any goat keeper should be to not inhibit such behaviour in any way that could compromise overall goat health and welfare.

Goats develop strong bonds with each other, particularly with siblings and other family members, and as a result, separation can have a negative impact on welfare. When kept in increasing numbers, they will develop close groups each with their own strong hierarchical structure, with regular confrontations (head to head butting, **Fig. 1.6**) to establish dominance by both males and females. For this reason, it is inadvisable to keep goats with horns and goats that have been dehorned/disbudded or are naturally

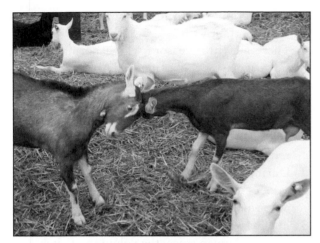

Fig. 1.6 Goats head to head butting. This may be playful or used to establish dominance.

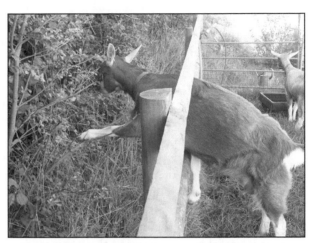

Fig. 1.7 A goat browsing through the fence.

polled together, to avoid potentially harmful confrontations. It follows, therefore, that goat groups need to remain fairly static where possible – constant movements and regrouping can be unnerving and lead to reduced milk yields, and may even predispose to illness. Goats should be moved in pairs or small groups (e.g. after kidding) so that they integrate into the herd faster and face significantly fewer interactions than if they were introduced individually.

Separating goats from the herd should be avoided whenever possible. If isolation is necessary, then as much as is practicable, locate the isolated goat in a pen nearby or adjacent to the herd or provide it with a companion. Keeping small groups of animals together when handling for veterinary procedures such as blood sampling will mean that they remain much calmer and easier to handle.

Goats also appear to develop an affinity for owners, and are often unnerved by changes in owner and environment.

There may be subtle breed differences in behaviour. In the UK, for example, British Alpine, British Toggenburg and Saanen goats appear to be more laid back and are not easily unnerved, whereas Anglo-Nubian and Golden Guernsey goats are more easily unsettled, although as ever there will be individual exceptions.

Goats are gregarious animals, can become easily bored and will constantly look for stimuli, hence their apparent desire to investigate anything in their environment by licking and chewing (including light switches, electric cables, gate fasteners). They can stand on their hind legs, reaching up to 2 metres above the ground, therefore any building, paddock or yard should be constructed in such a way that it is not simply stock-proof but 'goat proof'; they are masters of escape (**Fig. 1.7**).

Goats are good climbers and extremely agile, clambering into and over obstacles that are of interest, including trees. This natural behaviour, although to be encouraged, can also lead to misadventure as goats can get caught up in fencing, netting or other material with broken limbs a possible sequela, particularly in young kids, and strangulation at any age if an inquisitive head gets caught (**Fig. 1.8**).

This inquisitive and gregarious behaviour should be fostered at all times, avoiding barren

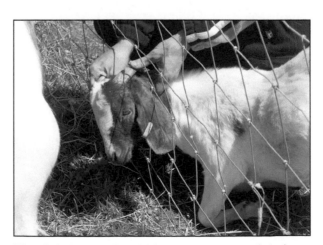

Fig. 1.8 A goat's inquisitive nature can result in its head becoming trapped.

environments and instead providing environmental enrichment. The following can be very simple fixtures for goats to climb onto:

- Mounds of earth, or a large stone (**Fig. 1.9a**).
- An old trailer (**Fig. 1.9b**).
- Straw bales (**Fig. 1.9c**).
- Large plastic drums open at one end to roll around.

Places to hide in or under are also important; goats have evolved as prey species and as such will seek out a place of safety if frightened.

When considering the individual goat as a clinician, it is useful to bear in mind that they are usually very quiet individuals, and it is not often that you will hear a goat vocalising for no reason. A goat starting to vocalise more is often a sign that something is wrong. In contrast, some goats make gentle noises when they are content and become quieter when something is wrong. Knowing your stock is vitally important.

There are three reasons why a normally quiet, placid goat may start bleating, and particularly bleating more constantly:

1 When they are hungry or thirsty. This is usually alleviated by giving food or water, with a quick return to normal behaviour.
2 During the breeding season, particularly when a doe is on heat, or during the latter part of pregnancy as kidding approaches.
3 Finally, when a goat is sick or in pain and, as with the human voice, the volume and pitch will change depending on the intensity of pain or discomfort. Conversely, as the animal deteriorates the sound will be of a lower intensity in a goat that is feeling really miserable.

Goats seem to have a relatively low pain threshold when compared with other farm animals such as cattle. They do not tolerate ill-health very well, and a diligent owner will be aware of this and the need to give plenty of TLC ('tender loving care') to any sick goat to ensure it continues to feed, is warm and comfortable, and maintains an interest in life.

In the wild, a pregnant doe will separate herself away from the main herd and attempt to hide as kidding becomes imminent. She may attempt this behaviour when confined, even attempting to build a nest in which to hide the kid after it is born. One consequence of this behaviour is the rapid ingestion of placenta and any other products of kidding

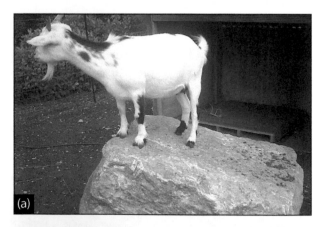
(a)

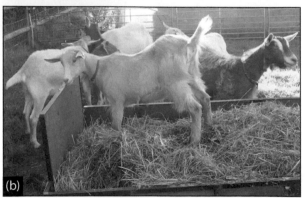
(b)

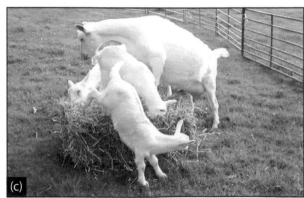
(c)

Figs. 1.9 Environmental enrichment. (a) Encouraging safe climbing (top). (b) Making hay feeding fun (left). One disadvantage is potential faecal contamination of feed. (c) Playing with a straw bale (right).

or abortion to conceal the birth; this can be particularly frustrating when investigating the causes of abortion. More information on kidding and care of the neonate can be found in the relevant chapters.

In summary, there are certain behaviours the goat needs or wants to perform. Allowing these can promote welfare, denying them can lead to stress, boredom and frustration. Secondly, physical and mental health can be expressed in behaviour. Understanding behavioural needs and assessing behavioural activities displayed can help prevent and solve health problems on the farm.

NUTRITION

Many generic aspects of the nutrition and feeding of goats are similar to other farmed species. Because they are ruminants, the principles of rumen function (and dysfunction) should be understood. Weight for weight, a dairy goat will produce considerably more milk than the equivalent dairy cow, but it will only achieve this potential if it is fed properly, with a daily intake of an adequate quantity of feed of the correct nutritional value and in a form that the goat will eat.

Goats have evolved into very efficient browsing animals (versus cattle and sheep who are grazers). They will readily eat grass, thistles and other weeds, hedgerow and leaves and branches from overhanging trees, often standing on their hind legs to achieve this (**Fig. 1.10**). When other sources of feed ('browse') are in short supply, they will eat the bark from around the tree base, and given the opportunity will also climb up into trees to continue their search for feed. When kept in confinement, goats are often very wasteful of their feed, as they sort through and discard even good quality forage. They are extremely fussy about the quality of their feed, readily refusing to eat spoiled or contaminated feed. Their preferred pasture sward height is similar to cattle (i.e. 7–8 cm).

The exact nature of the diet fed will vary between geographical regions dependent on what is available, but should consist of a source of forage (most commonly hay; **Figs. 1.11, 1.12**) for maintenance, balanced where necessary to allow for pregnancy, lactation and growth by additional compound, concentrate or cereal feed. Both grass and maize silage (often as part of a total mixed ration [TMR]) are widely fed to commercial herds and, as with other ruminant species, good silage making and subsequent storage are key factors, partly to ensure a good palatable and nutritious product, but also to reduce the risk of high levels of *Listeria* organisms, to which goats are very susceptible (**Figs. 1.13, 1.14**).

It is important to ensure that all goats can feed together when providing any feedstuff in which individual component parts are still visible (such as a course mix). If there is insufficient trough space available for all goats to feed simultaneously (recommended linear space is 0.75–0.95 metres per adult goat), then the dominant goats can selectively consume the best bits, leaving the poorer quality

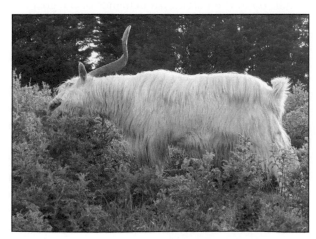

Fig. 1.10 Browsing and feeding behaviour extends to weeds and even thistles.

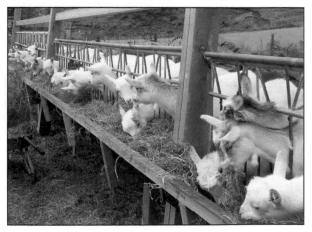

Fig. 1.11 Feeding dried lucerne (syn. alfalfa) in Norway.

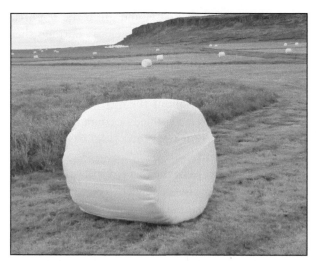

Fig. 1.12 Big-bale haylage in Iceland.

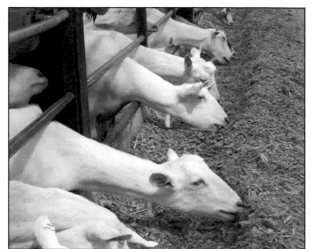

Fig. 1.13 Feeding a total mixed ration, based on maize silage, on a commercial dairy unit in the UK.

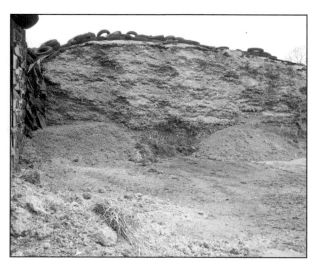

Fig. 1.14 A maize silage clamp. Aside from good techniques during harvest, ensiling and storage, good face management is important.

constituents for subordinate goats. Feeding a commercial pellet or other well milled product will overcome this problem. Overfeeding is common in goats, especially when fed titbits.

As with any ruminant feeding programme, it is important to ensure that any dietary change is made gradually to allow the rumen microflora to adjust and mitigate against any potential dietary disorders such as rumen acidosis, bloat or enterotoxaemia.

Baseline energy requirements are: 0.44 MJ of ME (megajoules of metabolisable energy)/kg body weight $^{0.75}$ for maintenance in the housed goat, which translates to about 8.5 MJ of ME for a 50 kg goat and 10.5 MJ of ME for a 70 kg goat. For animals at pasture, an additional 20–25% is allowed for increased activity levels. An additional 6 MJ of ME/day above maintenance is added in the last 2 months of pregnancy. Lactation requires 4.4 MJ of ME/kg of milk produced (at 3.5% fat).

To fulfil baseline dietary protein requirements, a maintenance ration should have 11% crude protein (CP) (averaged across the entire ration), and for lactation or growth 14% CP. Rumen undegradable protein should be increased for lactation (e.g. soya bean meal).

Monitoring body condition and balancing this condition to the nutritional demands of the goat and the available feedstuff is important. Goats are often described as looking thin when compared with sheep and cattle. They have evolved essentially as tropical and subtropical animals and, as such, have only minimal subcutaneous fat, their body fat stores being laid down internally, particularly in the abdominal cavity and omentum (**Fig. 1.15**). Due to the variation in rumen fill, body weights are less reliable in ruminants, hence the widespread use of condition scoring (**Fig. 1.16**). The lack of subcutaneous lumbar fat in goats, however, makes the procedure less reliable than in cattle and sheep, and a second assessment should be made by palpation of the fat pad overlying the sternum – this is convex in goats in good condition and progressively concave in thinner goats (**Fig. 1.17**).

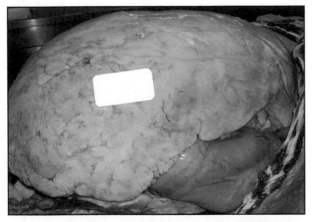

Fig. 1.15 Goat fat storage site – abdominal cavity.

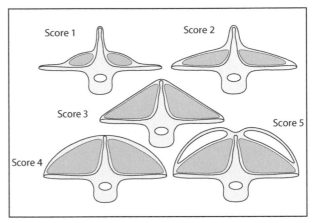

Fig. 1.16 Schematic illustration of the lumbar area for different body condition scores (in cross-section; muscles shaded pink, bone shaded nude, fat deposits shaded light blue).

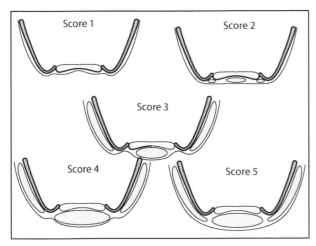

Fig. 1.17 Schematic illustration of the fat deposits (shaded grey) overlying the sternum (shaded turquoise) and ribcage (shaded pink).

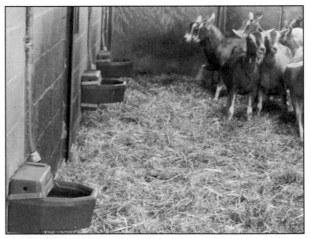

Fig. 1.18 Satisfactory water provision with multiple, largely clean drinking points. Automatic drinkers, such as these, must be checked regularly for full functionality. Note: Positioning water points at the back of the bedded area should be avoided, as wet and poached bedding invariably results.

In a commercial herd, it would be advisable to condition score all or a proportion of goats at:

- Drying off.
- Last 2 weeks of gestation.
- 6 weeks into lactation.
- Turnout onto pasture (if grazing).
- Beginning of breeding season.

Suggested target condition scores (on a scale of 1 to 5 with 1 = thin):

- Kidding: 3.0–3.5.
- Service: 3.0–3.5.
- During pregnancy: 3.0.

Water must be easily accessible, and also be kept clean and free from extraneous debris, or goats will refuse to drink (**Figs. 1.18–1.20**). A goat may drink up to 18 litres of water (4 gallons) each day, depending on climate and ambient temperature, type of diet fed and milk yield. A lactating goat requires 1.4 litres (0.3 gallons) of water per 1 kg (2.2 lb) milk produced. At least 10% of the goats in a group must be able to drink at the same time.

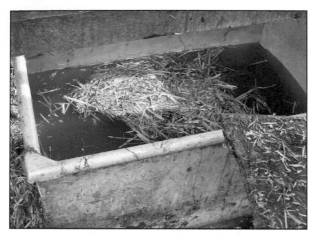

Fig. 1.19 Poor water provision. The water is dirty and access is partially obstructed by a board. Also, being placed in the bedded area means that the trough is unlikely to be emptied and cleaned regularly.

Problems related to vitamin or mineral disorders do occur in goats, but when outdoors their natural browsing activities do seem to result in fewer deficiencies than might be expected when compared with other ruminants (specific disorders are discussed in Chapter 15). A well balanced diet (with known nutritional values) is key to preventing deficiencies or toxicity, with problems more likely to occur when feeding forage alone, home mixed rations or by relying too heavily on *ad-libitum* mineral blocks or free access mineral, where individual intakes will be variable and haphazard.

It is important to remember some fundamental principles related to the safe storage and use of any composite feed or feed constituents, which can pose a potential risk to goat health if they are not followed. Owners and stock-keepers should be encouraged to:

- Obtain feed from safe and reliable sources.
- Store feed securely to prevent access (where possible) by rodents and wild birds in particular (**Fig. 1.21**).
- Recognise unexpected changes in colour, odour, texture or appearance.
- Know where in any rearing or production system there may be a potential for unacceptable feed risks to occur (e.g. change in dietary constituents or feeding programmes).

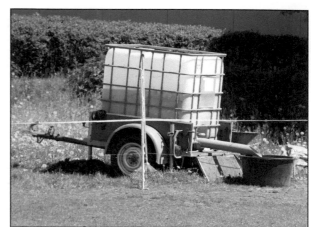

Fig. 1.20 A water bowser, here self-made using an intermediate bulk container on a trailer, provides a satisfactory way to get water to paddocks. The bowser, as well as the trough, should be cleaned regularly (e.g. with dilute bleach). Natural water sources for grazing animals are suboptimal. Water quality in stagnant bodies such as ponds is often poor, and rivers or streams may carry pathogens from upstream livestock farms.

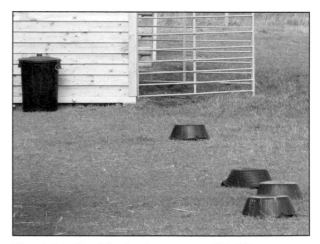

Fig. 1.21 Good feed safety on a small-holding: concentrates are stored in bins with secure lids, and the buckets are turned upside down after feeding to reduce the risk of contamination and attraction of wildlife.

- Ensure that feed labels are kept and notes made of dietary constituents contained therein.
- Ensure that all those involved in feeding goats have clear and concise feeding instructions (**Fig. 1.22**).

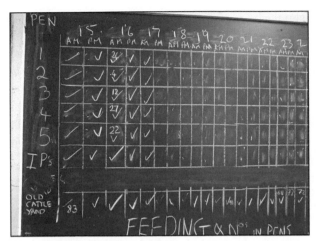

Fig. 1.22 Simple, but effective feed board for the kidding period, showing number of animals per pen and whether supplementary feed has been given on a particular day (dates along the top).

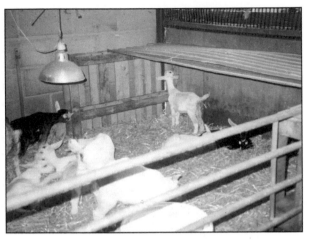

Fig. 1.23 A horizontal board provides protection from down draughts in a goatling pen.

ENVIRONMENT

Housing

The ideal housing environment for goats is very similar to that required for other livestock. It should provide as a bare minimum:

- Adequate ventilation free of draughts (**Fig. 1.23**).
- Temperatures not exceeding upper or lower critical levels in summer and winter.
- Plenty of light, including artificial lighting for the hours of darkness to meet physiological needs and allow inspection; however, an appropriate period of rest from lighting must be provided each day.
- Enough room to be able to move around freely (minimum 2.0–2.5 m² floor space/goat; **Fig. 1.3**).
- Good access to food and water (**Figs 1.3, 1.18**).
- A dry bed to lie on.

Effective ventilation removes heat, water vapour, microorganisms, dust and gases. It distributes air evenly and prevents draughts. These factors combine to reduce stress in housed goats, reduce the amount of bedding required, improve the environment leading to an improvement in productivity, and potentially reduce respiratory problems.

The target is to provide air changes (stale air out; fresh air in) of at least 30 m³/hr during the winter, and 120–150 m³/hr throughout the summer. For the majority of time (around 95%) in the UK, air speed is above 1 m/sec, which allows suitable ventilation provided there is sufficient air inlet and outlet. For the remaining 5% of time, ventilation is reliant on the 'stack effect' (i.e. warm air rises and is vented from the apex of the roof and in doing so pulls fresh air into the building). If the outlet is insufficient or the inlet area is too small or compromised by surrounding buildings or other features such as trees, then natural ventilation will fail. This results in the air cooling and collapsing back on to the bedding and goats. This stagnant air is damper, leading to greater levels of dust particles, bacteria and viruses. Stack effect ventilation depends on heat generated by the stock, temperature difference inside and out, height difference inlet to outlet, and the inlet and outlet areas.

Adequate air inlet can be provided by space boarding, or Yorkshire boarding in very exposed areas. Boarding is usually placed above a wall that is higher than head height to avoid potential draughts. An alternative to space boarding is the installation of curtain sides to the building, which allows the amount of air admitted through the inlets to be varied according to prevailing weather conditions. These curtains can be lifted and raised manually or automatically and provide greater environmental control. As a general rule of thumb, inlets should amount to 50% of the surface area of the side of the building, bearing in mind that neighbouring buildings and trees can potentially disrupt airflow.

Suitable outlet ventilation can be provided by an open ridge. Concern is often expressed about rain and snow falling on to the floor below. If the area beneath is a feed table, then this is unlikely to be a major issue – in reality very little rain does come through an open ridge in adequately stocked buildings. An alternative ridge design is the protected ridge, which still provides the correct area of air outlet, but minimises the chance of rain coming through.

Goats are homoeothermic animals and need to maintain a constant body temperature of between 38.7° and 40.7°C. Correct building design and ventilation take account of the goats' thermoneutral zone (i.e. the temperature range at which the animals operate most efficiently). The range of temperature of the comfort zone does vary according to breed and their habitat of origin, and is influenced by levels of body fat, thickness of coat and diet. However, as a generalisation, most breeds found in the UK have a lower critical temperature of 0°C (i.e. a temperature below which they need to convert feed into heat and where they feel cold). In extreme cases temperatures below the lower critical temperature can lead to reduced feed intake, potentially resulting in nutritional disorders such as pregnancy toxaemia. The upper critical temperature is around 30°C, at which temperature goats potentially become heat stressed, although this figure will depend on breed type and local environmental factors such as average daily ambient temperature and humidity. Heat stress in turn can lead to low-grade production problems through reduced feed intake, digestibility and rate of passage through the gut, to more serious consequences including death in extreme cases.

Relative humidity has an influence on the thermoneutral zone. In winter, it can make the animal's coat wet, which reduces the insulating properties. In summer, it reduces evaporation and limits heat loss.

Additionally, care should be taken to make the building 'goat proof'. As stated previously, goats are inquisitive animals, so electric cables and switches should be placed well out of reach. Door fasteners need to be of a type they cannot open, and any sharp or projecting objects should be removed or covered. Where possible there should be two openings to any building or section, to prevent any dominant goat from blocking others entering or leaving.

Some form of shelter should be available for goats when outdoors, to offer shade and protect them from inclement weather, in particular wetness and wind.

Fencing

There is no such thing as a 100% goat proof fence. Fences should be strongly constructed, preferably of a material that they cannot get their head caught in, and high enough that they cannot jump over (minimum 1.2 metres [4 feet]). Goats will often stand with their hind legs on top of a fence to reach overhanging branches, and if this is done repeatedly, then even a strong fence may sag or collapse in time. Some goat keepers use electric fencing or electric fence topping wire to good effect.

Tethering

Goats are occasionally kept on tethers when outdoors, and specifically when kept in areas that are difficult to fence around. It is important, however, to ensure that adequate care is provided at all times, as tethered goats are particularly vulnerable to attack by dogs, to getting caught up in the tether, to knocking over feed and water supplies out of reach, and to any extremes of weather from which they cannot escape.

HANDLING

Goats need to be handled to move them from one location to another, for management procedures such as medication or foot trimming, and for clinical procedures. Any such procedure should be undertaken in a manner that will keep stress levels to an absolute minimum.

There are a number of generic factors to consider when handling ruminants:

- They have excellent peripheral vision.
- They prefer to move towards light and do not like to enter dark buildings.

- They have a natural herding instinct, and can become distressed and agitated if they are separated from the rest of their group.
- They like to follow a leader.
- If a handling procedure is stressful or frightening, this unpleasant experience may well make any future similar experience even more stressful, so get it right first time round.

Additionally, goats' natural inquisitiveness for anything they encounter, together with their friendly disposition, can 'slow things up'. As with other ruminants, they will want to move as a group, but there are often complex mini or family groups that may lead to increased hesitancy when driven. Their ability to escape should never be forgotten. Gates and other barriers will need to be higher than those used for sheep, and any potential escape hole or gap will be explored. When stressed some goats will simply lie down and can become trampled and suffocated – for this reason, always keep groups to be handled small and manageable.

Individual goats should be caught by firmly placing an arm around their neck or torso, or by grabbing at a collar or horns (**Fig. 1.4**). The latter should be a last resort, as goats resent being pulled by their horns and it may encourage head-butting, even though it is tempting to use the horns as 'handles'. Once caught, tame goats will usually remain fairly calm, and can be trained to be haltered and lead around. Struggling goats are best backed into corners, and may be straddled for procedures such as drenching.

Foot examination and trimming is best carried out in the standing position, although there are handling crates designed to hold goats firm if large numbers are to be examined (see **Fig. 9.22**). Goats can be placed onto their haunches as with sheep but, unlike sheep, they rarely become passive and will often continue to struggle; however, this approach may be useful when examining the penis and prepuce of males.

Care should be taken at all times to protect the handler from injury, particularly when working closely with horned goats where there is a potential risk of injury to the face and eyes (safety goggles should be considered).

PHYSIOLOGY AND BODY FEATURES

Baseline physiological information is provided at the beginning of each chapter.

Lactation

Goats will start lactogenesis at the end of pregnancy, but unlike other ruminants some females can lactate spontaneously (so called maiden milkers). Milk production will vary tremendously between breeds, and will also be dependent on nutritional input. Dairy breeds typically produce around 1,000 litres per lactation, with some top females capable of 2,000 litres per lactation. Lactation lengths are often extended to 365 days or longer. Milk composition is similar to cattle, although milk taints are occasionally reported as a problem (*Table 1.2*).

Horns

Most goat kids are born with the horn bud already developing. Some kids can be born naturally polled, but in many dairy breeds, such as the Toggenburg, Saanen and Alpine breeds of European descent, this is linked genetically to an infertility trait. In these breeds the presence of horn buds is determined by a recessive gene. The polled trait is dominant, but is linked to a recessive gene for infertility. A female goat that is homozygous for the polled gene develops into a sterile intersex.

Coat

The coat of all goats is formed basically of primary follicles producing long coarse guard hairs, and secondary follicles producing undercoat or down. It is the secondary follicle in Angoras that has been selectively modified to produce mohair. In tropical regions, the undercoat is minimal or absent, while

Table 1.2 **Comparative average composition of goat and cow milk.**				
	DRY MATTER	**PROTEIN**	**FAT**	**LACTOSE**	**MINERAL MATTER**
Goat	12.1%	3.4%	3.8%	4.1%	0.8%
Cow	12.2%	3.2%	3.6%	4.7%	0.7%

secondary follicle undercoat production is greatly increased in colder climates. Cashmere is the fine downy undercoat of many goat breeds.

Wattles

Many goat breeds have 'wattles' found in the throat area (see **Fig. 2.3**, p. 22). They have no known function and consist of a central cartilage core, smooth muscle, connective tissue, a blood and nerve supply, and covering skin.

Weight

With more than 300 distinct goat breeds worldwide, there is a wide variation in body weight, but as a rough guide approximate goat weights are:

Adult dairy	Doe	55–105 kg (120–230 lb)
	Buck	75–120 kg (165–265 lb)
Adult Angora	Doe	33–55 kg (73–120 lb)
	Buck	70–85 kg (155–187 lb)
Adult Pygmy	Doe	22–27 kg (48–60 lb)
	Buck	28–32 kg (62–70 lb)

Longevity

When kept as pets or companion animals, goats can live well into their teens and occasionally beyond 20 years of age. Such geriatric goats may need special care.

HISTORY TAKING AND CLINICAL EXAMINATION

Relevant history is unique to each case; however, there are common important aspects to consider.

Farm related history of interest
Includes:

- Type and purpose of enterprise: meat, dairy, smallholding, pedigree, etc.
- Closed or open. If closed, soundness of policy/risk of breaches. If open, buying-in policy.
- Other species or enterprises managed concurrently (for example, arable contractor or farm shop).
- Routine preventive protocols.

- Recent disease or management problems and changes, including seasonal changes and weather events.
- Local disease occurrences.

For the individual animal, history of interest
Includes:

- Signalment: age, gender, breed, home-bred or bought-in (and when), value.
- Specific concern or complaint of owner, and atypical behaviour noted (in particular feed intake).
- Others in the group or herd affected, including other clinical signs that could be part of the same picture (e.g. salmonellosis causing abortion and diarrhoea). Where group problem, morbidity and mortality, and timeline.
- Production status of animal and interval to last major event: for example, drying-off, parturition, weaning.
- Production data for the animal: milk yield, weight gains, reproductive events.
- Gradual or sudden onset, and any potential triggering events.
- Health history of this particular animal, including routine treatments: for example, vaccination, anthelmintics, castration.
- Environment of animal: housed or at pasture, and recent changes to this.
- Diet and any recent changes to this (deliberate or accidental).
- Treatments administered by farm for current problem, and response seen. Also taking into consideration that recent treatments may mask clinical signs.

Basic clinical examination
Specific ancillary diagnostics will be highlighted in the relevant chapters.

Observations of the environment, and the patient at a distance, are important and include:

- Animal's environment: water availability and quality; feed types, availability and quality; space allowance; bedding quantity and quality;

ventilation, draughts and unpleasant smells; ambient temperature; exposure to inclement weather; signs of disturbance (for example, breakages, animals rubbing against structures); undesirable components (waste products, poisonous plants, injury risks, etc.).
- Group behaviour and interactions: bullying, crowding, restlessness or agitation.
- Patient behaviour: proximity to group, stance and gait, respiratory rate

The clinical examination itself may either address body systems one at a time, or follow a 'nose-to-tail' pattern. Aspects to observe include:

- **Vital signs:** respiratory rate, heart rate, rectal temperature, rumen rate.
- **Body condition score (BCS):** in particular poor or emaciated.
- **Mental state:** the normal goat is alert, bright and responsive to approaches.
- **Respiratory system:** airflow through nostrils, nasal or ocular discharge, respiratory effort and pattern, coughing, response to palpation of larynx and trachea, superficial lymph nodes, adventitious sounds over trachea or thorax, percussion of sinuses and thorax.
- **Cardiovascular system:** mucous membrane colour, capillary refill time, surface temperature of extremities, jugular filling and deflation and presence of jugular pulse, femoral pulse character, audibility of heart sounds, adventitious sounds, heart rate and rhythm, hydration status.
- **Digestive system:** oral mucosa integrity, dental health, abdominal shape, rumen fill and character of rumen contractions, borborygmi, percussion of abdomen, abdominal pain tests, trans-abdominal palpation (depending on size and BCS), defecation and character of faeces, perineal staining.
- **Urogenital system:** urination and character of urine, vulval discharge and/or staining of tail or perineum. Transabdominal palpation of kidneys (depending on size and BCS).
- **Mammary system:** colour, surface temperature, pain, swelling or oedema, milk character, teat or skin lesions, masses or nodules, supramammary lymph nodes.
- **Locomotor system:** stance and gait, stride length, weight-bearing, swellings, abnormal angulation or sounds, foot horn integrity.
- **Neurological system:** mental state and behaviour, ability to stand and rise, stance and gait, head position, skin sensation, reflexes.

In the neonate, particular attention should be paid to the presence of congenital defects.

ADMINISTERING MEDICATION

Oral administration

For administration via tube, the orogastric route is preferable over nasogastric administration. It is useful to indicate the distances to the larynx and ultimate end-point (cervical oesophagus in preweaned animals, rumen in weaned animals) on the tube with permanent marker.

In preweaned animals, drugs or fluids should be deposited into the cervical oesophagus (one-third to one-half down the neck) to trigger the oesophageal groove reflex, resulting in channelling of the medication into the abomasum. A lamb feeder tube (6 mm OD, 40 cm length) is suitable for kids up to about 4 weeks old, and a mouth gag is not necessary in this age group. The kid is held on the handler's lap with its back end towards the handler and its chin supported by the non-dominant hand (**Fig. 1.24**). After stimulating the suckle reflex for 30–60 seconds, the mouth is held open with a finger or thumb of the non-dominant hand. The tube is passed over the tongue and, when reaching the larynx, gentle pressure is maintained until swallowing occurs. Correct location is ascertained by observing fleece movement and palpating the tube in the oesophagus with the other hand.

In adult goats, a foal-size stomach tube (9–11 mm OD, minimum length 120 cm) is suitable, and the inner tube of a bandage roll makes a useful mouth gag to provide protection from the sharp molar teeth (**Fig. 1.25**). The goat is reversed into a corner, and the handler stands astride over the animal with their legs in front of the goat's shoulder (**Fig. 1.26**). The non-dominant hand holds the chin

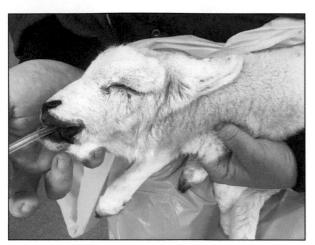

Fig. 1.24 Use of an oesophageal feeder (here shown in a lamb). The kid is rested on the handler's lap with its back end towards the handler. The dominant right hand holds the chin and oesophageal tube. The left hand is at the target level of insertion (halfway down the neck) and palpates the oesophagus for the tube.

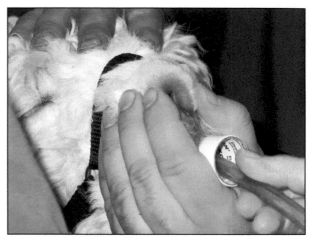

Fig. 1.25 The inner tube of a bandage roll can be used effectively as a gag and protector to pass a stomach tube in adults (here shown in an alpaca).

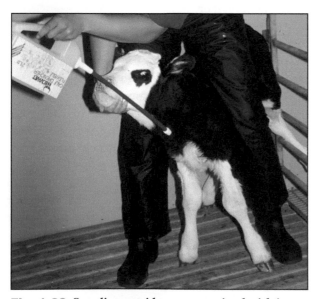

Fig. 1.26 Standing astride over an animal with its back end in a corner, and the handler's legs in front of its shoulders provides good restraint for stomach tubing and intravenous access (here shown in a calf).

of the goat and the mouth gag. The tube is passed over the tongue and, once the larynx is reached, gentle pressure is maintained until the animal swallows. Moderate resistance may be encountered as the tube passes the thoracic inlet and the cardia.

Correct location is confirmed by the presence of rumen smell and the absence of coughing or expiration through the tube.

Small approximate amounts of medication may be administered using a catheter-tip syringe. Its nozzle is inserted through the diastema, placed onto the tongue and aimed towards the larynx. It is important to hold the goat's head only just above horizontal and to administer slowly, to avoid accidental inhalation (especially in recumbent patients).

Subcutaneous injection

Suitable sites include the proximal or distal neck and the fleece-less area caudal to the elbow. The escutcheon is useful for injecting goats in the parlour (**Fig. 1.27**).

Intramuscular injection

The quadriceps muscle is suitable for all ages of goats, taking care to inject into the bulk of the muscle (thereby avoiding stifle joint, sciatic nerve, etc.; see **Fig. 1.4**).

Neck muscles may also be used, particularly in meat goats, thus avoiding a higher value cut of meat. However, injections into the neck muscles should be avoided in nursing kids, as inflammation secondary to the injection may reduce suckling. The ligament nuchae and spinal column must be avoided in this region (**Fig. 1.28**).

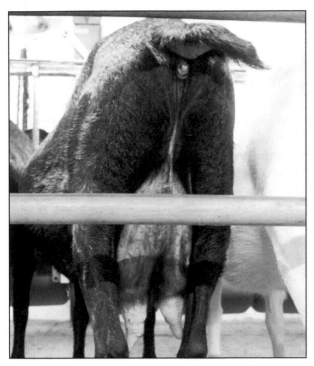

Fig. 1.27 The escutcheon is readily accessible in many parlours for subcutaneous injections.

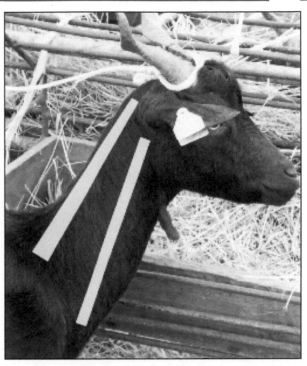

Fig. 1.28 When using the neck for intramuscular injections, the ligament nuchae and spinal column (shaded areas) must be avoided.

The gluteal muscles may be used in well-conditioned goats.

Intravenous injection and catheterisation

The jugular, cephalic and saphenous veins are all suitable in all ages and types of goat. The jugular vein is accessed in the upper third of the neck to reduce the risk of intra-arterial injection (**Fig. 1.29**). This is particularly important when administering sedatives – inserting the needle off the syringe allows confirmation that the vein has been entered prior to injection. The mammary vein should only ever be used for euthanasia.

Catheter placement is greatly aided by subcutaneous injection of 1–2 ml of local anaesthetic, followed by a small stab incision through the skin with a scalpel blade. Jugular catheters should be at least 50 mm

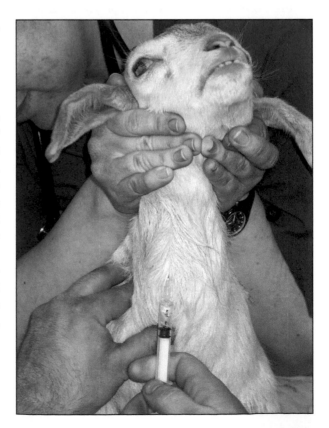

Fig. 1.29 Intravenous injection into the jugular vein. Note that the vein is entered in the upper third of the neck. Blood sampling is often easiest if the goat's head and neck are held straight (rather than towards one side).

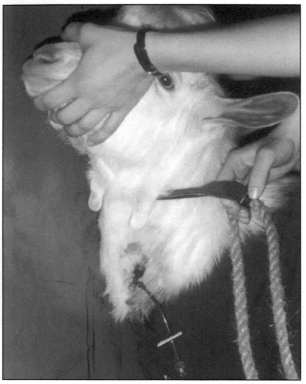

Fig. 1.30 An intravenous catheter held in place with sutures. Use of a T-port connector preserves catheter hygiene.

long, to accommodate skin movement over the jugular grove. For adult goats, 16–20 gauge is suitable, for kids 20–22 gauge. Short-stay catheters are suitable for a dwell time of up to 72 hours. For longer dwell times, a medium- or long-stay catheter is used. Super glue is a convenient alternative to suturing where the catheter remains in place for a few hours only (**Fig. 1.30**).

Needle sizes
Usually, a needle length of 2.5 cm (1 in) is suitable for subcutaneous, intramuscular and intravenous injections, both in adult goats and kids. For low viscosity drugs, 20 or 21 gauge needles are used; for more viscous drugs or large volumes, 18 or 19 gauge.

Intraperitoneal injection
Intraperitoneal injection of glucose may be employed in hypothermic or hypoglycaemic neonates (see Chapter 4). The recommended needle size is 18–20 gauge, 2.5 cm (1 in) long.

Using the non-dominant hand, the kid is held vertically by its front legs (hand placed near elbows), with its back to the handler's body (**Fig. 1.31a**). The needle insertion point is one finger-width lateral and caudal to the umbilicus (**Fig. 1.31b**). Long fleece in this area is clipped, and disinfectant applied (for example, povidone–iodine solution). The needle is inserted at an angle of 30–45 degrees to the skin (pointing towards the tail base) and advanced slowly into the peritoneal cavity up to its hub. After aspiration to check that no viscera have been entered, the fluid is injected steadily.

Subconjunctival injection
The head of the animal is rotated to expose as much sclera as possible. Using an episcleral vessel as reference point, topical anaesthetic is applied with a cotton bud to the scleral conjunctiva. A 23–25 gauge needle is inserted under the conjunctiva and advanced for a few millimetres parallel to the eye ball (**Fig. 1.32**).

ROUTINE PROCEDURES AND HEALTH PLANNING

The key to keeping goats healthy and productive, and ensuring that their welfare is not compromised, is to develop a health plan, and reference to this will be made throughout the book. Such a plan need not be complex, but should ensure that routine procedures such as vaccination, worming, disbudding and foot trimming are carried out in a structured manner, and that other information is readily available on disease recognition and management. Such a plan is relevant no matter whether goats are kept in large numbers commercially, or as two or more goats kept as pets.

Individual procedures will be outlined in the relevant chapter.

BIOSECURITY

Biosecurity is defined as 'the prevention of disease-causing agents entering or leaving any place where farm animals are present (or have been present recently)'. It involves a number of measures and protocols designed to prevent disease-causing agents

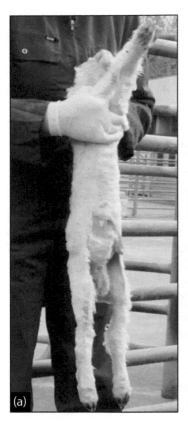 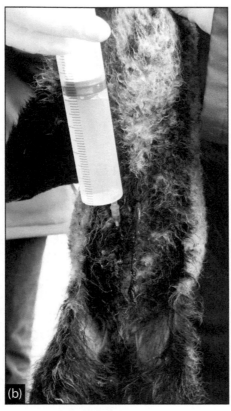

(a) (b)

Fig. 1.31 Intraperitoneal injection. (a) The kid is held by its front legs just above the elbows, with its back against the handler's body. (b) The needle is inserted at a 30–45-degree angle one finger-width lateral and caudal to the umbilicus.

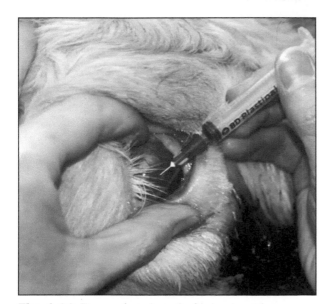

Fig. 1.32 For a subconjunctival injection (shown here in a bovine), the head is rotated to expose the sclera. After point application of topical anaesthetic, the needle is inserted parallel with the eye ball. The clinician's thumb is on the lower eyelid and index finger on the upper eyelid.

from entering or leaving a property and being spread. The word farm animal is emphasised in this paragraph because of the number of infectious agents shared with livestock species other than goats, and in particular other ruminants such as sheep and cattle.

Good general hygiene and biosecurity is essential to:

- Prevent the introduction of infectious diseases.
- Protect the health of goats, other susceptible animals in the vicinity and any humans in close daily contact.
- Reduce the risk of disease exposure to any members of the public who visit goat premises. This is particularly important if open days are held, especially involving young children or disease-vulnerable adults.

Farm animal diseases relevant to goats are mainly spread through:

- Animals, people and machinery moving between and within holdings.

- Outside visitors to livestock holdings – people and vehicles.
- Introducing new animals (of any species).
- Contact with neighbours' livestock over the fence or gate.
- Shared farm equipment – a particular problem with hobby goat keepers.
- Contamination by vermin and wild birds.
- Goats drinking from contaminated rivers and streams.

New goats moving onto a unit should be kept in quarantine for a minimum of 14 days, but ideally longer if possible. A building with a separate airspace to the main goat accommodation is ideal (**Fig. 1.33**), as is a separate paddock outdoors, providing goats do not have nose to nose contact with others in adjoining fields. They should not, however, be kept in social isolation, but should always be within sight, sound and contact of at least one other goat for company.

During this quarantine period, they should be examined for any clinical evidence of infectious disease such as ectoparasites, footrot and caseous lymphadenitis (CLA). A blood sample should be taken to assess, for example, the caprine arthritis encephalitis or CLA status. A tuberculin test should be considered if tuberculosis is a known local problem, and a quarantine anthelmintic treatment should be given to avoid the risk of introducing anthelmintic resistant nematodes. Any vaccinations relevant to the holding onto which they have been moved should be administered, together with any other prophylactic or therapeutic regime deemed necessary, based on history and clinical and laboratory test results.

LEGISLATION

Legislation relevant to the goat will vary widely depending on where and how they are kept, and as such any detailed description is beyond the remit of this book. However, legislation will for the most part be relevant to all goats, no matter why and how they are kept. In the UK, for example, all goats including those kept as pets are designated as farm animals, mainly because of their susceptibility to notifiable/scheduled diseases such as foot and mouth disease and the need for relevant authorities to be aware of their geographical location for possible disease control measures. Such legislation may include the requirement to:

- Be kept on a registered holding.
- Ensure individual goat identification such as an ear tag, electronic identification device, tattoo, pastern or collar mark.
- Keep a record of movements onto and off the premises.
- Maintain a medicines record of products administered, and be aware of the required meat and milk withhold times.
- Be aware of any mandatory codes of goat welfare.
- Be aware of those notifiable or scheduled diseases relevant to the country within which the goats are kept.
- Be aware of any relevant legislation covering minor procedures such as castration and disbudding, and also of on-farm emergency euthanasia.

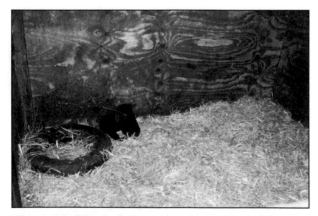

Fig. 1.33 **This isolation pen was constructed in a tractor shed. Wooden walls make disinfection more difficult, therefore should be avoided.**

CHAPTER 2

REPRODUCTIVE SYSTEM

THE DOE

NORMAL STRUCTURE AND FUNCTION

The goat has a bicornual uterus, with a short uterine body of about 30 mm, and curled-up horns (**Fig. 2.1**). The endometrium is grey–pink in colour (in older females sometimes brown–yellow) and bears the typical caruncles (**Fig. 2.2**). Pigmentation of the endometrium is rare in the doe.

The external cervical os lies close to the vaginal floor, with a transverse mucosal fold in front of it. The internal os is poorly developed. The cervical mucosa forms 5–8 circular folds (**Fig. 2.2**) and contains cervical glands that are unique to the goat and cat (in contrast, vestibular glands are absent in the goat).

The caprine ovary is oval to round, about 15 mm long and 10–18 mm high, weighs 1–2 g and is encased by the ovarian bursa. Twin ovulations may originate either from the same ovary or from both ovaries. Therefore, corpora lutea (CLs) from the same oestrous cycle may be present in one or in both ovaries.

The oviduct is 140–150 mm long.

FERTILITY

Goats are regarded as highly fertile, regularly achieving >90% overall pregnancy rate. Puberty starts at 5–10 months of age, when the goat has reached about 45% of its mature body weight. Most breeds are pubertal around 200–220 days (240 days for the Angora).

Nulliparous (maiden) animals should have achieved at least 60–65% of their expected mature body weight at the point of breeding. Fertility is reduced in small maidens. For example, the ovulation

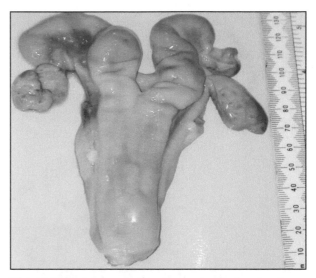

Fig. 2.1 **Normal reproductive tract of a doe (vagina at bottom, horns and ovaries at top of image).**

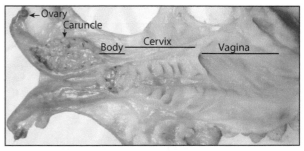

Fig. 2.2 **Partially opened reproductive tract, showing the circular folds of the cervix and caruncles. (Note: Endometrial pigmentation, as in this tract, is rare in the doe.)**

rate was 50% in Angora doelings <22 kg, compared with 90% when >27 kg. Doelings <27 kg showed a conception rate of only 50%, compared with 80% if >27 kg. Twin ovulations are rare in small maidens, yet reach 100% for females >45 kg.

FECUNDITY

Litter size varies with genotype due to differences in kisspeptides, which are major upstream regulators of gonadotropin-releasing hormone (GnRH). There is a positive correlation between prolificacy and the presence of wattles (**Fig. 2.3**).

OESTROUS CYCLE AND SIGNS OF OESTRUS

Goat breeds originating from mid- to high latitudes (temperate regions) are short-day seasonal

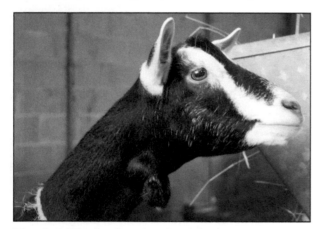

Fig. 2.3 Wattles, here in a British Alpine goat, are associated with prolificacy.

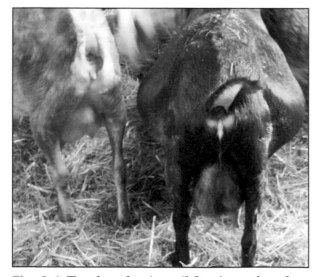

Fig. 2.4 Two does showing tail flagging, a sign of oestrus. Frequent urination may also be seen.

polyoestrus breeders. In Northern Europe they are typically in anoestrus between April and June, in the transitory phase in July and August, with full ovarian activity between September and January to February.

The oestrous cycle is 19–21 days long, with behavioural oestrus lasting 24–36 hours and ovulation taking place 24–36 hours after the start of oestrus. At the start and end of the breeding season, short oestrous cycles may occur. Equally, ovulation may occur without oestrus behaviour. Puberty and onset of ovarian activity is linked to body weight in the maiden female, and occurs when she reaches 40–50% of her expected mature body weight.

Signs of oestrus include flagging of the tail (**Fig. 2.4**), bleating (which can be very vocal), vulval hyperaemia and oedema, and frequent urination. Occasionally, does will mount each other, but this can also be a sign of dominance or hermaphroditism and, therefore, is not a reliable sign on its own. The doe will show interest in the male (**Fig. 2.5**) and, on farms without a buck, a 'scent cloth' (also

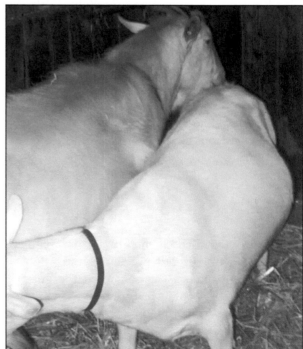

Fig. 2.5 The doe (animal in the foreground) expresses interest in the buck when in oestrus (and vice versa).

known as 'billy rag') may be used to detect this. The buck's reaction to the doe can also be used as an indicator of oestrus. Buck pens may be usefully placed at the exit of the milking parlour to detect receptive does.

CONTROL OF OESTRUS

Out-of-season breeding
Overview
There are four main options for manipulating the breeding season. The total period of ovarian activity in such stimulated females is often shortened. Use of progesterone typically results in the stimulated oestrus plus one other, before anoestrus sets in again. For natural service, sexual activity must be ensured in the buck – if necessary by lighting regime stimulation. The doe:buck ratio is reduced to 5–10:1 for synchronised does.

Technique
1 Artificial lighting: a change from exposure to long days (16–20 hours of light) to short days (8–12 hours) will induce ovarian activity. Long and short days are alternated every 60–90 days to achieve the desired breeding period. Alternatively, for spring mating does are exposed to long days from mid-winter. Exposure to 7 hours of light during the day, plus one hour of light 16–17 hours after dawn is sufficient to mimic a long day. Light intensity should be about 300 lux (equivalent to illumination in an office).
2 Presence of male: exposure to a sexually active male (including vasectomised) before or after the normal breeding period shortens and delays, respectively, the anoestrus period of does by around 1.5 months. In addition, the continuous presence of photostimulated males prevents seasonal anoestrus in the majority of does, and the introduction of such males can trigger ovarian activity during the normal anoestrus period.
3 Melatonin: exposure to melatonin mimics a short day. It may be administered either in the early afternoon, orally or by i/m injection, or as a slow-release implant (e.g. Regulin®, containing 18 mg melatonin). In Northern European breeds, the season can be advanced by up to 1.5 months. For earlier onset or higher response rates, a combination of lighting regime mimicking long days and melatonin is required.
4 Progesterone in combination with equine chorionic gonadotropin (eCG):
   - Megestrol acetate (MGA), given orally at a total daily dose of 0.25 mg for 8–14 days, either mixed into TMR or divided into two daily doses 12 hours apart.
   - Intravaginal progesterone-impregnanted sponges: for example, ones containing fluorogestone acetate (minimum dose 20 mg [some authors prefer 40–45 mg] for 11–18 days), or CIDR® Sheep and Goat Devices (0.3 g progesterone) for 18–21 days. Two days before the device is removed, 400–800 IU of eCG are given. Prostaglandin-F 2 alpha ($PGF_{2\alpha}$) is not necessary during the anoestrus period. Natural mating or artificial insemination (AI) is carried out 40–48 hours after device removal (or 30 and 48 hours for double insemination).
   - 3 mg norgestomet as an ear implant (using half of the available cattle implants) for 11 days. Twenty-four hours prior to removal, $PGF_{2\alpha}$ and 500 IU eCG are given. Oestrus follows within 24 hours of implant removal.

The dose rate of eCG depends on age (doelings receiving a lower dose) and gap to natural breeding season (the wider, the higher the dose). The higher dose rates may stimulate moderate superovulation, resulting in larger litters.

Synchronisation during the breeding season
Indication
Synchronisation can facilitate batch kidding or the use of AI, although pregnancy rates to AI are often lower than to natural service following synchronisation.

Technique
1 Use of progesterone sponges or CIDR® Sheep and Goat Devices (as above) for 14–16 days. 400 IU eCG plus $PGF_{2\alpha}$ are either given 2 days before or at the time of sponge removal. Most animals are in oestrus 30 hours later,

with single service or insemination at 40–48 hours, or double at 30 and 48 hours.

2 Two doses of 2.5 mg of PGF$_{2\alpha}$ given 11 days apart. Does may be bred to observed oestrus after the first injection or at a fixed time after the second injection (double insemination recommended). In either case, mean interval to oestrus is 44–50 hours after injection.

OVARIAN DISORDERS

Anoestrus

Nulligravid animals (maiden, doeling):

- Prepubescent because of suboptimal growth (see above).
- Intersex:
  - Overview. A recessive gene with incomplete penetrance, and closely linked to the polled gene, resulting in genetically female animals (60 XX chromosome complement), of which most are male hermaphrodites. Sterility in males results from blocked epididymes.
  - Clinical presentation. Varying degrees of phenotypic appearance, including abnormally long (>3 cm) anogenital distance, and an enlarged clitoris (**Fig. 2.6**) or penile structure ventral to the anus in the female. The vulva may appear normal. In the male, a shortened penis, hypospadias (**Fig. 2.7**) and testicular hypoplasia may be present. Depending on the abnormalities present, urine scalding may result.
  - Diagnosis. If no outward signs, check vaginal length in infertile or anoestrus doelings. Also useful is ultrasonography of the reproductive tract. Affected males are often aspermic.
- Freemartinism (XX and XY chimera) is relatively rare in goats.
- Partial aplasia of reproductive tract unrelated to intersex.

Age-independent causes of anoestrus include:

- Season: breeding attempts out of season.
- Pregnancy: unobserved mating, especially if male kids weaned later than 4 months of age.

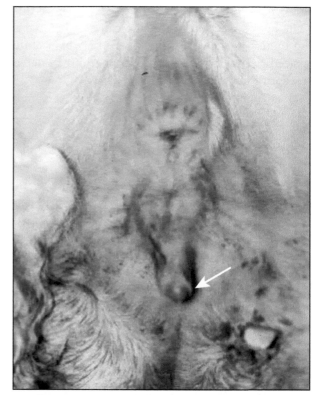

Fig. 2.6 An enlarged clitoris (arrow) may be seen in intersex females.

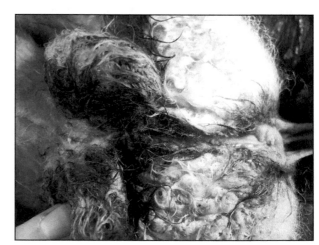

Fig. 2.7 Hypospadias may be present in intersex males, shown here in a lamb lying in right lateral recumbency.

- Lactational anoestrus.
- Negative energy balance resulting in suboptimal luteinising hormone (LH) surge.
- Poor heat detection.

- Failure to stand: not being in oestrus; fear of the buck, especially in maiden animals.
- Old age: ovarian activity will progressively wane from teen years onwards.

Cystic ovarian disease

There is limited information on the prevalence or incidence of cystic ovarian disease (COD). One abattoir study showed 12% of goats had COD.

Clinical presentation

Luteal cysts typically result in anoestrus or prolonged inter-oestrus intervals. Follicular cysts may result in anoestrus, irregular inter-oestrus intervals and, occasionally, nymphomania.

Diagnosis

Ovarian ultrasonography allows the most definitive diagnosis (**Fig. 2.8**). Milk or blood progesterone levels may be used to confirm the type of cyst (luteal cysts resulting in high levels, and follicular cysts in low levels).

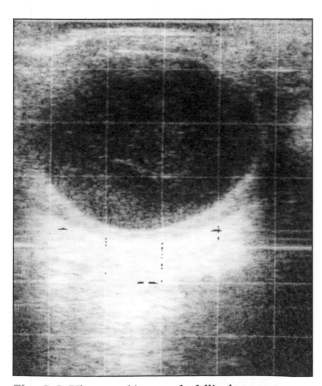

Fig. 2.8 Ultrasound image of a follicular cyst. Characteristic are the thin wall and anechoic fluid.

Treatment/management/control

Options mirror those used in cows: $PGF_{2\alpha}$ for luteal cysts and GnRH for follicular cysts, or intravaginal progesterone for either type. It should be noted that goats appear to be less responsive than cows to treatment of COD. In valuable does, physical destruction via laparoscopy may be considered.

For treating follicular cysts, the dose rates are:

- 8–10 µg buserelin;
- 25–50 µg gonadorelin.

BREEDING

Natural service

Male behaviour

The male's reaction to a doe in oestrus consists of sniffing her urine (**Fig. 2.5**), flehmen, striking with the front leg, tongue flicking and vocalisation (snorting- and clicking-like sounds). Copulation takes place in the standing position. Thrusting, often with simultaneous throwing back of the head, indicates ejaculation. Sperm is deposited into the cranial vagina.

Technique

Hand mating is commonly employed, providing control over the mating process and allowing accurate recording of breeding date and sire. The AM-PM rule applies, meaning that a doe first seen in oestrus in the morning is presented to the buck in the evening and vice versa. Alternatively, the doe may be bred every 12 hours until going out of oestrus. Sexual performance, including time to mounting and ejaculation, is shortened in bucks that have observed another male mating a doe.

For single-sire group mating, a doe:buck ratio of 50:1 is acceptable for a mature buck. The ratio is 10:1 for a yearling (or where does are synchronised) and 25:1 for a 2-year-old male. After 6 weeks, the buck should be moved to a different group of females to maintain sexual interest. On farms with multiple buck–doe groups, fighting along the fence line is avoided either by wide alleyways between paddocks or, less effectively, solid fence panels.

Multiple sire groups afford the easiest management. However, sire and breeding dates will be unknown, and dominance and fighting often lead to suboptimal pregnancy rates (**Fig. 2.9**). Horned and polled bucks should not be mixed in the same paddock.

If raddles are used, the harness must be well-fitting and the bucks checked regularly for harness-induced trauma.

Artificial insemination

Overview

AI allows effective use of the best male genetics, reduces biosecurity and disease risks and is independent of the geographical proximity of the male and female. Pregnancy rates between 40% and 60% are achievable, in part influenced by type of semen (fresh, chilled or frozen-thawed) and insemination method (transcervical or laparoscopic). In contrast to several other species, yearling females appear to have a lower pregnancy rate following AI than older does. Pregnancy rates also decline by about 5% in does that have received several hormonal treatments or where cryopreservation of the semen exceeds 9 years. Sexed semen is reported to achieve about a 40% pregnancy rate, with 83% accuracy of gender of the kids.

Technique – semen collection

Semen is collected into an artificial vagina. Either the buck is allowed to mount a female in oestrus, or they are trained to use a dummy. For the latter technique, the presence of a teaser female appears to increase sperm output. An insemination dose of $60–120 \times 10^6$ spermatozoa is common. Bucks may be light-stimulated to allow collection throughout the year.

After dilution, fresh semen is kept at 30°C in tris-buffer or ultra-high temperature (UHT) skimmed milk, and used within 30 minutes of collection. For chilled semen, the sperm needs to be washed if egg yolk is used as buffer (to remove the phospholipase A enzyme from the seminal plasma). The semen is then gradually cooled to 5°C and used within 24 hours of collection. For cryopreservation, standard freezing methods are used as for other species, again washing the sperm if egg yolk is used.

Technique – insemination

For frozen-thawed semen, the AM-PM rule applies (see above). Fresh and chilled semen have a longer survival time in the doe, making insemination timing in relation to ovulation less critical.

Suppliers' guidelines on thawing frozen semen should be followed (**Fig. 2.10**). If not stipulated, semen is thawed at 35–37°C for at least 40 seconds. Chilled semen does not require warming prior to use.

Insemination via laparoscopy has replaced laparotomy, and allows precise placement of semen into the horn ipsilateral to the corpus luteum (**Fig. 2.11**). The fasted doe is either anaesthetised (e.g. with a

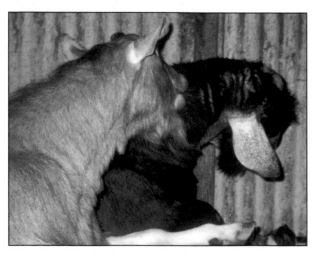

Fig. 2.9 Fighting between bucks is common in multiple sire groups.

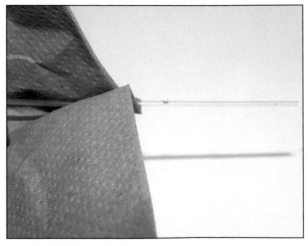

Fig. 2.10 After thawing an AI straw, all water must be removed from its outside prior to insemination.

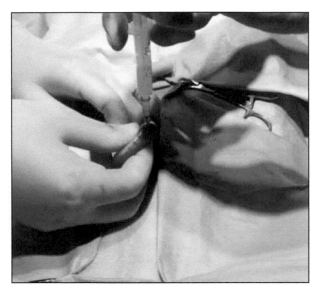

Fig. 2.11 **Insemination via laparotomy. (Image courtesy Angelika von Heimendahl.)**

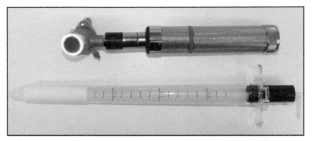

Fig. 2.12 **A human sigmoidoscope with a ring light source is invaluable for transvaginal procedures. A head with a ring-shaped light is obtainable for most ophthalmoscope base units (e.g. Welch Allyn, Buckinghamshire, UK).**

xylazine–ketamine combination) or sedated followed by local anaesthesia, and placed in dorsal recumbency with the head tilted slightly downwards.

Transcervical intrauterine insemination is often more practical and yields acceptable, if up to 20% lower, results. It may be used in does that have kidded at least once. Semen is deposited deep into the cervix. A straight insemination pipette is warmed by vigorous rubbing. An air-bubble is drawn up into the syringe prior to filling with the semen dose. Sedation and epidural anaesthesia are recommended. The doe's hindquarters are lifted up high and the perineal area dry-wiped. Using a human sigmoidoscope with a ring-light source (**Fig. 2.12**), the external os is visualised and the pipette advanced into the cervix. The doe is kept in the elevated position for 1–2 minutes.

Embryo transfer
Overview
Embryo transfer (ET) allows proliferation of genetically superior females or expansion of small breed populations. Just as with AI, additional applications include biosecurity and disease control, and inter-country exchange. This technique is not as reliably developed in goats as in other species, although pregnancy rates of 50% have been achieved. The doe's response to the hormonal programme can

be variable, and costs may be deemed prohibitive by the producer, with ET costing about ten times more than AI per kid produced. In addition, the repeated use of large molecule hormones carries a hypersensitivity reaction risk.

Technique
The superovulation programme is best started after a natural or induced reference heat (= day 0). A progesterone sponge is inserted on day 0 for 11 days. A luteolytic dose of $PGF_{2\alpha}$ is given on day 9. A total dose of 16–20 mg follicle stimulating hormone (FSH) is administered every 12 hours in a tapering dose from day 9 (e.g. 2 × 4 mg on day 9, 2 × 2 mg on days 10 and 11; **Fig. 2.13**). FSH is preferred over eCG; however, with both hormones premature luteal regression may be observed leading to the loss of the embryos. The use of GnRH, LH, human chorionic gonadotropin (hCG) or flunixin meglumine after the onset of oestrus is variably successful in reducing this risk.

Flushing is carried out 6–7 days after oestrus in the anaesthetised or sedated (plus local anaesthetic) doe. Laparoscopy is the conventional method, but transcervical collection is also possible. For the latter, administration of $PGF_{2\alpha}$ 8–16 hours prior to flushing makes catheterisation of the cervix easier and results in good embryo recovery rates.

For freezing, ethylene glycol is a suitable cryopreservant.

The recipient's oestrus should be synchronised to occur within 12 hours either side of the donor's oestrus. Transfer is by laparoscopy.

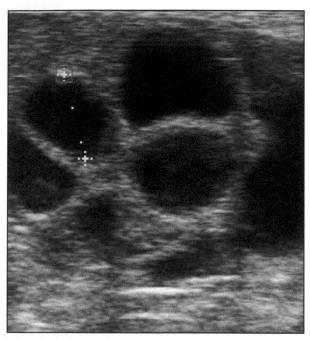

Fig. 2.13 Multiple follicles on an ovary after a superovulation programme.

Pregnancy diagnosis
See Chapter 3.

Misalliance
Administering PGF$_{2\alpha}$ up to day 90 after breeding will quite reliably induce abortion 42–76 hours later. There are no data on misalliance after day 90, but a similar effect would be expected.

UTERINE DISORDERS

Abattoir study-based prevalence of acquired reproductive tract abnormalities (such as salpingitis or endometritis) is reported in the region of 2%. To reduce the number of potential differential diagnoses, it is useful to group disorders into congenital versus acquired.

Anatomical abnormalities – congenital
Overview
Abnormal embryological development of the female reproductive tract may lead to incomplete perforation, canalisation, duplication or partial or complete agenesis or aplasia.

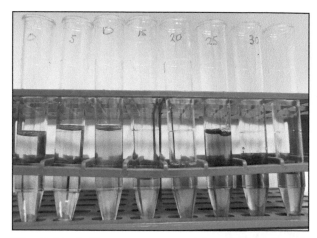

Fig. 2.14 Oviduct patency test. After placing phenol-sulphonthalein (Phenol red) into the uterus, the dye passes into the peritoneum via the oviduct, enters the peritoneal circulation and is excreted via the kidneys. Urine is collected every 5 minutes via a Foley catheter (under epidural anaesthesia). Dye in the urine after 10 minutes indicates both oviducts are patent; dye after 20 minutes indicates one oviduct is patent; no dye after 30 minutes indicates both oviducts are blocked. Best performed 14 days after oestrus.

Clinical presentation
Nulligravid (maiden) females are affected. Disorders affecting the uterus or oviduct (syns. fallopian tube, salpinx) will lead to failure to conceive. Ovarian aplasia or hypoplasia will present as anoestrus if bilateral or irregular oestrous cycles if unilateral. Agitation during mating on either the maiden female's or buck's part may indicate a persistent hymen.

Diagnosis
Transrectal ultrasonography is the best method to detect uterine and ovarian abnormalities. Sedation and the use of an epidural is recommended to reduce the risk of trauma. A persistent hymen may be confirmed with the aid of a speculum (e.g. a human sigmoidoscope). An oviduct patency test may be necessary to rule out fallopian tube abnormalities (**Fig. 2.14**).

Differential diagnosis
Other causes of failure to conceive and irregularities of the oestrous cycle, as discussed elsewhere.

Treatment/management/control

A thin, membrane-like persistent hymen may be broken down with the aid of forceps and a vaginal speculum. Removal of a thick, flesh-like hymen is usually unsatisfactory and may result in substantial haemorrhage. Doelings with unilateral ovarian or oviduct abnormalities could, in theory, be bred from, either with ultrasonographic monitoring of activity on the normal ovary or using oocyte aspiration and *in-vitro* fertilisation techniques. However, a genetic base to the abnormalities must be considered, and such doelings are best removed from the breeding pool.

Anatomical abnormalities – acquired

Overview

Primi- or multiparous does may acquire abnormalities such as scarring, incomplete vulval or cervical seal (**Fig. 2.15**), rectovaginal fistula or salpingitis.

Aetiology

Trauma may result from the mating process, parturition or reproductive manipulations such as transrectal ultrasonography, vaginal examination and AI or ET techniques. Infectious aetiologies are also common, typically involving opportunistic or commensal pathogens.

Clinical presentation

Disorders of the vulva and perineum are obvious on clinical examination. Vulval discharge, failure to conceive, oestrous cycle abnormalities and signs of abdominal discomfort (such as back arching, tail lifting, squatting) should prompt examination of the reproductive tract. Frequent squatting and straining may give the appearance of dysuria (**Fig. 2.16**).

Diagnosis

Vaginal examination with the aid of a speculum (e.g. human sigmoidoscope; **Fig. 2.12**) will reveal abnormalities involving the vestibulum, vagina and external cervical opening. Oviduct abnormalities may be detectable on transrectal ultrasonography. Sedation and the use of an epidural are recommended for both methods.

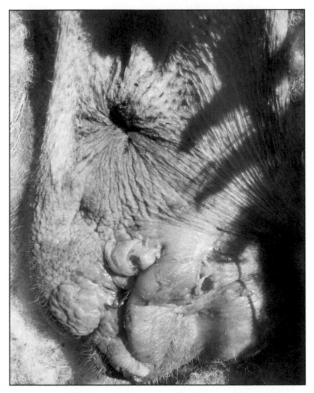

Fig. 2.15 Vulval sutures to address a prolapse have caused marked tissue trauma, inflammation and distortion, potentially leading to a poor vulval seal.

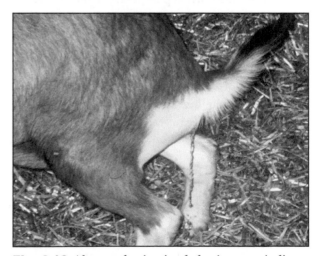

Fig. 2.16 Abnormal urination behaviour can indicate an acquired uterine tract abnormality.

Differential diagnosis

For signs of abdominal discomfort, these include disorders of the urinary or gastrointestinal tract that result in pain.

Treatment/management/control

Surgical correction of traumatic lesions may be considered. Surgery is either conducted within a few hours of the trauma occurring or after several weeks when healing by secondary intention has occurred and tissues have remodelled. Incomplete seal of the vulval lips may be addressed by Caslick surgery or vulvoplasty. Where the Caslick technique is used, mating must be supervised or AI used to avoid trauma, and the seal opened surgically prior to parturition. Vaginal trauma leading to urine pooling may be corrected by vaginoplasty.

Infectious lesions are treated with a course of antimicrobials.

For both groups of lesions, anti-inflammatory drugs are strongly recommended, and the doe must be sexually rested until complete resolution of the problem.

Endometritis

Overview

Endometritis is mild to moderate inflammation of the endometrium only, with or without infection and without systemic effects. Clinically, the term is often used to describe chronic endometritis (i.e. beyond the normal puerperal period [i.e. present after 14–21 days post partum]). Occurrence tends to be occasional in the doe.

Aetiology

A variety of gram-positive and gram-negative pathogens, including anaerobes, may be involved, including *Trueperella pyogenes*, *Fusobacter necrophorum*, *Escherichia coli* and *Streptococcus* spp. Occasionally, fungal pathogens are involved.

Affected does often have a history of dystocia (**Fig. 2.17**) or retained fetal membranes (RFM).

Clinical presentation

Mucopurulent to purulent vaginal discharge is present, often noticed on the tail or hind legs, but sometimes only apparent on vaginal examination or during oestrus. Uterine involution is often delayed. The cervix typically remains open; however, if it is closed, the sub-form 'pyometra' results. Frequent return to oestrus is common, but anoestrus or other irregular oestrous patterns also occur.

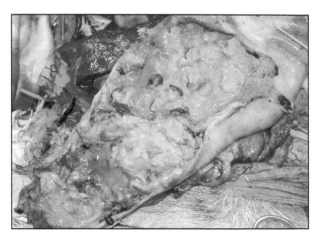

Fig. 2.17 Dystocia is a risk factor for endometritis, as in this ewe that required a caesarean section.

The doe is not systemically affected.

Diagnosis

Excessive uterine fluid, typically echodense, is detected during ultrasonography (**Fig. 2.18**). Establishing the presence of a corpus luteum is important for treatment decisions. Vaginal examination using a speculum or

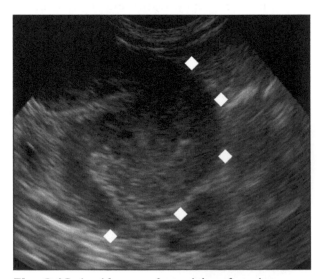

Fig. 2.18 A mid-tone echogenicity of uterine fluid suggests the presence of debris. This, together with uterine horn enlargement, is a common finding in endometritis or pyometra (as in this image of a 10-year-old Pygmy goat). The outline of the uterus is indicated by the white diamonds.

endoscope shows mucopurulent fluid exiting through the cervix.

Definitive diagnosis requires either culture or uterine biopsy. These are rarely performed in practice, but should be considered in protracted cases. To obtain a sample for culture, a double-guarded pipette is used to avoid contamination from the more caudal tract.

Differential diagnosis

Uterine neoplasia frequently presents with vulval discharge (ultrasonography and biopsy are used to confirm). The discharge present in metritis typically has a haemorrhagic and malodorous element to it and the doe is often systemically affected. It is important to establish that the discharge originates in the uterus, not the urinary tract.

Treatment/management/control

The aim of hormonal treatment is to exert oestrogen influence. This is achieved by a luteolytic dose of $PGF_{2\alpha}$ if a corpus luteum is present, or use of exogenous oestrogen if available for veterinary use (e.g. oestradiol benzoate).

Hormonal treatment may be combined with antimicrobials, typically given systemically because of the impracticality of intrauterine administration in the doe. Suitable groups include penicillins (from week 5 post partum), tetracyclines (at minimum 10 mg/kg) and cephalosporins. Not suitable are trimethoprim–sulphonamide, aminoglycosides, streptomycin and enrofloxacin, because of a combination of presence of necrotic material, low oxygen tension, acidic pH and presence of anaerobic pathogens.

No goat-specific treatment studies of fungal endometritis are available. In the mare, lufenuron has been found useful.

Plasma and colostral whey intrauterine infusions are being investigated in the cow.

The mainstays of control are avoidance of predisposing factors, such as dystocia, unhygienic intervention and RFM, and, if they do occur, prompt treatment. Routine post-partum administration of $PGF_{2\alpha}$ has shown ambiguous results in the cow. Immunosuppression (e.g. caused by endoparasitism) should be ruled out.

Uterine neoplasia
Overview

No firm data on incidence or prevalence exist. As with most neoplasia, older does are more commonly affected.

Aetiology

A variety of tumours have been reported, including adenocarcinoma, leiomyoma or leiomyosarcoma, and lymphoma (**Figs. 2.19, 2.20**). These may affect any part of the tubular reproductive tract and also the broad ligament. Squamous cell carcinoma of the vulval lips has occurred. Vaginal papillomas may be seen, which are typically benign.

Clinical presentation

Affected does often present because of chronic vaginal discharge. Failure to conceive may also be reported.

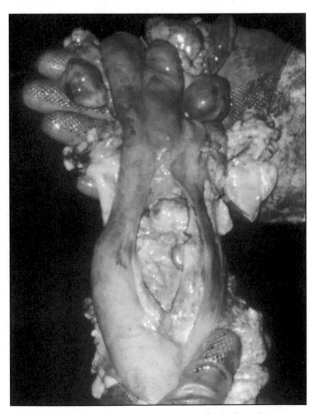

Fig. 2.19 Reproductive tract neoplasia in a 9-year-old Toggenburg doe presented for return to oestrus. A follicular cyst and purulent vaginal discharge were present.

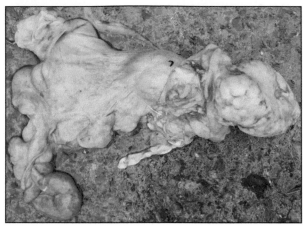

Fig. 2.20 Cervical tumour in an elderly doe. (Cervix to the right, uterine horns to the left.)

Diagnosis

Ultrasonography combined with uterine biopsy is most useful. Where treatment is attempted, a thorough clinical examination combined with thoracic and abdominal ultrasonography and radiography is advisable to rule out metastasis.

Differential diagnosis

For vaginal discharge, endometritis. For failure to conceive, multiple differentials are possible, as discussed elsewhere in this chapter.

Treatment/management/control

Ovariohysterectomy may be attempted if metastasis is not present. This may be followed by chemotherapy, although very limited clinical experience exists in the goat.

HERD INFERTILITY PROBLEM

Areas to investigate include:

- Female to male ratio (max. 50:1, or 5–10:1 if synchronised).
- Out-of-season breeding (where used): males not sexually active.
- Oestrus detection rate and accuracy poor; wrong timing if hand-mating used.
- No male contact provided.
- Negative energy balance and/or suboptimal body condition in does.

- Concurrent disease (e.g. endoparasite burden).
- Nutritional deficits (possibly including phosphorus, copper, selenium, iron).
- Excessive stress levels (e.g. frequent re-grouping, bullying).
- AI technique (where used): poor storage, handling and insemination technique, wrong timing.
- Presence of venereal or abortive pathogens.

INFECTIOUS DISEASES

Caprine herpesvirus 1
Definition/overview

Caprine herpesvirus 1 (CpHV-1) infection is associated predominantly with a venereally transmitted vulvovaginitis and balanoposthitis. The virus can also cause early embryonic death or abortion and a fatal viraemia in newborn kids. The condition has been reported in the USA, Australia and New Zealand, but also more recently in a number of European countries. Its presence has often been confirmed only by serological surveys, with little or no evidence of known clinical infection.

Aetiology

A DNA virus, one of a closely related group of alphaherpesviruses known to cause a spectrum of diseases in ruminants (e.g. bovine herpesvirus 1 causing infectious bovine rhinotracheitis infection in cattle). Although cross-species infection with these viruses can occur experimentally, natural cross infection is uncommon.

Pathophysiology

Infection is acquired either via the intranasal route, resulting in a viraemia and localisation in the genital tract, or the venereal route whereby infection appears to remain localised without systemic spread. One of the features of herpesvirus infection is latent infection and subsequent recrudescence of clinical disease, and this feature is recognised in goats with CpHV-1 infection. Recrudescence can occur during oestrus, potentially resulting in the rapid spread of infection during the breeding season.

Clinical presentation

Both males and females are susceptible to the genital form of the disease, which tends to occur as an outbreak during the breeding season, rather than in a sporadic form. Vulval lesions begin with swelling and congestion of the vulval lips; some does may develop a vaginal discharge (there are usually no systemic signs). Over the next few days, small shallow multiple erosions appear over the vulval and vaginal mucosa, and the discharge becomes more copious and mucopurulent in appearance. These lesions gradually develop superficial scabs before healing spontaneously, although recrudescence often occurs during the next breeding season. Infected males may be asymptomatic or develop hyperaemia and congestion of the penile and preputial mucosa, followed by the emergence of small superficial erosions and a penile discharge. In severe cases, males may be reluctant to serve. Infection via the intranasal route, resulting in viraemia, may lead to early embryonic loss and abortion, otherwise the overall effect on reproductive performance is minimal. Many infected goats may remain completely asymptomatic.

Diagnosis

Diagnosis is based on the presenting clinical signs during the breeding season. Paired serology may give further confirmation, although any test employed must be able to distinguish between CpHV-1 and other alpha-herpesviruses. Definitive diagnosis is based on a demonstration of the virus either in cell culture or by means of other available tests such as polymerase chain reaction (PCR).

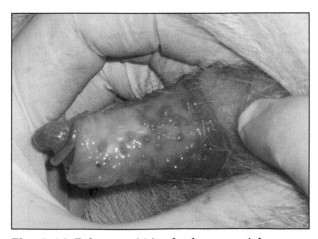

Fig. 2.21 Balanoposthitis of unknown aetiology. (Image courtesy Yoav Alony-Gilboa.)

Differential diagnosis

Other causes of vulvovaginitis and balanoposthitis (**Fig 2.21**), including some *Mycoplasma* and *Ureaplasma* spp., and *Corynebacterium renale* in males.

Treatment/management/control

There is no treatment for the primary viral infection, although topical or parenteral antibiotic may be useful if secondary bacterial infection has occurred. Most cases regress spontaneously. Any attempt to eradicate disease must be based on a repeated test and cull policy, although this can be a slow process due to latency and recrudescence of infection. Vaccines have been developed and are available in some countries.

EMBRYONIC LOSS AND ABORTION

Once implantation has taken place, there are a number of infectious and non-infectious insults that may challenge the viability of the developing embryo and fetus, resulting in embryonic loss or abortion.

Early embryonic losses may go unnoticed, merely resulting in an apparent failure to conceive with return to oestrus, or may be evident at scanning when one or more fluid-filled areas may be apparent in the uterus where implantation had originally occurred.

Infectious causes of early embryonic loss include:

- Toxoplasmosis: if a naive doe is exposed to heavy field infection in early pregnancy.
- Border disease virus (BDV).
- Schmallenberg virus.
- Caprine herpesvirus.
- Tick-borne fever.
- Any infectious agent causing pyrexia in the critical early stages of implantation and establishment of the developing embryo in the uterine wall. Also subclinical endometritis.

Non-infectious causes of early embryonic loss include:

- Nutrition: goats will breed successfully in arid areas even when nutritional input is very low, and carry kids to full term. Overt starvation would need to be extreme to cause embryonic or fetal loss. Specific vitamin and trace element deficiencies, imbalances and excesses have all been cited as causing embryonic loss in goats, but any underlying mechanisms are poorly understood, and any association is rarely proven.

- Genetic abnormalities affecting either the autosomes or the sex chromosomes.
- Failure of the maternal body to recognise the presence of the embryo (interferon tau) or failure of hormonal support (especially progesterone).
- Environmental stress such as extremes of temperature.
- Trauma, including AI of a pregnant doe and forceful early pregnancy diagnosis.
- Inadvertent use of $PGF_{2\alpha}$ causing luteolysis.
- Inadvertent overdose with a wide range of pharmacological agents in early pregnancy has been cited as leading to embryonic loss.
- Sheep and goat hybrids: when run together, inadvertent matings between sheep and goats may occur. If a male sheep fertilises a female goat, then the resulting embryo rarely survives beyond the second month of pregnancy.

ABORTION

Ascertaining the cause of abortion in goats requires a thorough, well-structured investigation including an assessment of the environment and any nutrition and management factors, in addition to gathering material for laboratory examination. Many of the infectious causes of abortion in goats also cause abortion in sheep (and vice versa).

At what stage intervention is necessary will depend on the size of the unit and the number and timescale of losses. Occasional abortion is an inevitable risk of every pregnancy, often related to physiological or anatomical abnormalities of the fetal–maternal unit. As abortions escalate in number, and in particular if 'abortion storms' occur, the likelihood of a common underlying cause will rise, and an investigation becomes necessary.

History taking should include the current management of the cohort, the diet fed and recent diet changes, recent purchases or other introductions to the group (including both goats and sheep), any

evidence of contact with sheep, particularly if pregnant/breeding, the ages of does affected and an estimate of the current abortion rate. A good recording system enables comparisons with previous years.

Clinical examination may identify relevant factors such as pyrexia or septicaemia, or any intercurrent disease problem such as enterotoxaemia.

Material should be collected from aborting does for laboratory examination – this includes:

- Placenta.
- Fetus.
- Maternal blood sample.

If fetuses cannot be sent directly to a laboratory, the following samples should be submitted:

- Aseptically collected fetal stomach content (e.g. using a sterile vacutainer). In the absence of free fluid, an aseptically taken swab.
- Free abdominal or thoracic fluid.
- Portion of placenta to include a cotyledon.
- Maternal blood sample.

It may also be useful to collect fresh fetal spleen, brain and lung and store them in a freezer, together with similar tissue in fixative, for submission for further more specific testing after routine testing has been completed.

Blood samples can also be collected from other goats at the same stage of pregnancy, which can be retained as stored serum for serology pairing if any does do subsequently abort. Material from more than one aborting doe is gathered, if possible, to reduce the chance of selecting an atypical sporadic abortion case.

Goats do present the investigating veterinary surgeon with a dilemma, however, as they are fastidious about clearing up any evidence that they have either aborted or kidded. As such, the placenta will often be consumed rapidly and may not be easily obtainable for submission. It is the single most useful specimen to collect, so its importance should be stressed to the owner or stock-keeper, who should remain vigilant, swiftly harvesting any that may appear (and, most importantly, from representative cases).

Management advice to minimise any further subsequent spread of infection includes:

- The rapid removal and safe disposal of any aborted material including fetus and placenta.
- The removal and safe disposal of any contaminated bedding (e.g. by incineration).
- The isolation of any goat that has aborted.

It is important to remember that many of the infectious causes of abortion in goats are potential zoonoses, including Q fever (*Coxiella burnetii*) and enzootic abortion (enzootic abortion of ewes [EAE]; *Chlamydia psittaci*), the latter organism presenting a particular risk to pregnant women.

Common infectious causes of abortion

Toxoplasmosis
Definition/overview
Toxoplasmosis is an important cause of abortion in both goats and sheep and has a worldwide distribution. Although widespread tissue distribution of oocysts may occur in a susceptible goat after ingestion, clinical disease other than abortion is rare. It is a potentially zoonotic disease, with risk to humans associated with the potential excretion of tachyzoites in the milk and the presence of tissue cysts in the meat of recently infected goats, killed by pasteurisation and adequate cooking, respectively.

Aetiology
Toxoplasmosis is caused by the obligate intracellular protozoal parasite *Toxoplasma gondii*, of the Family Sarcocystidae, of which there are a number of recognised genotypes that are useful in epidemiological surveys.

Pathophysiology
The cat (both wild and domestic) appears to be the definitive host for this parasite, and becomes infected by eating small rodents, undercooked meat or aborted ruminant material. It can also become infected congenitally from an infected dam. Oocysts are first seen in the faeces at around 3 days after infection and may be released for as long as 20 days, when many million oocysts will have contaminated the environment. Oocysts sporulate when voided within 1–5 days, depending on aeration and temperature, and remain viable in the environment for several months. It is suggested that cats generally develop immunity to *T. gondii* after the initial infection, but may continue to shed if re-exposed.

Goats become infected by eating forage, bedding, cereals or concentrate contaminated by cat faeces (**Fig. 2.22**). Cats nesting in amongst straw or hay bales are considered a particular risk. If the goat is pregnant at first exposure, invasion of the fetus and placenta follows haematogenous spread. Exposure at any other time results in widespread tissue distribution and immunity. Immunity after exposure is usually strong and protective, although there are reports of repeat abortion in subsequent pregnancies.

Clinical presentation
Infection in early pregnancy may result in fetal loss, with no other clinical signs evident. Infection in later pregnancy may result in the death of one or more developing fetuses, which may or may not be instantly voided. Therefore, kids of different sizes and of apparently differing gestational lengths can be encountered. It is also possible to have live healthy kids born alongside smaller (often mummified) kids. Infection in late pregnancy may also result in the birth of acutely infected, weak kids.

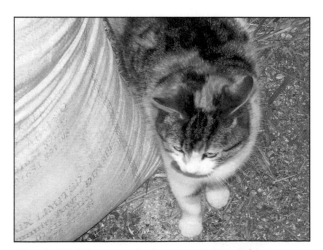

Fig. 2.22 The control of cats on farm, and in particular preventing their faecal contamination of feed, forage and bedding, is important in the control of *T. gondii*.

Diagnosis

Although not pathognomonic, the appearance of aborted kids of differing sizes, including smaller mummified kids, is highly suggestive of toxoplasmosis (**Fig 2.23**). The placental cotyledons may show small foci of necrosis (**Fig 2.24**), although anecdotally these are less well pronounced than those described in aborted lambs.

Laboratory diagnosis may include demonstration of antigen in placental material by indirect fluorescent antibody test (IFAT) or PCR, and the demonstration of antibody in immunocompetent fetuses voided in late pregnancy by IFAT (this requires goat-specific antigen). Surveys have shown that *T. gondii* antibody can be widespread in goat populations regardless of abortion rates, therefore single maternal seropositive results from aborting dams may give misleading results, although a seronegative result will probably rule out infection. Histological examination of brain and other organs, including placenta, may demonstrate non-specific necrosis, aided by specific immunohistochemistry.

Differential diagnosis

Other potential causes of abortion.

Treatment/management/control (including prognosis)

Successful control is based predominantly on reducing environmental exposure to the infective oocyst. The cat population should be managed where possible, and ideally all cats neutered, because pregnant cats and young kittens can shed at higher levels and entire tomcats are likely to roam between farms. Where possible cats should be kept away from feed stores, and feeds stored securely. Bales of hay or straw that show signs of cat faeces or of recent kittening activity should be discarded. Placental material and/or aborted fetuses should be made inaccessible to cats.

Toxoplasmosis vaccines are available in some countries, most of which will have been licensed for use in sheep, with minimal data as to efficacy in goats. Prophylaxis in the face of an abortion storm has also been suggested using, for example, ionophore preparations. In the UK, decoquinate (Deccox 6% premix) has a marketing authorisation for toxoplasmosis control in sheep at a dose rate of 2 mg/kg daily in feed, and has been used off-licence and with unvalidated results in goats. Care should be taken to avoid overdosing.

Chlamydiosis (syns. enzootic abortion, ovine enzootic abortion)

Definition/overview

Chlamydiosis, also referred to as EAE or OEA (ovine enzootic abortion), is a worldwide cause of abortion in ruminants, particularly sheep and goats, between which infection can be readily transmitted. Infection can also be linked occasionally to ocular and respiratory infections.

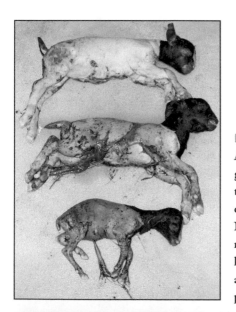

Fig. 2.23
Aborted Boer goat kids with toxoplasmosis confirmed. Note the small mummified kid (and absence of placenta).

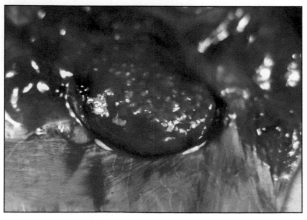

Fig. 2.24 *Toxoplasma* infection. Note the focal cotyledonary necrosis.

It is an important zoonotic pathogen, particularly for pregnant women exposed to infective material such as placenta, uterine fluids or kids from aborting does. It is generally advised that during pregnancy women should not be involved in lambing or kidding or in the rearing of sick or ailing neonates.

Aetiology
The causative agent of chlamydiosis is *Chlamydia abortus* (previous nomenclature *Chlamydophila abortus* and *Chlamydia psittaci*), which is a gram-negative, intracellular organism containing both DNA and RNA.

Pathophysiology
The organism can be carried in the intestinal tract and potentially introduced to a clean unit by faecal shedding, although the main route of transmission between goats (or goats and sheep) is via the products of abortion and the oral route. Multiplication occurs intracellularly in the gut wall, resulting in a septicaemic episode, which in turn leads to colonisation of the fetus and placenta, with particularly severe damage to the placental unit resulting in fetal death and expulsion.

Whereas in sheep abortion tends to occur in the pregnancy following ingestion, it is recognised that goats can become infected while pregnant and abort in that same pregnancy, thus leading to some quite dramatic 'abortion storms'.

The role of the male is poorly understood in goats - in rams cases of chlamydial orchitis have been reported. The potential faecal carriage of infection by a newly purchased buck into a high health status herd may be a possibility.

Clinical presentation
Abortions tend to occur during the second half of pregnancy, although earlier abortions have been reported. The doe is not usually ill, although in abortion storms individual goats may become febrile due to weight of infection. The fetus and placenta are often voided as a single unit, often with a normal appearing well-formed kid. The main pathology is associated with the placenta, which shows a severe intercotyledonary placentitis, with thickening and congestion of the

membranes, often covered in a purulent exudate. Infection in late pregnancy can result in the birth of live kids that can be congenitally infected and themselves abort when first pregnant following a period of latency.

Diagnosis
The appearance of the placenta is not pathognomonic and laboratory confirmation is required (**Fig. 2.25**). Staining impression smears prepared from the placental surface using a modified Ziehl–Neelsen (MZN) technique will demonstrate intracellular acid-fast inclusions, although these can be difficult to distinguish from *Coxiella* and *Brucella* spp. Some laboratories may use other staining methods (e.g. Giemsa). More specific PCR tests are now available to aid in confirming a diagnosis. In the absence of a placenta, smears or PCR testing can also be undertaken on fetal stomach content.

Serological testing of aborting does with a specific ELISA test gives further confirmatory evidence.

Differential diagnosis
Other potential causes of abortion.

Treatment/management/control
The generic principle of isolating any goat that aborts and removing the products of abortion promptly is significant in the control of this highly

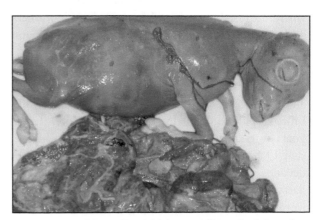

Fig. 2.25 **Chlamydia abortion confirmed, although the stage of pregnancy and gross appearance of the placenta is atypical. This demonstrates the importance of laboratory investigation.**

infectious cause of abortion. Shedding may continue for as long as a vaginal discharge is evident, and this may continue for up to 2 weeks after abortion. It is not known whether goats can continue to shed infection at subsequent pregnancies, even if they kid successfully. On a commercial unit, culling of aborting does is generally recommended, although after any discharge has dried up, they may be allowed to complete the lactation.

A number of vaccines are licensed worldwide for use in sheep, and have been used in the face of infection in goats in the UK with unvalidated results. The use of tetracyclines in outbreaks in sheep has been shown to be of economic benefit, and may be considered in goats at a recommended dose rate of 20 mg/kg i/m q3–10d.

The aim should be to maintain an EAE-free herd. Biosecurity is important, and incoming breeding females should be tested for antibody. A number of country-specific health schemes are available, giving local advice on achieving and maintaining freedom from infection.

Q fever

Definition/overview

Q fever has a worldwide distribution and a wide host range including mammals (humans, farmed and wild species), birds and arthropods. It is extremely infectious, with only a single colony-forming unit needed to produce infection. The organism *Coxiella burnetti* was first discovered in Queensland, Australia, in 1937 where it caused unexplained fever in abattoir workers. This so called 'query' fever led to the common name used today.

Q fever is an important zoonotic infection, with a particularly serious human outbreak (in excess of 3,000 cases) in Holland between 2007 and 2009, linked epidemiologically to a number of infected goat units nearby. Seroprevalence studies suggest that Q fever had been endemic in Holland several decades before clinical disease was confirmed in dairy goats and dairy sheep, and Q fever abortions were registered on 30 dairy goat and dairy sheep farms between 2005 and 2009. Fifty-nine percent of human cases in 2009 lived within 5 km of a farm that had tested positive by bulk milk PCR. Serological studies of at-risk groups also showed that over 80%

of practising veterinarians and 83% of farmers were seropositive to *C. burnetii*, compared with 2.4% in the general population.

Infection with Q fever is undoubtedly more widespread than its clinical appearance suggests, as many infected ruminants can carry a fetus to full term, producing a live viable offspring, yet still shed the organism in fetal fluids and placenta, thus posing an ever present occupational risk on many livestock units.

Because of the zoonotic risks, the organism must be handled in containment level III facilities in the laboratory. It is classed as a Category A biological substance (International Air Transport Association).

Aetiology

Q fever is caused by *C. burnetii*, a pleomorphic, weakly acid-fast, variably gram-negative bacterium (**Fig. 2.26**).

Pathophysiology

In animals infection is mainly subclinical, but abortion may occur in ruminants. *C. burnetii* has a tropism for the reproductive tissues and mammary gland. It is shed in milk, faeces and semen, and is present in fetal fluids and placenta of both aborting females and infected females at normal parturition. The organism has two forms, one of which is a highly stable spore-like form that can persist in the environment and is resistant to cleansing and disinfection. In this form the organism is tolerant of acid pH and is unaffected by UV light. It is also resistant

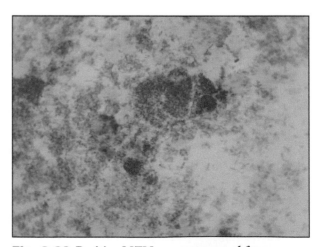

Fig. 2.26 **Positive MZN smear prepared from placental exudate.** *Coxiella* **was confirmed.**

to many disinfectants, including 0.5% hypochlorite and 5% formalin. Temperatures reached during pasteurisation are effective at killing *C. burnetii*.

Environmental contamination with the spores can be high on infected units, particularly in bedding as it is removed from buildings (occupational risk to those working in the vicinity), but also as this material dries out, with spore carrying dust particles being distributed by the wind into local communities. Abortions are most likely to occur after infection is introduced into a naive herd (or subgroup within a herd) or in times of stress such as overcrowding, environmental extremes or nutritional shortfalls.

Clinical presentation

Abortion is associated with a progressive placentitis: the placenta shows a generalised thickening often covered with an abundant thick discharge (**Fig. 2.27**). There are no obvious lesions in the fetus, other than some post-mortem autolysis. The doe is not affected clinically unless there is intercurrent disease.

Q fever abortions tend to present at a significantly high level in year one, but in a stable herd reduce dramatically by year two.

Diagnosis

Examination of MZN-stained placental smears will demonstrate acid-fast pleomorphic organisms, but these can be difficult to differentiate from *Chlamydia*

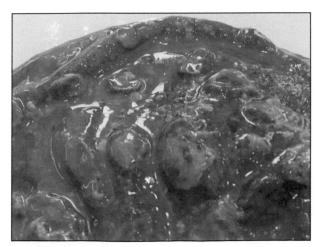

Fig. 2.27 Q fever abortion. Note the thickened necrotic appearance overall.

and *Brucella* spp. Confirmatory specific *C. burnetii* PCR tests are now available. Serological testing of dam's blood using an ELISA test is useful, particularly as a screening tool alongside PCR testing of bulk milk, although serological results should be interpreted carefully if vaccine has been administered.

It is important to bear in mind that *C. burnetii* can be shed heavily at the time of a normal kidding, therefore demonstration of the organism may not necessarily confirm disease.

Differential diagnosis

Other potential causes of abortion.

Treatment/management/control

There is good evidence to suggest that prophylactic antibiotic administration in the face of an abortion storm is beneficial (e.g. using tetracyclines). This likely reduces the number of abortions, but does not prevent shedding or the underlying zoonotic risk.

The products of abortion should be removed and aborting goats segregated to reduce lateral spread. There is likely to be heavy environmental contamination when a herd becomes infected, so test and cull strategies are unlikely to be very effective overall.

The overall management and nutrition of the affected group should be reviewed, and improved if found to be deficient, to reduce overall stress factors.

There are a number of vaccines available, some of which are licensed locally for use in goats. There are differences in the notifiable or reportable status of Q fever between different countries. For example, in the UK Q fever is not notifiable. In the Netherlands the disease was made notifiable in small ruminants in 2008, and in Australia it is notifiable.

Brucellosis
Definition/overview

Brucellosis is endemic in many areas of the world such as the Middle East, India, China and some southern Mediterranean countries, but many other countries, such as the UK (in which it is a notifiable disease), are completely free of infection.

Brucellosis is a recognised zoonotic infection, being associated with Malta fever in humans, contracted most commonly from milk or dairy products originating from infected goats and sheep. There is also an occupational risk to those handling infected products of abortion.

Aetiology

The majority of cases of brucellosis in goats will be associated with infection by *Brucella melitensis*, a small, faintly acid-fast coccobacillus. The cattle pathogen *Brucella abortus* has been described in goats, but is extremely rare.

Pathophysiology

Once a goat becomes infected (mainly by the oronasal route), the organism becomes widely distributed through the body, with trophism for placental tissue, if pregnant, and the udder. Abortion tends to be more likely if infected in late pregnancy, but can occur at any stage, particularly as a 'storm' following introduction into a naive herd. Abortion often results in a persistent vaginal discharge rich in the infective organism. Shedding can also occur in urine, faeces and milk. Kids born alive to infected does may themselves be infected and continue to shed the organism.

Clinical presentation

Abortion is the most common presenting sign in goats, and there are usually no characteristic signs evident. Asymptomatic disease can be identified by serological surveying either for brucellosis disease surveillance or following epidemiological tracing from a human case of Malta fever.

Diagnosis

The organism can be demonstrated in MZN-stained smears from placenta, but is difficult to differentiate from other similar staining organisms such as *Coxiella* and *Chlamydia* spp. *B. melitensis* can be cultured using specialist media such as Farrell's. A number of serological tests have been developed for both diagnostic and surveillance testing of blood samples. Bulk milk testing by either PCR or ELISA is a further diagnostic tool.

Differential diagnosis

Other potential causes of abortion.

Treatment/management/control

As stated, many countries are free of infection, and great efforts are taken to maintain this status by rigorous pre- and post-import testing of blood samples, coupled with post-import quarantine.

In endemic areas, a test and cull policy may be beneficial in low prevalence herds, and such an approach has underpinned control strategies for geographical area clearance of infection.

In herds where this is not practical because of widespread infection coupled with a lack of infection-free replacement stock, the use of available vaccines allows such units to continue in production. The administration of a parenteral antibiotic, such as long-acting tetracycline, may also be considered, although there is limited evidence of its impact.

Abortions are more likely to occur in goats under stress due to concurrent problems such as inadequate or unsuitable nutrition and overcrowding, and, in the face of an abortion storm, a review of husbandry and management could be beneficial.

The continuous environmental occupational risk to human health should be emphasised, particularly on heavily infected units.

Listeriosis

Definition/overview

Listeriosis is a disease of goats causing a variety of clinical signs, including abortions, encephalitis, septicaemia and sudden death – these other presentations will be dealt with in the relevant chapters.

It is a potential zoonosis, linked either directly or indirectly to contamination of dairy products such as cheese, with the added problem of multiplication within the infected product at fridge temperature.

Aetiology

The causative organism is *Listeria monocytogenes*, a ubiquitous organism in soil and the general environment including harvested forage such as silage. It is a gram-positive, predominantly rod-shaped organism, which is able to survive and multiply at low temperatures and has a number of distinct serotypes.

Silage becomes contaminated mainly due to excessive soil contamination during harvesting and ensiling. This is often associated with mole activity in fields or setting the cutting blades too low. A poor

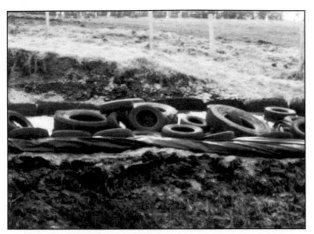

Fig. 2.28 Poorly made silage – this clamp was the source of a severe outbreak of listeriosis in goats.

ensiling process encourages multiplication of the organism, particularly when secondary fermentation occurs and the pH rises above 5.0 (**Fig. 2.28**). Silage ash levels can give a good indication of likely soil contamination. Silage should be kept under anaerobic conditions until use. Once spread out as a feed, low levels of *Listeria* organisms can rapidly multiply to dangerous levels. Therefore, the advice is to remove any uneaten silage after 24–36 hours and replace with fresh silage.

Miscellaneous sources of infection have included wet pea straw bales that were heavily contaminated with soil, and thistle and bramble trauma to the mouths of goats browsing around manure heaps or old spoiled forage.

Pathophysiology
Abortions usually develop as one of a series of differing clinical manifestations in an outbreak, and most often follow a septicaemic episode as a result of either maternal illness and pyrexia, or because of colonisation of both fetus and placenta causing fetal death and expulsion.

Clinical presentation
Aborting does are often, but not always, systemically ill with pyrexia and inappetence prior to abortion occurring. Recovery after abortion can be rapid (aided by antibiotic therapy), although a persistent vaginal discharge (rich in *L. monocytogenes*) can be a sequela, causing udder contamination and

the potential for transfer into milk during the milking routine.

Diagnosis
Abortions will often occur during a herd episode of listeriosis in which other clinical manifestations have been identified. Unlike other causes of abortion described, the doe is often sick shortly before or at the time of abortion. Laboratory diagnosis is based mainly on the isolation of *Listeria* organisms from fetal stomach content or placenta.

Differential diagnosis
Other potential causes of abortion.

Treatment/management/control
In commercial units, control is based on avoiding soil contamination when making silage or other conserved forage, and ensuring a good ensiling and feeding process.

Clinical cases in which encephalitis or septicaemia are presenting signs may respond to an intravenous antibiotic such as potentiated sulphonamides or benzylpenicillin sodium and supportive therapy with non-steroidal anti-inflammatory drugs (NSAIDs), which may have a beneficial effect on reducing the overall abortion rate. Vaccination in the face of an outbreak may be effective if commercial vaccines are available. Autogenous vaccines have been utilised with variable results.

Less common infectious causes of abortion

Salmonellosis
Salmonellosis is an unusual cause of abortion in goats, and most fetal losses result from systemic infection in the doe. Serotypes involved have included *S. dublin*, *S. typhimurium* and *S. montevideo*. Infection is often the result of environmental contamination by other clinically infected livestock such as cattle, or by wild bird or rodent carriers contaminating feed, water and bedding. Sewage spills or overflows contaminating pastureland or watercourses are other potential sources. Confirmation of infection is normally achieved by isolating the organism from aborted material supported by other associated clinical signs such as severe fibrinonecrotic diarrhoea and systemic illness.

Neosporosis

Neospora caninum is a microscopic protozoan parasite with worldwide distribution, and is recognised as a major cause of abortion in cattle. Sporadic abortions associated with infection in goats have been confirmed, but its presence has also been confirmed by serological surveys in goat herds with no associated clinical signs.

Dogs, including some wild canids, are the definitive hosts of *N. caninum* and are capable of shedding oocysts in faeces after eating placental tissues of infected animals. *Neospora* oocysts have an impervious covering that enables survival in soil and water for prolonged periods after canine faeces have decomposed. Goats may become infected by ingesting these oocysts, but just how susceptible they are is unclear. Confirmation of infection is by histological examination of the brain and myocardium of aborted fetuses and immunohistochemistry.

Tick-borne fever

Anaplasma phagocytophilum, previously referred to as a rickettsial organism, causes an acute febrile condition that can result in abortions in immunologically naive goats and other ruminants in a number of countries including the UK and parts of Europe, Africa and India. It is transmitted from animal to animal by the feeding activities of the hard tick *Ixodes ricinus* and possibly other tick species.

Diagnosis is based on demonstrating the pathogen in polymorphonuclear leucocytes in Giemsa-stained smears or by demonstrating a rising antibody level in paired blood samples.

Pregnant, previously unexposed does should not be grazed in known tick infested areas during the tick activity seasons where possible. In endemically infected areas, however, it is likely that most goats will have been exposed in early life and hence will be immune. If clinical infection is suspected, the organism is susceptible to tetracyclines, which can be used either therapeutically or prophylactically.

Arbovirus infections

Arthropod-borne bunyavirus infections reported to have been associated with abortions (and birth defects in kids) include:

- Akabane virus (Australia, Israel, Japan, Korea, and parts of Southeast Asia, the Middle East, and Africa).

- Schmallenberg virus (Europe).
- Cache Valley virus (USA, Canada and Mexico).

Each of these infectious agents is transmitted between susceptible species, including goats, by a wide variety of biting flies and midges. If infected while naive and pregnant in the first trimester, the virus crosses the placenta after a period of viraemia, and causes a variety of fetal abnormalities that may result in immediate abortion or the later birth of a deformed kid. The dam is usually unaffected clinically. Fetal abnormalities described include:

- Severe damage to or absence of the cerebral cortex, leading to microencephaly and hydrocephalus.
- Neurogenic atrophy of fetal muscles, such that limbs develop arthrogryposis and are fused at abnormal angles, often leading to fetal dystocia.
- Mummification.

Laboratory confirmation is based on demonstration of the virus or maternal antibody. Vaccines are available in affected countries for Schmallenberg virus and for Akabane virus.

Campylobacter infection

Although *Campylobacter* infection is a common cause of abortion in sheep worldwide, its involvement in goat abortion appears to be more sporadic, and variable between countries. Infection most often involves *Campylobacter fetus fetus* and *Campylobacter jejuni*, both of which can be carried in the gut of healthy carrier sheep and goats who can introduce infection into a clean herd.

Infection in naive pregnant does, particularly during late pregnancy, can lead to abortions. The placenta may be thickened and oedematous, and occasionally characteristic focal liver necrosis can be seen in expelled fetuses. Confirmation is based on the demonstration of the causative organism in fetal stomach content.

In the face of an outbreak, prophylactic use of long-acting tetracyclines may be of benefit. Control should be aimed at preventing introduction and spread of *Campylobacter* infection, particularly by keeping each group of late pregnancy goats as a stable unit, thus minimising the impact of any clinically healthy carrier animals. Any re-grouping of animals should be done at another time.

Leptospirosis

There are occasional (and often anecdotal) reports of abortion associated with infection by *Leptospira interrogans* serovars including *hardjo*, *icterohaemorrhagiae*, *sejroe* and *pomona*. Confirmation is often based on the demonstration alone of antibody in the aborting doe's blood.

Border disease virus/bovine viral diarrhoea virus (BDV/BVDV)

These antigenically similar viruses are associated predominantly with disease in sheep and cattle, respectively, although there is cross susceptibility between both viruses and goats. However, reports of reproductive failure in goats are scant.

Infection with BDV has been linked to early embryonic loss, reports of increased barren rates at scanning, or returns to oestrus after apparent pregnancy. Fetuses that survive this early insult can show a variety of congenital abnormalities depending on the stage of pregnancy when first infected. If the insult is severe, then the fetus may be aborted; mummification is often described, and gross abnormalities may be visible. Some fetuses will survive to term and be born alive (with abnormalities described in other chapters), or may show no visible abnormalities yet be persistently infected with the virus.

Caprine herpesvirus

CpHV1 can cause sporadic outbreaks of late-term abortions, often with no other clinical signs in the dam. The virus is also potentially associated with vulvovaginitis, balanoposthitis and respiratory disease in adult goats, and enteric and systemic disease in neonates. Aborted fetuses may be fresh or autolysed, and show no gross lesions. Presumptive diagnosis is by microscopic identification of necrosis with the presence of intranuclear inclusion bodies in the fetal liver, lungs and other organs, or by demonstrating the virus in fetal tissue and/or maternal antibody. (See earlier in chapter for more details.)

Rift Valley fever

Rift Valley fever is a mosquito-borne viral infection causing sporadic outbreaks of disease among domestic and wild ruminants, including goats, in Africa. During an outbreak, the characteristic pattern is for numerous abortions to occur with increasing mortality among young animals, together with disease in humans (it is an important zoonotic infection). Pregnant animals affected by this disease will almost always abort (80–100%).

Maceration – non-specific

Maceration is the result of fetal death accompanied by loss of the CL, opening of the cervix and entry of autolytic and other bacteria into the uterus. The fetus decays *in utero*: soft tissues break down and are passed as malodorous vaginal discharge; bones may be too large to pass through the cervix and remain *in situ*.

Indication is a malodorous vaginal discharge in an animal thought to be pregnant. Ultrasonography or radiography is used to confirm the diagnosis. Prognosis is guarded, with treatment – consisting of physical removal and lavage – often unsatisfactory because of the difficulty in removing all bone fragments from the uterus. If the cervix is largely closed, a combination of oestrogen injections and prostaglandin E pessaries placed into the cervix may cause relaxation. Hysterotomy can be employed if economically justified.

Non-infectious causes of abortion

Pharmacological products

Prostaglandins (administered throughout pregnancy) and corticosteroid products (administered in later pregnancy) can each result in a termination of the pregnancy and resultant abortion.

There are a number of reports of many other products potentially causing abortions, but these are often anecdotal. The pharmacological safety data necessary for modern products to receive a marketing licence are robust, and as such will result in a reasonable safety margin. The greatest risk will be from the gross overdosing of a licensed product, the use of unlicensed products or stress induced by handling and administration.

CHAPTER 2

Toxicity

Plants and shrubs are often recognised locally as potential causes of abortion. These are impossible to confirm by laboratory examination of aborted material, and diagnosis often relies on circumstantial evidence that consumption has occurred.

Chemical toxicity has also been incriminated, with abortions most often associated with widespread organ failure and other clinical signs rather than a specific effect on the pregnancy itself.

Vitamin/mineral deficiencies

A number of deficiencies have been linked to abortions in the literature, but are often difficult to reproduce experimentally, and as such may be components of a multifactorial cause. These include:

- Retinol (vitamin A).
- Selenium.
- Copper.
- Manganese.
- Iodine.

There are often other clinical manifestations, such as stillborns or weak kids (retinol [vitamin A] and iodine) or congenital abnormalities (copper and manganese).

Malnutrition/pregnancy toxaemia

If goats are severely malnourished in late pregnancy or, conversely, are overweight and develop pregnancy toxaemia, late abortions or the birth of weak kids may occur.

Angora goats appear to be particularly susceptible to late abortions if placed under nutritional stress in late pregnancy (see below).

Habitual abortion in Angora goats

In South Africa, where marked genetic selection for fine-quality mohair has been undertaken, there has been an apparent parallel selection for genetic habitual abortion. It is thought that the nutritional stress associated with producing this high-quality mohair results in chronic hyperadrenocorticism. This in turn interferes with the normal regulation of the water and electrolyte balance of the body, causing placental dysfunction and thus the progressive accumulation of excessive intrauterine fluids and fetal oedema, a retarded fetal heart rate and eventually congestive heart failure and fetal expulsion. It is now recognised that this same physiological process may also occur in other stressful situations in pregnant Angoras, such as cold inclement weather shortly after shearing.

Mummification – non-specific

Mummification is a result of fetal death *in utero*, with the cervix remaining closed. Resorption of fetal and body fluids leads to mummification (**Fig. 2.29**). The CL normally remains active and thus the dam does not return to oestrus. Only part of the litter may be affected.

Clinical suspicion may arise because the doe is overdue or does not show as much abdominal distension as expected for the stage of pregnancy. On abdominal palpation, mummification may be confused with an intra-abdominal mass. Ultrasonography aids diagnosis. Luteolysis is induced with $PGF_{2\alpha}$. (**Note:** Because no active placenta is present, corticosteroids are ineffective in inducing abortion.) The fetus typically enters the vagina 2–3 days later and must be removed with great care and plenty of lubrication. Caesarean section is a possible approach, but difficult to perform satisfactorily.

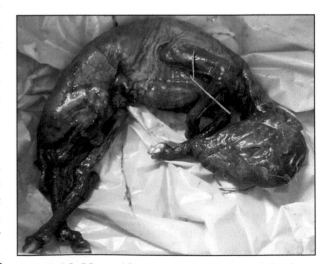

Fig. 2.29 Mummification results from fetal death while the cervix remains closed and the corpus luteum is maintained.

THE BUCK

NORMAL STRUCTURE AND FUNCTION

Male kids are precocious, and puberty commonly starts around 4 months of age. It is important, however, not to confuse onset of puberty with sexual maturity. The latter will follow some months later and result in sperm production of satisfactory quantity and quality.

Bucks are not fully seasonal, although in breeds from temperate regions sexual behaviour, testes size and sperm production is markedly reduced during the females' anoestrus period.

Testicles are oval-shaped, paired and arranged in a vertical orientation in a pendulous scrotum (**Fig. 2.30**). The epididymis is arranged such that its head lies dorsal to the testicle and its tail ventral. Some breeds (e.g. Somali) have a split scrotum. The accessory sex glands consist of seminal vesicles, prostate gland and bulbourethral glands. The ductus (vas) deference widens into an ampulla prior to merging with the urethra.

The penis is fibroelastic and has a sigmoid flexure, and there is a urethral process (syn. filiform appendage; **Fig. 2.31**) extending beyond the glans penis.

The buck produces about 30 million sperm per gram of testicular tissue per day. Spermatogenesis takes about 48 days, resulting from 4.5 cycles of seminiferous epithelium each of 10.6 days duration. Maturation and progression along the epididymis takes another 10 days or so.

OUT-OF-SEASON BREEDING

Indications
Out-of-season breeding may be desirable to put young bucks to use early (including for progeny testing), allow breeding soundness examination before the natural breeding season, in AI centres or to have sexually active bucks available for doe synchronisation.

Technique
Artificial lighting regimes or melatonin may be used, as discussed under oestrus manipulation in the female.

EXAMINATION FOR BREEDING SOUNDNESS

Indications
Ideally, all bucks should undergo a physical health check 8–10 weeks prior to being used (to allow for

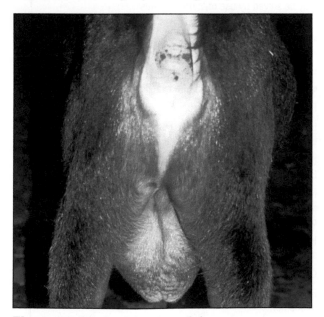

Fig. 2.30 The buck has a pendulous scrotum. The testicles are arranged vertically.

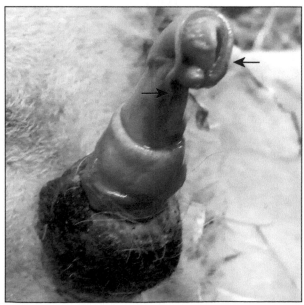

Fig. 2.31 Extruded penis showing the glans penis and urethral process (syn. filiform appendage; indicated by arrows).

resolution of any general health issues and a full cycle of spermatogenesis), plus a breeding soundness examination about 1 month prior to being used. The timing of this examination in relation to the buck's natural breeding season must be taken into account when interpreting findings. Other indications include unsatisfactory pregnancy rates or return to oestrus in the does, and examination for insurance purposes or prior to entering a buck into an AI facility.

Aetiology

The causes of failed breeding soundness components are shown in *Table 2.1*.

Table 2.1 Aetiology of failed breeding soundness components.

COMPONENT	CAUSES	COMMENTS
Deficient libido	Hormone deficiency	Negative energy balance may affect LH pulsatility
	Age related factors	Natural decrease from 5–7 years of age. Sexual maturity may not be reached yet if under 1 year of age
	Breed	Differences recognised in other species, but little known in goats. Estimated heritability is 0.59 in cattle, suggesting that selection is possible
	Over- or underuse	Difficult to control in multiple sire groups. (See earlier in chapter for buck:doe ratios)
	Systemic disease	Especially those affecting body condition, causing a systemic inflammatory response or pyrexia, or affecting the locomotor system
	Psychological factors	Fear or pain experienced during previous mating attempts. Selective libido in group-mating systems may occur
Inability to mount	Problems of the musculoskeletal system or spine, or neurological deficits	Potential problems include: degenerative joint disease, arthritis, spondylitis, foot disorders, ataxia
Inability to achieve intromission	Size disparity	May be solved by use of 'service crates'
	Conformation	Poor conformation (e.g. straight-legged or sickle hock) may result in poor positioning of buck relative to the doe's perineum
	Anatomical defects	Persistent frenulum or other penile deviation. Erection failure caused by hereditary or acquired vascular shunt
	Injury, adhesions, neoplasia	For example, penile haematoma, phimosis, papillomatosis
Inability to fertilise	Aspermia	Infectious disease of genital system, congenital or acquired obstruction of vas deference, testicular degeneration. Rarely, anti-sperm antibodies
	Low sperm count	Excessive use, testicular hypoplasia or atrophy, cryptorchism
	Poor motility	No recent mating activity ('stale sample'), sperm tail abnormalities, handling error during semen evaluation (such as cold shock, exposure to water or other spermicidal agents)
	Morphological abnormalities (**Fig. 2.32**)	Heat or cold stress, testicular abnormalities including epididymis, seminal vesiculitis
	Venereal disease	CpHV-1 and certain *Mycoplasma* spp.
	Urethral process abnormality	Failure to detach from penis or absence may affect sperm deposition
	Genetic defect	Lethal gene preventing fertilisation or causing early embryonic death

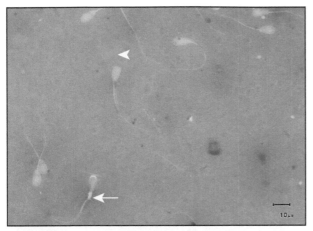

Fig. 2.32 Morphological abnormalities of spermatozoa, such as proximal droplets (arrow) or detached heads (arrowhead), may render a buck subfertile.

History

Knowing the buck's history will influence the list of differential diagnoses and interpretation of results. Of particular interest is whether the buck has bred successfully before or is a maiden, is currently with a group of cycling females, is presented within the breeding season, has had any recent illnesses or treatments and whether libido and mounting ability have been observed.

Physical examination

Bucks are often poorly cared for outside the breeding period, potentially resulting in poor foot health and body condition, and heavy ecto- and endoparasite burdens. In addition to the feet, joints are examined for arthritis, in particular the elbows. The target body condition score is 3–3.5 (scale 1 to 5). Overconditioning may negatively affect libido, as well as sperm quality, with fat deposition increasing scrotal temperature. Scrotal mange may also lead to increased scrotal temperature. Negative energy balance affects LH pulsatility.

The cardiovascular and respiratory systems are examined to determine physical fitness. Vision and smell are important, especially where group mating is used. Where bucks are kept together, the poll and horns are examined for signs of fighting injuries. The brisket area is checked for trauma, especially if a raddle harness is used. Attention is paid to urinary tract health.

The buck should display a strong scent. While this does not reflect on the buck's fertility, it influences standing oestrus in the doe.

Karyotyping may be used to identify specific genetic abnormalities.

Genital tract examination

In the normal buck, the scrotal skin is soft and undamaged. Attention is paid regarding vasectomy scars. The testicles are freely mobile within the scrotal sac, roughly of equal size, and have the consistency of a ripe tomato. The head, body and tail of the epididymis are palpated for presence, normal size and closeness to the testes. No pain should be elicited when palpating scrotal contents.

A minimum scrotal circumference of 25 cm is expected in dairy breed bucks weighing more than 40 kg (**Fig. 2.33**).

Examination of the penis and prepuce may be performed with the buck sitting on its haunches (but is less tolerated in goats than in sheep) or in the standing position (elevated on a table or bale of straw for ease of examination). The penis, including its sigmoid flexure, is palpated through the prepuce; it should be mobile, without any swelling or enlargement and pain free. After extrusion, the glans penis and urethral process are examined. In the prepubescent male, normal preputial adhesions prohibit extrusion. The integrity and health of the prepuce and parapreputial abdominal skin is established (**Fig. 2.34**). Preputial hair should be moist, with no evidence of urolithiasis or discharge.

Assessment of the accessory sex glands is limited in the buck. While the prostate gland is within digital reach, its diffuse nature prevents meaningful examination. However, pain may be elicited on digital rectal palpation if severe pathology of any accessory gland is present.

Further diagnostic aids include ultrasonography of the testicles (transcutaneous) and accessory sex glands (transrectal), and culture or other pathogen isolation of either a preputial wash or a semen sample.

Semen evaluation

Semen may be collected using either an artificial vagina or electroejaculation (EEJ). When using EEJ,

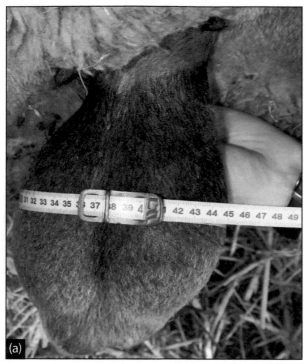
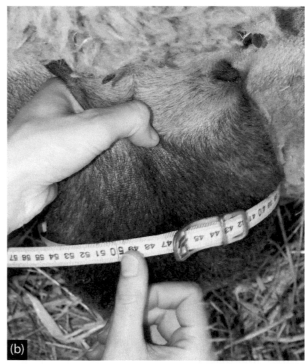

Fig. 2.33 Scrotal circumference indicates sperm output capacity. (a) Measured correctly: testicles fully descended and held in place by tightening the scrotal skin in the neck area, with the measurement over the widest part of the scrotum. (b) Incorrect holding of the testicles: the thumb of the left hand pushes the testicles apart, resulting in an elevated measurement.

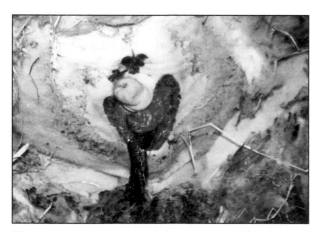

Fig. 2.34 Lesions around the prepuce will reduce libido and mounting willingness.

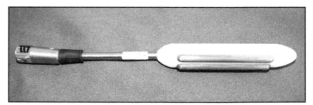

Fig. 2.35 For electroejaculation, a 3 cm diameter probe with ventrally placed electrodes is suitable. (Probe shown is by Lane Manufacturing, Denver, Colorado.)

the ejaculate is commonly diluted by accessory gland fluid. This will result in reduced density and lower apparent gross motility, but not affect other semen evaluation parameters. For EEJ, a ram probe (circa 3 cm diameter; **Fig. 2.35**) is used. A probe with ventrally placed electrodes is preferable to a ring-electrode one, and the unit should allow gradual increase of stimulation. EEJ is a veterinary procedure and heavy sedation is recommended. (**Note:** Anaesthesia is a requirement in some countries.)

Semen evaluation parameters include (**Fig. 2.36**):

- Volume: typically 1.0–1.5 ml.
- Colour and appearance: a rough estimate of density can be made based on appearance (beware EEJ dilution effect). In a creamy

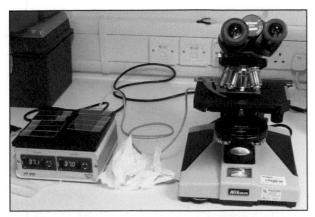

Fig. 2.36 Handling errors, like cold shock, must be avoided when assessing semen quality. Note the use of a hotplate to pre-warm slides and the heated stage on the microscope. The procedure should be carried out in a draught-free, warm environment.

sample, the presence of pus must be ruled out (e.g. by examining a stained smear). No blood contamination should be present.
- Sperm concentration: varies from 2–10 $\times$ 10^9 spermatozoa/ml (beware EEJ dilution effect).
- Gross motility: 2.5 or higher (on a scale of 0 = no movement, to 5 = strong swirling waves; beware EEJ dilution effect).
- Progressive motility: minimum targets are 30% for natural service in a multiple sire group, 50% for a single sire group, and 70% for AI.
- Morphology: target is >70% morphologically normal, with no one abnormality exceeding 20% (taking into account whether defects are compensable or not).
- Live-to-dead ratio: for routine examinations, this step may be omitted. Gross and progressive motility will indicate proportion of live sperm. Where performed, strict adherence to protocol is important to obtain meaningful results (quality of reagent, correct temperature maintained throughout, accurate timing).
- pH: target is 6.8–7.0.
- Cellularity and bacterial contamination: Gram stain or Diff-Quik® are suitable to assess excessive cellular debris or bacterial count.

TESTICULAR AND EPIDIDYMAL ABNORMALITIES

Testicular hypoplasia

Definition
Testicular hypoplasia is a congenital defect with a genetic basis.

Clinical presentation
Unilateral or bilateral underdevelopment of testicle, recognisable from puberty onwards.

Diagnosis
Suboptimal scrotal circumference. For unilateral cases, also unevenness between testes size.

Differential diagnosis
Testicular degeneration developing later in the buck's life.

Treatment/management/control
Moderately high hereditability, therefore selection against is possible.

Testicular degeneration or atrophy

Definition
This acquired reduction in testicle size is one of the common testicular problems seen. The buck typically has been fertile before, and continues to show normal service behaviour.

Aetiology
Testicular degeneration or atrophy is often a result of elevated scrotal temperature (e.g. secondary to heat stress or pyrexia). Other possible insults include trauma and genital tract infections leading to regional inflammation or vascular compromise, frostbite and a systemic illness-induced inflammatory response. Toxic damage, high oestrogen diet, gonadotrophin deficiency and autoimmune disease are rarer causes. Testicular degeneration has been observed as part of caprine contagious agalactia (see Chapter 12).

Clinical presentation
Testicular consistency is soft and fibrosis may be palpable. Scrotal circumference is often reduced.

Diagnosis

Systematic clinical and reproductive tract examination, together with history (e.g. exposure to extreme weather). The exact cause may be difficult to identify. Ultrasonography is useful to establish the extent and type of changes within the testes.

Differential diagnosis

Testicular hypoplasia, which is present from a young age.

Treatment/management/control

Addressing the underlying cause, including NSAID therapy. Prognosis is generally guarded to poor, but depends on type and length of insult. Gonadotrophin treatment may be tried. Monitoring for resolution should take into account the 58 days required for spermatogenesis.

Orchitis and epididymitis

Definition

Orchitis and epididymitis are more commonly recognised in the buck compared with some other species, but often not detected until severe pathological changes are present. May be unilateral or bilateral.

Aetiology

Post-traumatic invasion with opportunistic pathogens may occur, typically as an ascending infection. Specific pathogens associated with orchitis and epididymitis include *Corynebacterium pseudotuberculosis*, *Brucella melitensis*, *Actinobacillus seminis*, *Staphylococcus pyogenes*, *Chlamydia abortus*, *Escherichia coli*, *Pseudomonas* spp. and *Besnoitia* spp.

Pathophysiology

Infection causes rapid damage to seminiferous tubules, reducing sperm output. The inflammatory response may result in heat insult of the unaffected testis, and pressure build-up in the tunica albuginea leading to internal tissue necrosis. Infection may spread to the epididymis and accessory sex glands.

Clinical presentation

Pyrexia is common in the early stage. The testicle is enlarged and painful (**Fig. 2.37**), often resulting in reluctance to move and an abnormal stance.

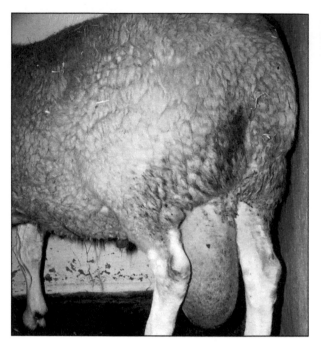

Fig. 2.37 Noticeable scrotal enlargement in a ram with epididymitis.

Testicular mobility within the scrotum is reduced. If accessory glands are affected, pain on rectal palpation may be present. Gangrenous changes are occasionally present in the scrotal skin.

Diagnosis

Clinical signs, combined with ultrasonography showing tissue oedema and irregular echogenicity (**Figs. 2.38**).

Differential diagnosis

Inguinal herniation (**Fig. 2.39**), testicular haematoma, spermatic cord torsion, neoplasia.

Treatment/management/control

If only one testicle is affected, unilateral castration is a viable option. Sperm output in the remaining testicle may reach 80% of normal total output. However, the client should be advised that the inflammation may have caused secondary damage to the unaffected testicle. For bilateral cases, aggressive antibiosis (e.g. macrolides) combined with anti-inflammatory therapy, and emollient cream if the scrotal skin is affected. Prognosis for suppurative cases is guarded.

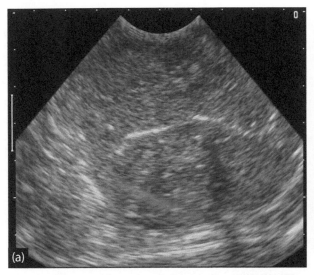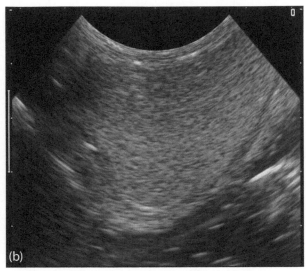

Fig. 2.38 Irregular echogenicity indicates testicular pathology (such as orchitis, degeneration or neoplasia, as in [a]), compared with the homogeneous appearance of normal testicular tissue (b).

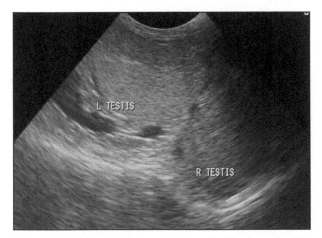

Fig. 2.39 A loop of intestine (longitudinal section) is apparent on the left-hand side in this ultrasonography scan of the scrotum. This indicates an inguinal hernia as the cause of scrotal enlargement.

The epididymis and deferent duct may become obstructed secondary to the inflammation.

Cryptorchism (syn. retained gonad)
Definition
Cryptorchism is the absent or incomplete descent of one or both testicles. Subfertility often results, mainly due to a lower sperm count. Exposure to higher than normal temperatures of the retained gonad may increase the risk of neoplastic changes. Prevalence in the goat appears to be low.

Aetiology
Likely to have a genetic component, with irregular transmission by parents and their offspring. Insufficiency in testosterone and Müllerian-inhibiting hormone may be involved. Cryptorchism is frequently seen in intersex animals. In the goat, testicular descent is usually complete at birth.

Clinical presentation
One or both testicles are absent from the scrotal sac. They may be located at any point along their normal migration path between the external inguinal ring and the kidneys. Occasionally, they are positioned cranial to the scrotum along the ventral abdominal wall.

Diagnosis
Palpation confirms absence from the scrotal sac and may reveal the position along the abdominal wall or near the inguinal ring. Ultrasonography is used to locate intra-abdominal gonads (**Fig. 2.40**) or to confirm the testicular nature of any mass detected on palpation. The retained gonad is typically smaller than normal and the parenchyma often appears less uniform.

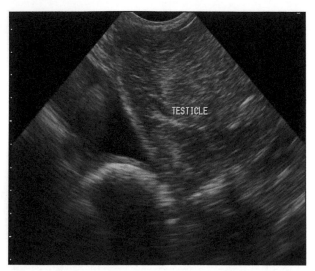

Fig. 2.40 Intra-abdominal testicle, with intestinal loops visible to the left. The normal, homogenic appearance is often lost in retained gonads, and they are often smaller than normal (about 3.5 cm length in this case).

Differential diagnosis

Monorchism is much rarer than cryptorchism, but may be ruled out by a LH stimulation test 2 months after surgical removal of the testicle that is present.

Treatment/management/control

Because the retained gonad may produce fertile sperm, and because of the increased risk of neoplasia, surgical removal is recommended in males destined to be kept into adulthood or housed with does. A scrotal approach is usually successful for gonads lying near the inguinal ring. The gubernaculum testis can be used as a guide towards a gonad lying in the inguinal canal. A laparotomy is usually necessary to remove gonads located near the kidney.

ACCESSORY SEX GLAND DISORDERS

Definition

The most widely recognised accessory sex gland disorder is seminal vesiculitis. This is caused by inflammation or infection, either as part of a wider genital tract infection or just affecting this accessory sex gland, and may be unilateral or bilateral. Cysts in the bulbourethral gland have also been reported.

Clinical presentation

The animal may display dysuria or stranguria. Pain is elicited during digital rectal examination. The ejaculate contains inflammatory cells and bacteria, and sometimes outright pus. Very rarely, the affected seminal vesicle may rupture, causing peritonitis, or fistulate into the rectum.

Differential diagnosis

Urolithiasis or urinary tract infection for dysuria or stranguria. Pelvic trauma for pain on rectal examination.

Treatment/management/control

Aggressive antibiosis (e.g. macrolides) in the early stages, but prognosis is guarded with often remission rather than cure being achieved. Aspiration of cysts may be attempted.

PENIS AND PREPUCE ABNORMALITIES

Penile deviation
Overview

Persistent frenulum in a young buck and acquired deviation in older males are the main causes of penile deviation.

Aetiology

A persistent frenulum results from failure of the preputial attachment to break down fully, leaving a remnant connecting the ventral penis with the prepuce (**Fig. 2.41**). A lack of testosterone exposure may be responsible.

A loose attachment of the dorsal penile ligament to the dorsal surface of the tunica albuginea results in lateral deviation during erection. The penis may adopt a corkscrew shape (spiral deviation) in severe cases. Degeneration or trauma to the ligament are possible precursors.

An hereditary component has been postulated for both conditions. Affected bucks should not be used to sire offspring destined for a pedigree breeding pool.

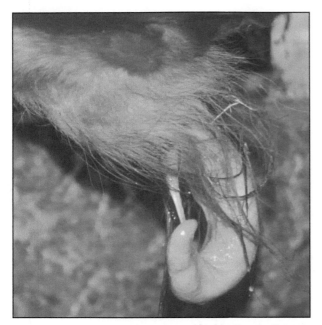

Fig. 2.41 Persistent frenulum in a yearling bull.

Clinical presentation

The buck fails to achieve intromission. Close observation of mating activity is required to detect this, as sexual behaviour is normal including possible ejaculation and thrusting outside the vagina.

Differential diagnosis

Spiral deviation during semen collection using EEJ can occur, but this does not mean that deviation also occurs during natural service.

Treatment/management/control

A persistent frenulum can be surgically corrected. After digital or EEJ stimulation to cause an erection, the penis is 'snared' (e.g. with a loop of gauze bandage). The frenulum is ligated and cut at both ends. For lateral or spiral deviation, suturing the dorsal ligament onto the tunica albuginea may be attempted. However, improvement is often only temporary.

Penile trauma
Overview

In fibre breeds, careless shearing may result in injury to the penis or prepuce. Penile haematoma (syn. broken penis) is reported much less in small ruminants compared with bulls.

Aetiology

Penile haematoma is usually caused by the male thrusting without having achieved intromission, thereby deflecting the fully erected penis ventrally. This results in a tear in the dorsal tunica albuginea, often around or anterior to the sigmoid flexure, with subsequent haemorrhage into the surrounding tissues.

Clinical presentation

Initially a soft, fluctuant, typically bilateral symmetrical swelling develops on the ventral abdomen cranial to the scrotum. Pain may be present on palpation. Over time, the swelling becomes harder and may reduce in size. If presentation is delayed, it may be difficult to exteriorise the penis because of adhesions.

Diagnosis

Palpatory findings and history of recent mating activity. Ultrasonography confirms the presence of a haematoma associated with the penis.

Differential diagnosis

Ruptured urethra secondary to urolithiasis, with subcutaneous accumulation of urine. The swelling is more extensive and the condition more common in a castrated male, rather than in an entire male. Also, history of dysuria or anuria and elevated blood urea and creatinine levels.

Treatment/management/control

Routine wound management principles are applied to shearing injuries.

For penile haematoma, conservative treatment consists of cold or hot packing, if discovered early, combined with anti-inflammatory therapy.

Surgical repair of the rent may be attempted, either under epidural, local infiltration or general anaesthesia and with the buck in dorsal recumbency. After blunt dissection to expose the penis, the blood clot is removed and the defect in the tunica repaired with absorbable suture material. Routine antibiosis and anti-inflammatory therapy is given.

To avoid adhesions, the buck is teased without being allowed to mate, starting from 2 weeks after surgical repair and 4 weeks after conservative treatment.

Prognosis is about 50% with either approach, with recurrence and adhesions the most common problems.

Phimosis and paraphimosis

Overview

Phimosis and paraphimosis are an inability to extend the penis or withdraw the penis back into the prepuce, respectively. Both are relatively rare in the buck, but result in marked loss of libido and fertility.

Aetiology

Causes include hair rings, trauma and balanoposthitis.

Clinical presentation

Phimosis presents as failure to extrude the penis when sexually stimulated. With a traumatic aetiology, adhesions may prevent manual exteriorisation. Paraphimosis presents as a continuous extrusion of the penis, with secondary inflammation, swelling and trauma (**Fig. 2.42**).

Differential diagnosis

Urolithiasis or urinary cystitis, if dysuria or stranguria is present.

Treatment/management/control

The buck is sedated. For phimosis, any hair rings are removed and the penis manually exteriorised to check for trauma. Where penile adhesions prevent this, treatment becomes unrewarding. Any traumatic lesions found are treated along the same principles as

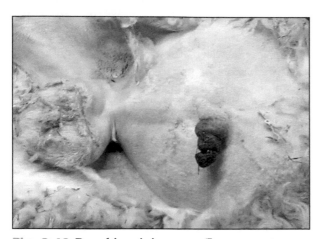

Fig. 2.42 **Paraphimosis in a ram. (Image courtesy Daniel Scovenna.)**

for paraphimosis: extruded parts are cleaned, if necessary using surgical debridement. After thorough lavage with saline or a mild disinfectant, an antibiotic ointment, with or without corticosteroids, or udder cream is applied, and the penis is replaced. If a risk of re-prolapse is perceived, a purse-string suture may be placed into the preputial orifice, encasing a tube to facilitate urination. The penis is manually exteriorised every 1–3 days, with repeated lavage and ointment application.

Phimosis carries a poor prognosis, in part because of loss of libido. Prognosis for paraphimosis is poor if presentation is delayed or the swelling continues to prevent withdrawal of the penis after a few days.

Where hair rings are the cause, regular shearing of the hair just cranial to the prepuce may prevent the problem.

Balanoposthitis

Overview

Two main forms of balanoposthitis are recognised in goats: infectious and enzootic (syn. 'pizzle rot').

Aetiology

Pathogens associated with the infectious form include CpHV-1, contagious ecthyma (orf) and *Mycoplasma* and *Ureaplasma* spp.

The enzootic form is associated with high dietary protein (e.g. in bucks on lush spring pasture or during feeding-up for shows or sales). This leads to high urea levels in the urine, which is hydrolysed to ammonia by the commensal *Corynebacterium renale*. Both very short and very long preputial hair are recognised as risk factors. The condition is more common in castrated males. Early castration may increase the risk, with lack of exposure to testosterone leading to failure of the frenulum to detach and subsequent urination into the prepuce.

Clinical presentation

The irritation leads to severe inflammation of the penile shaft, parapreputial skin and preputial mucosa, often with pustules, ulceration and scab formation. Secondary bacterial infection is common. Dysuria and stranguria may be observed. Complete occlusion may result, leading to death.

Venereal transmission of the infectious form will result in infectious vulvovaginitis in the does.

Differential diagnosis
Urolithiasis if dysuria or stranguria is observed.

Treatment/management/control
Topical and systemic antibiosis, combined with anti-inflammatories, emollient cream and sexual rest. For the enzootic form, penicillin against *C. renale* and reduction of dietary protein.

Neoplasia of the male reproductive tract
Overview
Various tumours may affect any part of the reproductive tract, but overall neoplasia is rare in bucks. Unlike in bulls and boars, there is no specific virus-associated neoplastic disease in bucks.

Aetiology
Both benign and malignant tumours of a variety of tissues may occur, including squamous cell carcinoma, Leydig or Sertoli cell tumours, adenoma/adenosarcoma, teratoma, seminoma and haemangioma/haemangiosarcoma. Metastasis into reproductive tract tissues from other sites is very uncommon.

Clinical presentation
Proliferative penile lesions may interfere with intromission, and bleeding is often observed during or after mating activity. Associated pain often leads to loss of libido.

Tumours affecting the testes may lead to disruption of spermatogenesis (**Fig. 2.43**). Epididymal or accessory gland neoplasia often leads to secondary sperm abnormalities.

Behavioural changes may be apparent with either Leydig (aggression) or Sertoli (feminisation) cell tumours.

Diagnosis
A definitive diagnosis is achieved with histology of tissue biopsies.

Treatment/management/control
Unilateral castration may be an option for unilateral testicular neoplasia. Penile tumours sometimes can be excised, with optional cautery or cryosurgery (**Fig. 2.44**).

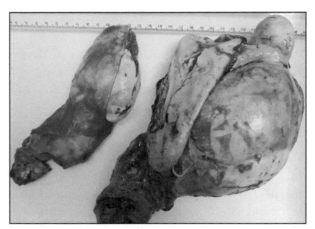

Fig. 2.43 Marked enlargement caused by unilateral testicular neoplasia affecting both germ and stromal cells. Severe adhesions necessitated scrotal ablation during surgical removal.

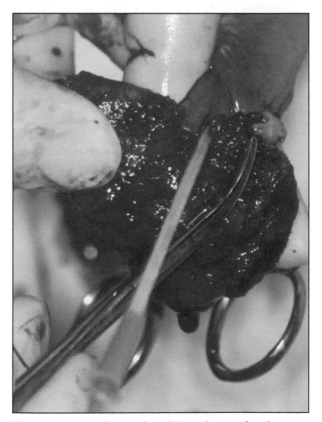

Fig. 2.44 A catheter placed into the urethra is useful during penile surgery to avoid accidental trauma to the urethra. (Image courtesy Peter G.G. Jackson.)

CASTRATION

A rubber ring may be used in kids up to 7 days of age (**Fig. 2.45**). Under UK regulations, anaesthesia must be used in animals over 2 months of age, but is recommended in animals of any age.

Indications
Easier management of pet goats and fibre breeds, in particular allowing cohabitation of males and females. Avoidance of meat taint if reared to a more mature age for slaughter.

Preparation and equipment
Tetanus cover (vaccination or antitoxin), routine antibiosis and NSAIDs. If performed with goat in recumbency, preoperative starvation. Simple procedure kit, absorbable suture.

Restraint
Typically performed in the standing animal under local infiltration of the scrotum and/or spermatic cord and/or testicle. Sacrococcygeal epidural is also suitable (2% lidocaine HCl at 1 ml/45 kg, possibly combined with 0.07 mg/kg xylazine HCl).

Technique
The scrotum is incised on both lateral aspects with a J-shaped incision, starting one-third to halfway up the scrotal sac and ending close to the median raphe. For open castration, the tunica vaginalis is incised (**Fig. 2.46**) and the testicle exteriorised. The attachment of the tunica near the epididymis is broken (**Fig. 2.47**) and the tunica pushed back into the scrotal neck. For closed castration, the tunica vaginalis is kept intact (**Fig. 2.48**). The cord is either ligated with absorbable suture material or clamped for 2 minutes above the pampiniform plexus (**Fig. 2.49**). The cord may also be broken by the 'twist and pull' method in young animals. The skin incision is left open.

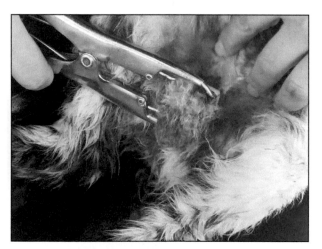

Fig. 2.45 **Castration using a rubber ring (here shown in a lamb).**

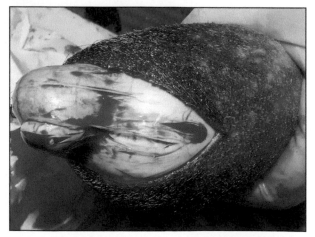

Fig. 2.46 **Maintaining firm pressure on the scrotal sac aids exteriorisation of the testicle. Incision of the tunica vaginalis has been started in this image.**

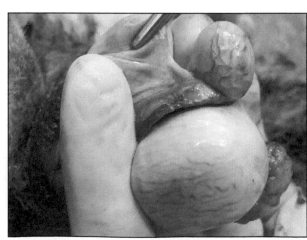

Fig. 2.47 **Breaking the tunical attachment near the epididymis with an instrument (rather than manually) reduces contamination of tissues to be retained.**

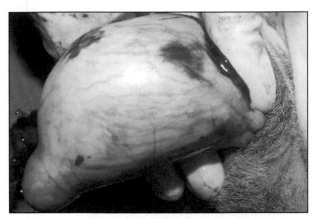

Fig. 2.48 The tunica vaginalis is kept intact for closed castration.

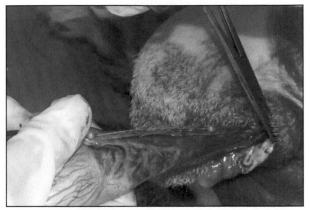

Fig. 2.49 Clamping or ligation must be done proximal to the pampiniform plexus.

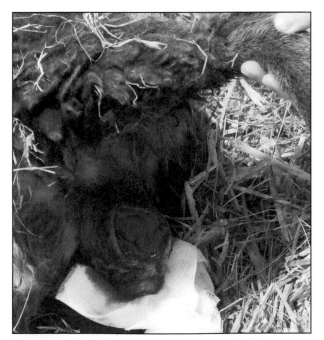

Fig. 2.50 Postoperative haemorrhage addressed by packing the scrotal sac with gauze swabs.

Aftercare

Clean bedding, encouragement and space to move around. Fly repellent if necessary.

Complications

Postoperative haemorrhage is addressed by locating the stump of the spermatic cord (in severe cases, via a laparotomy) and renewed ligation. Packing of the scrotal sac is less effective, as bleeding may continue intra-abdominally (**Fig. 2.50**). Occasionally, part of the tunica vaginalis prolapses through the skin incision; this is cut off at the level of the scrotal skin. Abscess formation is dealt with by drainage and lavage.

VASECTOMY

Indications

Creating a teaser buck that is sexually active, but incapable of fertilisation. Mainly used to advance the breeding season. (**Note:** Other techniques to create a teaser male, such as penile diversion or amputation, are banned in the UK.) Anaesthesia must be used for vasectomy in the UK.

A sexually mature (>1 year of age), physically fit male showing good libido should be used.

Preparation and equipment

Tetanus cover (vaccination or antitoxin), routine antibiosis and NSAIDs. If performed with goat in recumbency, preoperative starvation. Simple procedure kit, absorbable suture.

Restraint

Performed with the buck sitting on its haunches or in dorsal recumbency. Mild sedation, if necessary. Local infiltration over the cranial neck of the scrotum.

Technique

A 3 cm long, longitudinal skin incision is made on the cranial aspect of the scrotal neck over each spermatic cord (**Fig. 2.51**). Using blunt dissection, the cord is freed and lifted into the incision (e.g. by placing a pair of tissue forceps underneath it). The vas deference, lying slightly medial to the cord's midline, whitish in appearance and feeling firm under digital palpation, is identified (**Fig. 2.52**). Rotating the

cord slightly facilitates identification. The tunica is incised over the vas (**Fig. 2.53**) and the latter grasped. Haemorrhage from the tunica incision readily obscures the surgical field, therefore identification of the vas prior to incision greatly aids its location after the incision. The vas is ligated with absorbable suture at either end, and a section of at least 3 cm removed (**Fig. 2.54**). A few simple interrupted sutures are placed into the subcutaneous layers, and the skin is sutured in a routine way (**Fig. 2.55**).

Aftercare

Clean bedding, fly repellent if necessary, sexual rest for 1 month.

To confirm removal of the correct structure, the contents of the removed section of vas can be squeezed onto a slide and examined for spermatozoa. Alternatively, the removed sections are placed into formal saline, providing the option to perform histology should a dispute arise.

Complications

Haemorrhage tends to be minimal. A post-vasectomy spermatocoele is a common complication, occurring in a large proportion of teasers within 2 years of surgery, seen or palpated as distension of one or both testes within the scrotum.

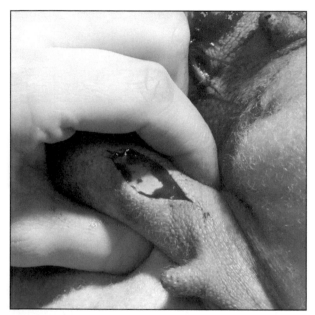

Fig. 2.51 Holding the spermatic cord firmly through the skin, a 3 cm long incision is made over the cranial aspect of the scrotal neck.

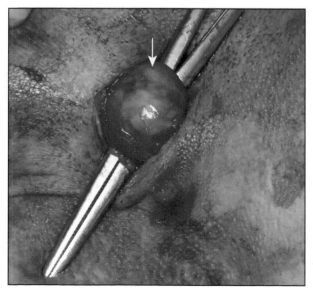

Fig. 2.52 The spermatic cord is freed and brought into the incision. The vas deference lies medially (arrow).

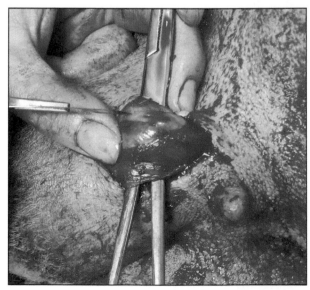

Fig. 2.53 The vas becomes visible (here underneath the point of the scalpel blade) after incision of the tunica.

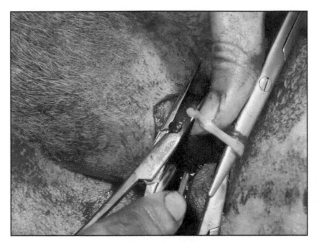

Fig. 2.54 The vas is clamped and ligated at either end, making sure a minimum of 3 cm length is removed.

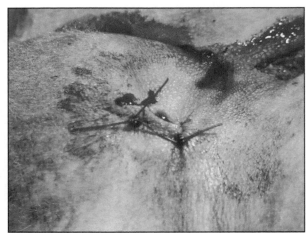

Fig. 2.55 The incision is closed in a routine manner.

TEMPORARY SUPPRESSION OF FERTILITY

Indications

This may be asked for by smallholders, where either housing of the buck separate from non-pregnant does may not be possible or where owners wish to suspend breeding activity for 1 year.

Technique

A commercial anti-GnRH vaccine was effective in 90% of Australian bucks, resulting in temporary suppression of spermatogenesis and male odour and behaviour for up to 1 year. Some regions use canvas or leather belly-aprons to prevent intromission.

Alternatively, progesterone may be administered to the female goats, either daily in feed or as an implant (not in UK).

OTHER MALE DISORDERS

Gynaecomastia

Commonly seen in males of heavily milking strains, especially in the British Saanen breed (**Fig 2.56**).

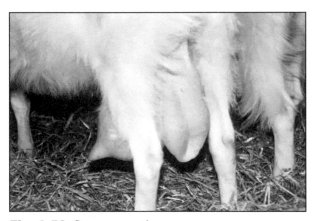

Fig. 2.56 Gynaecomastia.

Treatment is generally unsatisfactory, although cabergoline therapy has been tried with some success. The problem usually resolves with time.

Venereal disease

Vulvovaginitis and balanoposthitis can be associated with the venereal spread of both CpHV-1 (see above) and certain *Mycoplasma* spp. (see Chapter 10).

PREGNANCY

Fertilisation occurs in the ampulla of the oviduct several hours after ovulation. The conceptus reaches the uterus 4–5 days after conception. Fixation occurs around day 18 to day 22.

Gestation is on average 150 days' duration (range 147–155) and is corpus luteum (CL) dependent throughout. The doe has an epitheliochorial cotyledonary placenta. The maternal caruncles and fetal cotyledons form multiple concave placentomes (**Fig. 3.1**).

In the UK, the kidding period is typically from January (Anglo-Nubians) or February until March.

Pregnancy diagnosis

Indication

Confirming pregnancy and identifying non-pregnant animals for re-breeding or culling are of equal importance. Additional uses include determination of litter size, fetal gender, gestational length and fetal viability.

Technique

Pregnancy diagnosis methods include real-time (syn. B mode) ultrasonography transrectally from day 25 to day 30 and transabdominally from day 40 to day 45 (**Figs. 3.2–3.5**), blood or milk oestrone sulphate from day 45, and abdominal radiography from day 70 to day 80. A caprine pregnancy-specific protein (interferon tau) has been identified and could be used from day 25, but field testing kits are not currently available. The fetus may be detected on abdominal palpation in the second half of gestation. Supportive signs include non-return to oestrus, elevated milk or blood progesterone levels from day 18 to day 21 and, least accurate, live weight gain.

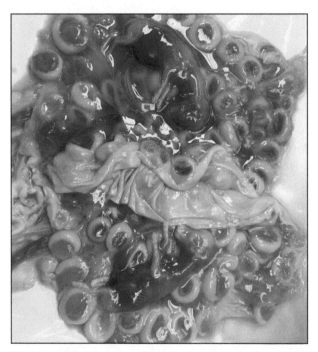

Fig. 3.1 The concave placentomes typical of the doe's placenta.

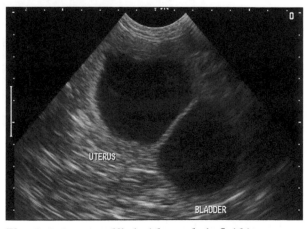

Fig. 3.2 A uterus filled with anechoic fluid is indicative of pregnancy. A single, fluid-filled structure may be the urinary bladder, therefore both uterus and bladder must be visualised to avoid misdiagnosis.

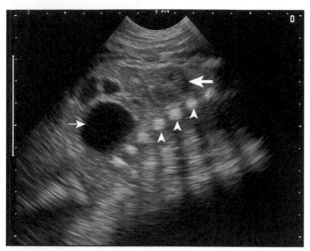

Fig. 3.3 As pregnancy progresses, fetal structures become apparent, such as the stomach (arrow), heart (wide arrow) and ribs (arrowheads; with reverberation artefacts below).

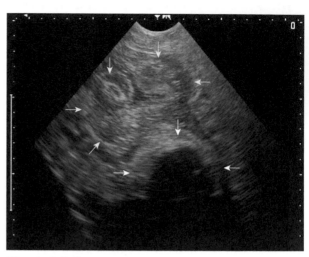

Fig. 3.4 In late-stage pregnancy, there is often little obvious free fluid. Yellow arrows = outline of placentomes; white arrows = outline of fetal head.

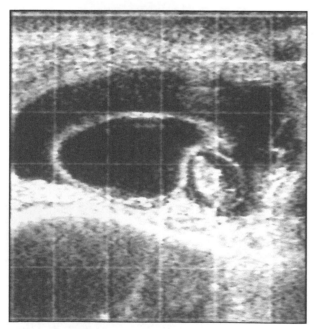

Fig. 3.5 Ultrasonography is useful to confirm fetal health. Here, two amniotic vesicles are present, but only the right-hand one contains a conceptus.

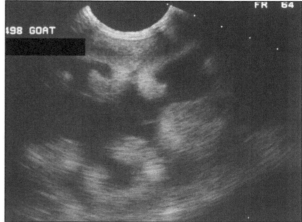

Fig. 3.6 Mushroom-shaped placentomes become visible from day 40.

from day 40, and reach 2–3 cm in length by day 60 (Fig. 3.6). In dairy breeds, fetal age can be calculated between 40 and 100 days using the biparietal diameter (BPD; Fig. 3.7) of the head and the formula:

Gestational age (days) = 1.71 × BPD (mm) + 14.6

Sexing may be attempted by ultrasonographically assessing the position of the genital tubercle at 60–69 days.

Ultrasonographic determination of litter size is best performed with a 3.5 MHz 170-degree sector probe between 40 and 75 days of gestation. Placentomes become visible on ultrasonography

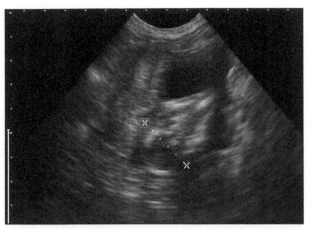

Fig. 3.7 The biparietal diameter is the distance between the eye sockets (indicated by the dotted line between the two white crosses [×]). The nose of the fetus points towards the 2 o'clock position in this image.

PREPARTUM PROBLEMS

Hypocalcaemia and pregnancy toxaemia
(See Chapter 14)

Mummification, maceration and fetal maldevelopment
(See Chapter 2)

Pseudopregnancy (syns. cloudburst, hydrometra)

Definition/overview
Pseudopregnancy is an abnormal accumulation of sterile uterine fluid in the absence of a fetus. A mean herd incidence of 9% has been reported (range 3–30%).

Aetiology
The exact cause of pseudopregnancy is unknown. Incidence appears to increase with age, and it may be more common after oestrus has been induced and in certain family lines. It can occur in both mated and unmated does.

Clinical presentation
Following oestrus (with or without mating), abdominal distension slowly increases, giving an external

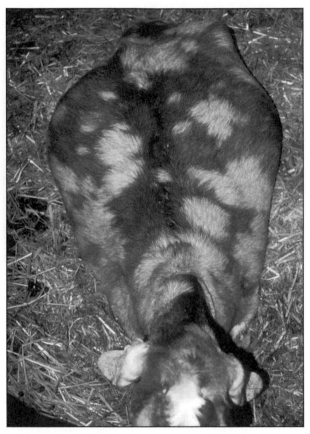

Fig. 3.8 Abdominal distension in a doe with pseudopregnancy.

appearance of pregnancy (**Fig. 3.8**). In non-lactating does, mammary development sometimes follows in the later stages. Lactating does may show a drop in milk yield.

Sudden loss of fluid occurs (giving rise to the colloquial term 'cloudburst'), usually near or beyond normal term (150 days) in mated does and before normal term in unmated does. Indirect signs that fluid loss has occurred include the abdomen returning to a normal size, damp bedding and a moist vulva and perineum.

Diagnosis
Transabdominal ultrasonography shows clear fluid in the uterus in the absence of a fetus, placenta or amniotic vesicle. A 'honeycomb' appearance may be present (**Fig. 3.9**). Other pregnancy diagnostic tests are equally negative (including oestrone sulphate levels, abdominal palpation, radiography).

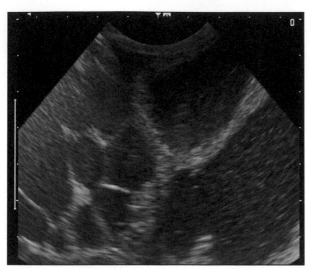

Fig. 3.9 Honeycomb appearance of the uterus on ultrasonography - here in a case of pyometra. The same appearance is commonly found in pseudopregnancy, although then the fluid will be anechoic.

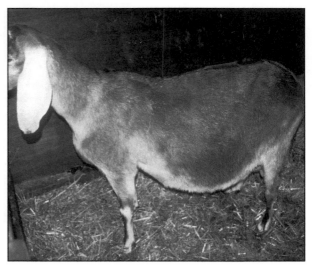

Fig. 3.10 Marked abdominal distension, excessive for the stage of pregnancy, in a doe with hydrops allantois.

Differential diagnosis

Normal pregnancy or pregnancy accompanied by hydrops allantois or hydrops amnion are ruled out by real-time ultrasonography.

Treatment/management/control

Prostaglandin-F 2 alpha ($PGF_{2\alpha}$) given i/m usually results in loss of fluid within 36 hours (e.g. 10 mg dinoprost or 62.5–125 µg cloprostenol; dinoprost may have a beneficially more direct action on the myometrium). A repeat dose of $PGF_{2\alpha}$ after 12 days is recommended. Oxytocin may aid involution. Affected does that remain unbred are likely to have the problem repeatedly, therefore mating, culling or spaying should be considered.

Hydrops uteri
Overview

Hydrops uteri is a rare condition in the goat, but often life-threatening to both dam and fetus, especially hydrops allantois, which is the more common form.

Aetiology

Excessive accumulation of either amniotic or allantoic fluid leads to hydrops amnion or hydrops allantois, respectively. It is unestablished in goats whether there is an association between hydrops allantois and an abnormal placenta and hydrops amnion and fetal malformation, as in cattle.

Clinical presentation

Hydrops amnion tends to be insidious in onset from the second half of gestation. The condition often goes unnoticed until parturition, when excessive fluid is noticed. Hydrops allantois shows a rapid development, leading to marked abdominal distension (**Fig. 3.10**). This may lead to respiratory distress, discomfort and recumbency.

Should pregnancy continue to term, contractions may be weak and the fetus may display oedema, anasarca, hydrothorax or ascites with both conditions, all potentially leading to dystocia.

Diagnosis

Ultrasonography to detect excessive fluid and placental, cotyledonary and fetal abnormalities. Centesis may be used to confirm the type of fluid, with sodium and chloride levels much higher in amniotic fluid (bovine values: sodium 120 versus 50 mmol/l, and chloride 90 versus 20 mmol/l, respectively).

Differential diagnosis

Large litter and pseudopregnancy for uterine distension. For hydrops allantois, also other causes of abdominal distension and respiratory distress, in particular rumen tympany, peritonitis or ascites.

Treatment/management/control

If the doe is not unduly affected, pregnancy may be allowed to continue to term, but assisted delivery is typically required, as well as intensive care for the neonate. If the doe is close to term, induction of birth and an elective caesarean section are options. In both, the rapid loss of abdominal pressure may trigger splanchnic disturbances, and fluid replacement therapy is advisable. If the doe is affected but far from term, abortion should be induced and occasionally euthanasia is indicated. Neither diuresis nor uterine drainage are effective long term.

Prognosis is guarded to poor, and recurrence in subsequent pregnancies cannot be ruled out.

Vaginal and cervical prolapse
Overview

Vaginal and cervical prolapse is an important problem in the prepartum doe, requiring careful management. While usually only seen sporadically, herd 'outbreaks' may be encountered. Occasionally, it is seen in the post-partum doe.

Aetiology

Principally, excess relaxation or weakness of pelvic tissues, possibly combined with increased intra-abdominal pressure. Predisposing factors include genetic predisposition, high body condition score (BCS), ageing, oestrogenic diet and bulky feeds (e.g. turnips). A sloping environment aids development. However, the exact aetiology remains unclear, and two herds with equal genetics and management may have a very different incidence rate.

Clinical presentation

Eversion of the vagina (sometimes including cervix), leading to exposure of the mucosal surface (**Fig. 3.11**). The prolapse may be intermittent, and partial or complete. The exposed tissues quickly become dry and traumatised. The doe often displays a raised tail and moderately arched back. Rupture

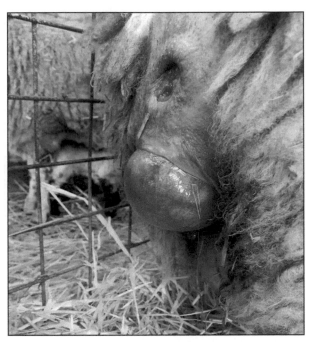

Fig. 3.11 **A recent vaginal prolapse in a ewe.**

of the vaginal wall with intestinal prolapse is a rare complication.

Diagnosis

Clinical examination confirms the condition and allows assessment of tissue viability. Pregnancy status should be confirmed.

Differential diagnosis

Rectal prolapse may be confused with vaginal tissue, and sometimes both occur concurrently.

Treatment/management/control

Mild or intermittent cases may be dealt with by cleaning, lubricating and replacing the prolapse, followed by one of several retention methods. In more severe cases, substantial trauma is addressed (e.g. by suturing) and a sacrococcygeal epidural given. It is useful to add 0.07 mg/kg xylazine HCl to the epidural to suppress straining for several hours. Retention methods include:

- Plastic retainer (**Fig. 3.12**) or body truss (**Figs. 3.13**). (**Note:** While not advisable, kidding is possible without removing these devices.)

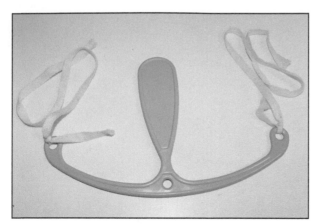

Fig. 3.12 A plastic spoon-shaped retainer for vaginal prolapse.

- Retention sutures placed in the vulva, such as Bühner or simple mattress. Careful placement is required to avoid discomfort and tissue trauma. Use of suture buttons is advised.
- Vulvoplasty, such as Caslick's, may be considered in chronic cases that are far from term.

Any sutures must be removed and the vulvoplasty reversed by an episiotomy prior to stage 2 of labour.

NSAIDs should be routinely given and antibiosis is strongly advised. Parturition must be supervised in affected does. Whether prepartum prolapse is recurrent in the doe (like in the ewe or cow) is not known, making culling advice difficult. Both pre- and post-partum prolapse leads to reduced fertility.

For post-partum prolapse, the Farquharson technique (submucosal resection) or Winkler's cervicoplasty (external cervical os secured to prepubic tendon) may be considered.

Rupture or herniation of the uterus
Overview
The gravid uterus may rupture prior to term or herniate through an existing or acquired body defect (including inguinal, umbilical, diaphragmatic, perineal, prepubic tendon). While rare, these are life-threatening conditions.

Aetiology
External trauma appears to be the most common reason for uterine rupture. Herniation through a rent in the prepubic tendon has been reported secondary to

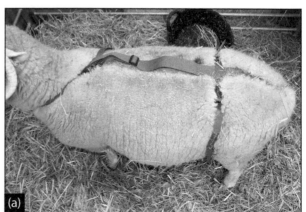

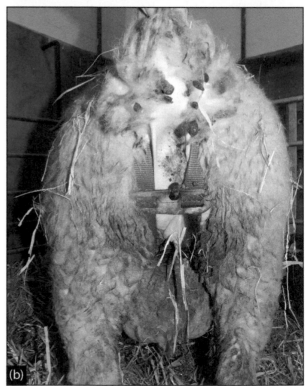

Fig. 3.13 A sheep prolapse harness or truss is also suitable for goats with a vaginal prolapse (a). It exerts pressure over the perineal area (b).

hydrops uteri in a goat. In general, abnormally high uterine weight contributes to herniation.

Clinical presentation
With herniation, the abdominal contour appears abnormal, and gait and stance may be altered. Prepubic tendon rupture is often accompanied by painful oedema just cranial to the udder.

Rupture of the gravid uterus may go unnoticed, as the sterile fetal fluids will not induce a septic peritonitis. However, haemorrhage may be substantial, leading to dyspnoea, weakness, anaemia and collapse. If caused by external trauma, other signs such as body wall haematoma and fractures may be apparent.

Diagnosis
Observation and palpation of abdominal contour. Ultrasonography to confirm fetal parts in an abnormal location.

Differential diagnosis
Other causes of dependent oedema (e.g. congestive heart failure), haemorrhage and abdominal distension (e.g. rumen tympany).

Treatment/management/control
Ventral herniation rarely breaches the abdominal skin, and if the doe is reasonably comfortable, she may be allowed to carry to term, potentially aided by a belly bandage. Blood loss is assessed and addressed as usual. Alternatively, the pregnancy may be terminated.

Assistance at parturition is invariably required, with surgical delivery if the fetus fails to present at the pelvic canal. Repair of an acquired hernia is often not rewarding long term. The udder may be inaccessible for suckling by the kid, necessitating supplementation with colostrum and milk.

Great care should be exercised when handling heavily pregnant does to avoid uterine or body wall ruptures.

Induction of parturition
Indication
Reasons for induction include prolonged gestation with risk of feto-maternal disproportion, prepartum metabolic disease in the doe (e.g. pregnancy toxaemia), injury or trauma in the doe. Elective induction may be indicated if the sire is found to produce large offspring, thereby avoiding potential dystocia.

Technique
$PGF_{2\alpha}$ (5–10 mg dinoprost or 62.5 µg cloprostenol) given i/m after day 140 typically results in parturition 30–72 hours later. Dexamethasone (16 mg)

has equally been used successfully, with parturition 90–150 hours later.

Aftercare/prognosis
Retained fetal membranes (RFM) are not a common problem after induction, rarely exceeding 10% of induced animals. Kids born more than a few days prematurely are unlikely to survive.

Ante-natal preparation
The doe is dried off 6–8 weeks prior to term at the latest. A clostridial vaccine booster is given 4–6 weeks prior to the doe's due date. Exercise opportunities should be made available in late pregnancy. Dietary protein and energy are increased to account for fetal growth, and post-natal dietary feeds introduced to allow for adaptation of the rumen microflora.

PARTURITION

Normal parturition
The fetus controls the time of parturition. In the goat, $PGF_{2\alpha}$ secretion by the mammary gland is important for initiation of normal parturition, with dystocia resulting in goats that underwent udder removal as a young female.

Labour has a normal duration of: first stage 6–12 hours, second stage 0.5–1 hour (**Fig. 3.14**), and third stage 3–4 hours. Cervical dilation appears to be of relatively short duration in the doe, with closure commonly starting 2–3 hours after onset of stage 2.

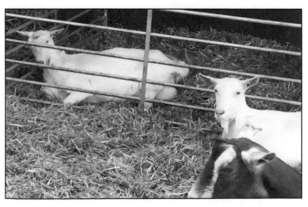

Fig. 3.14 Second stage labour typically lasts 0.5 to 1 hour. Not all does adopt lateral recumbency, as in this case. Straining and abdominal contractions are seen.

Anterior longitudinal presentation is the norm in the goat. Posterior longitudinal presentation occurs in up to 10% of births, but almost always involves multiple births and typically the first-born kid is presented correctly (i.e. anteriorly).

Dystocia

Overview

Average reported dystocia rates are 4–17%, but may reach 50% in individual herds. Fetal maldisposition and obstruction of the birth canal are common causes worldwide. Prompt attention is warranted, with the life of the fetus and dam at risk. Dystocia is always costly, even if both neonate and dam survive.

Aetiology

In common with other species, the incidence of dystocia is higher in primiparous does and those carrying a single male fetus.

The reported incidence of maternal causes ranges from 30% to 58%. A frequent maternal cause is obstruction of the birth canal. This may be bony (e.g. skeletal immaturity or secondary to pelvic trauma), but more often is a soft tissue obstruction and in particular failure of cervical dilation or cervical closure in delayed parturition. Primary uterine inertia appears to be rare. Other maternal causes include secondary uterine inertia ('exhaustion' of uterine and abdominal musculature), concurrent illness, rupture or herniation of the uterus, or neoplastic growths in the birth canal.

Fetal causes most commonly involve maldispositon. In single births, lateral deviation of head and neck or bilateral shoulder flexion is common. With multiple fetuses, simultaneous presentation is common. Feto-maternal disproportion accounts for about 20% of dystocia cases. Other fetal causes include fetal monsters or fetal death (**Fig. 3.15**).

Clinical presentation

Indications of dystocia include:

- During stage 1, no progression to stage 2 after several hours (i.e. fetal parts not becoming visible or labour signs subsiding) or doe showing marked restlessness or discomfort.

- During stage 2, unproductive straining for over 15 minutes or failure of the kid to be delivered after 1 hour.
- Obvious maldisposition.
- Malodorous fetal fluids, haemorrhage or premature separation of fetal membranes.

History

The two main aims of history taking in obstetrical cases are establishing a prognosis and narrowing down possible causes, both of which will influence management of the case. Prognosis is generally negatively influenced by previous dystocia, recent or concurrent illness of the dam, attempts at assisted delivery and time elapsed between onset of labour and attention. An obstruction is unlikely if one kid has already been delivered, whereas an overdue dam is likely to carry a large fetus.

General approach

The general health status of the dam is established with a brief clinical examination, paying particular attention to any respiratory distress, metabolic disease, position and trauma.

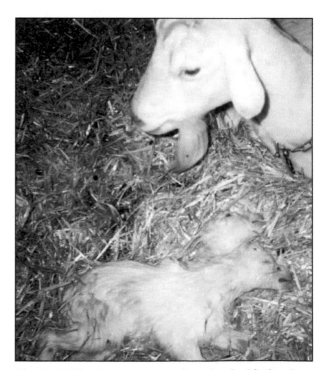

Fig. 3.15 Fetal monsters, such as the double-head formation in this kid, often lead to dystocia.

If necessary, the doe is moved into a clean, well-lit and well-bedded area. Manual restraint is usually sufficient in does. If low-level sedation is desired, detomidine HCl or butorphanol are preferable over xylazine HCl, which has a direct oxytocin-like myotonic action, making the uterus more friable.

The birth canal of the doe is tight and fragile, and great care must be exercised during vaginal manipulations (**Fig. 3.16**). A sacrococcygeal epidural (1 ml/45 kg 2% lidocaine; see Chapter 18) is strongly recommended. A smooth muscle relaxant (e.g. clenbuterol) may be useful. Plenty of obstetrical lubricant should be used and can, if necessary, be applied to the birth canal with the help of a lamb feeder tube and catheter-tip syringe (**Fig. 3.17**).

Both the perineal area and the obstetrician's hands and forearms must be clean throughout, using either a mild disinfectant (povidone–iodine or chlorhexidine) or soapy water. After gentle insertion of the well-lubricated hand into the vagina, the degree of relaxation (especially cervical) and fetal disposition (presentation, position, posture, singleton or multiple) are established, and a decision made on the correction method (vaginal delivery, fetotomy, caesarean section, euthanasia of dam). As a general rule, vaginal delivery is possible if there is room for one finger to be passed all around the fetus once it is engaged in the dam's pelvis. Oversize should be suspected if the head fails to stay aligned despite use of a rope or snare, the fetus's front legs are crossed over or bilateral shoulder flexion is present.

Fetus alive versus dead

Signs of fetal life include movements visible in the dam's flank, spontaneous limb movements and a variety of positive reflexes. In anterior presentation, these include suck, deep pain (interdigital space or tongue), palpebral and corneal. In posterior presentation, the anal and deep pain reflex can be used. It is important to remember that absence of reflexes is not a definite sign of death; the fetus may be unable to move (being wedged in) or too depressed to respond. If in doubt, the fetus should be assumed to be alive.

Feeling for a pulse in the umbilical cord can sometimes be useful, but in general the presence of a pulse is difficult to establish.

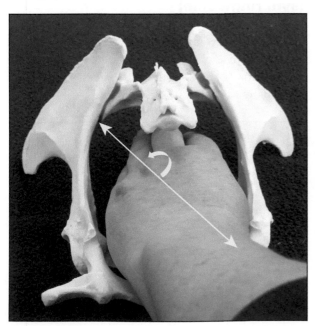

Fig. 3.16 The pelvis and birth canal are narrow in the doe (for reference, the person's hand shown in the image takes surgical glove size 7.5). One to two cm extra space may be gained by rotating the fetus 30–45 degrees clockwise or anticlockwise.

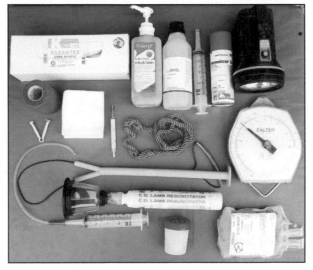

Fig. 3.17 Both owners and veterinarians should have a fully stocked parturition kit readily available. It usefully contains (from top left in a clockwise direction): rectal gloves, iodine or chlorhexidine disinfectant, obstetrical lube, catheter-tip syringe to aid lubricant application, disinfectant for navel, torch, weighing scales, plasma, colostrum, oesophageal feeder tube, resuscitator, lambing snare and ropes, navel clip, tail bandage, swabs, thermometer.

If the equipment is available, other techniques include detection of a heart beat by Doppler or B-mode ultrasound, fetal ECG, PO_2 levels on fetal blood gas or pulse oximetry.

Signs of fetal death include corneal opacity and collapse of the eyeball, emphysema or autolysis, separation of the placenta and a fetid discharge.

Signs of fetal distress include excessive movements visible in the dam's flank, breathing or vocalising, or a heart rate consistently below 120 bpm or above 180 bpm.

General principles of vaginal correction and delivery

In multiple births, it is important to allocate limbs and head to the correct fetus.

Correction of a maldisposition is usually a combination of repulsion of one fetal part while applying traction to another. Where this needs to be done simultaneously, a rope on the relevant fetal part is used for traction with the obstetrician's hand carrying out repulsion. Repulsion is often easier if a rocking movement, rather than continuous pressure, is used on the fetus. Sharp pointed extremities of the fetus are covered with a hand as much as possible during traction to avoid trauma to the reproductive tract. In the goat it is sometimes possible, with great care, to deliver a small fetus in an uncorrected maldisposition (e.g. unilateral shoulder flexion). As a rule of thumb, if correction is not possible or no progress in delivery is made within 20 minutes, a caesarean section should be considered.

Failure of vaginal or vulval dilation can typically be addressed with gentle manual stretching for 10 minutes or so. A true persistent hymen is easily broken down manually, but one should rule out a rare case of vaginal stenosis. Where the vulva fails to relax fully, an episiotomy is useful; an incision is made with a scalpel blade at either the 10 or 2 o'clock position, followed by post-partum closure with an absorbable suture.

Once correction has been achieved, the natural birth posture should be observed as much as possible. For the goat fetus in anterior presentation this is elbow flexion, with the nose resting on the feet. Therefore, traction on the limbs must be accompanied by expulsion of the head. A lambing snare (**Fig. 3.18**) or gentle digital pressure behind the poll (if necessary via gentle insertion of a finger into the rectal canal) can be used to achieve this.

In both anterior and posterior presentation, the fetus may be rotated by 30–45 degrees around its longitudinal axis to make best use of the widest diameter of the dam's pelvis (**Fig. 3.16**).

The natural arc of expulsion is followed and the fetus's head or hip aided through the vulva by gently pushing the vulval lips over the fetus. Traction is applied in synchrony with the dam's contractions and straining as much as possible.

Control

Prevention of dystocia relies on suitable matching of sire and dam, adequate growth of doelings prior to breeding, dams being in target body condition, nutritional and health status, and close supervision with knowledgeable intervention of parturition. Unsuitable dams (e.g. ones with pelvic abnormalities) should be promptly removed from the breeding pool.

Failure of cervical dilation (syn. ringwomb)
Overview

Insufficient cervical dilation is the commonest maternal cause of dystocia in the goat, reported to account for 12–23% of all dystocia cases, or 45% of maternally caused dystocia.

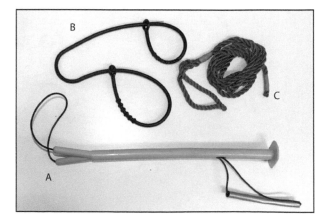

Fig. 3.18 A lambing snare (A) is easy to apply and ensures that the head stays in its normal position during traction. Leg snares (B) or lambing ropes (C) should be used with care, as they easily disrupt the normal elbow flexion with which the caprine fetus presents.

Aetiology

The normal cascade of hormonal factors and physical dilation by the fetal sacs (or fetus itself, for example in breech presentation) fails. It can also occur secondary to fibrosis after previous cervical trauma, and has been linked to hypocalcaemia and hypophosphatemia.

Clinical presentation

Stage 2 of labour has commenced, but no fetal parts become visible. Vaginal examination reveals a partially opened cervix.

Differential diagnosis

Premature births or abortions may present with a lack of cervical dilation. It is important to establish that parturition has commenced and abdominal straining is not caused by urinary tract disease, colic or another cause.

In delayed parturition, or missed cases of dystocia, the cervix may be in the process of contracting down again. A uterine torsion may present as an apparent failure of cervical dilation.

Treatment/management/control

For manual dilation, the fingers of a clean, well-lubricated cone-shaped hand are inserted into the cervix and gently opened and closed, repeatedly, for several minutes.

Response to medication is variable. A smooth muscle relaxant (clenbuterol, 30–60 µg slow i/v; or butylscopolamine bromide 4 mg and metamizole 500 mg combination product, 0.05–0.1 ml/kg) may help. Using valethamate bromide (15 mg) and cloprostenol sodium (250 µg) has been successful in 33% of cases. If no immediate effect is seen, one can wait for 30–60 minutes, providing the fetal membranes are intact and there are no signs of fetal distress. Otherwise, a caesarean section is indicated. Oxytocin must not be used, as it carries a high risk of resulting in uterine rupture.

Uterine torsion

Overview

This occasional disorder (average 2% incidence) may not be recognised even by experienced breeders. It almost always occurs during stage 1 or stage 2 of labour in the goat.

Aetiology

The aetiology remains unclear but causes may include an unstable suspension of the uterus in multiparous animals, a singleton occupying mainly one horn, vigorous fetal movements and possible reduced exercise in late pregnancy. The torsion may be up to 360 degrees, with a clockwise (towards the right) rotation possibly more common.

Clinical presentation

Unproductive straining without fetal membranes becoming visible. Any signs of parturition may cease altogether after some time. In the majority of cases, the point of torsion is the anterior vagina, and the deviation is detectable on vaginal examination (manually or visually via a speculum). Occasionally, a precervical torsion occurs, in which case there are no detectable signs on vaginal examination. Rectal examination is a challenge in goats, but may be possible in a large framed doe: the broad ligaments are palpable as tight bands across the pelvic inlet.

Differential diagnosis

As for failure of cervical dilation above.

Treatment/management/control

Caesarean section is often the best approach. Failure of cervical dilation may occur once the torsion is corrected, not least because the dystocia has often gone unnoticed. In addition, the uterine wall may have become fragile because of compromised blood supply.

The technique for non-surgical correction is as follows: for an anti-clockwise torsion, the doe is cast into left lateral recumbency. While kneeling at a right angle to the doe's ventral abdomen, one person folds their hands and pushes their parallel-held lower arms onto the fetus through the abdominal wall (**Fig. 3.19**). Two assistants slowly and carefully rotate the doe over her back into right lateral recumbency, while pressure on the fetus is maintained. The process is repeated for torsions of more than 180 degrees. For a clockwise torsion, the technique is reversed (i.e. the doe is rotated from right lateral recumbency over her back into left lateral recumbency).

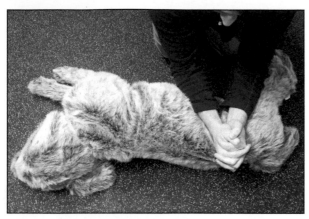

Fig. 3.19 Position adopted by veterinarian to fix the fetus in position through the abdominal wall during correction of a uterine torsion (shown here on a dog mannequin). The doe is rolled underneath onto her other side.

Caesarean section

Indications

In approximate order of importance, reasons for emergency caesarean section in the doe are: obstruction of the birth canal, feto-maternal disproportion, uterine torsion, rupture and tears to the reproductive tract, malpresentation and, rarely, abortion or fetal monsters. Not surprisingly, does with male kids and primiparous ones are overrepresented in case reviews.

As an elective procedure, it may be indicated where disproportion is suspected, gestation is prolonged, or the doe is suffering from disease. Induction is carried out whenever possible prior to an elective caesarean section. A combination of corticosteroids, followed 12–24 hours later by $PGF_{2\alpha}$, works well to support neonatal lung function, release of placental attachments and luteolysis. The ideal time for surgery is at the start of cervical dilation. Note that kids more than 5 days premature have a slim chance of survival.

Preparation and equipment

Preoperative medication includes antibiosis, NSAIDs, tetanus cover if not vaccinated and a uterine relaxant (e.g. clenbuterol). Intravenous fluids are indicated in a compromised patient.

For a left flank approach, the left flank is clipped from the penultimate rib to the tuber coxae, and from the transverse processes to near the midline. In long-haired breeds, duct tape can be usefully employed around the edges of the clipped area to keep the fleece away from the surgical site. The surgical site is aseptically prepared.

The owner or assistant is briefed on neonatal resuscitation (see Chapter 4), and relevant equipment for this laid out.

A full caesarean section kit includes: razor blade for shaving or clippers, povidone–iodine or chlorhexidine disinfectant and methylated spirit, local anaesthetic (with syringes and needles), nail brush, sterile gown and gloves, sterile lavaging fluid, large instrument kit, suture material; and, optionally, sedative, sterile drape, intra-abdominal antibiotics.

Restraint

Sedation and local anaesthesia is favoured for this procedure, as the rapid recovery of the dam allows her to nurse her offspring, and there is generally less effect on the neonate from the anaesthetic drugs used.

Suitable sedative drugs include detomidine HCl, butorphanol and xylazine HCl. For local anaesthesia, options include line block, inverted L-block, paravertebral block and lumbosacral epidural (see Chapter 18).

The goat is placed into right lateral (for left flank approach) or dorsal recumbency (for paramedian or ventral midline approach; **Figs. 3.20**). If the fetus is emphysematous, the ventral midline approach offers good access, allowing exteriorisation of the uterine horn prior to incision, thereby reducing abdominal contamination. From the dorsal position, the patient is leant 30–45 degrees towards the surgeon to aid this. The uppermost hind leg of the doe may be tied-out, if necessary.

Steps to reduce the risk of aspiration and hypothermia are taken (see Chapter 18).

Technique – left flank approach

A vertical flank incision of about 20 cm length is made in the centre to slightly caudal left flank, starting approximately one hand-width below the transverse processes (**Fig. 3.21**). The incision must be undertaken with care, as the patient

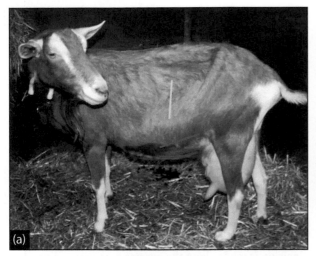
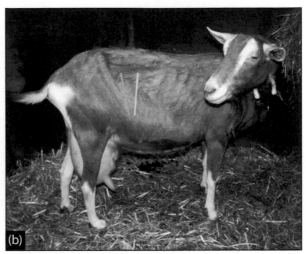

Fig. 3.20 Possible incision sites for a caesarean section in the left (a) or right (b) flank. Yellow = vertical sublumbar; green = angled sublumbar; blue = paramedian; red = ventral midline.

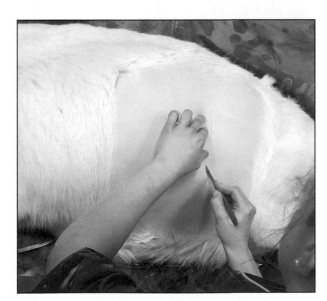

Fig. 3.21 A 20 cm long incision is made in the centre to caudal flank. The scalpel blade is held as parallel to the flank as possible, to avoid accidental puncture of deeper structures should the goat move. In this case, the goat was placed onto a tarpaulin to provide a reasonably clean surgical environment. (Image courtesy Adelle Isaacs.)

is conscious and therefore liable to move occasionally, the tissue layers are relatively thin and a distended viscus (rumen, uterus) may be present adjacent to the body wall. Remembering the direction of the muscle fibres in the various layers greatly helps to ascertain depth and level of incision. These are:

- Head to hind foot for the external oblique muscle.
- Hip to front foot for the internal oblique.
- Vertical for the transverse abdominis muscle.

Haemostasis is achieved with artery forceps, all of which are removed prior to exploring the abdominal cavity.

A hand is inserted into the abdomen and the pregnant uterine horn nearest the flank incision found and manoeuvred into the incision (**Fig. 3.22**). Orientation within the abdomen is often helped by initially placing the hand into the pelvic inlet, feeling the fetus within the uterus in that location and then following the fetus and uterus down onto the horn. Usually, it is possible to exteriorise the horn containing the fetal extremities. The uterine incision is started between the claws of the fetus and extended to the hock (if hind leg) or carpus (if front leg). To minimise blood loss, the incision is made along the greater curvature where blood vessels are minimal (**Fig. 3.23**), and care is taken to avoid incising into placentomes. The incision should be made reasonably close to the uterine body to aid delivery of any additional fetus from the other horn through

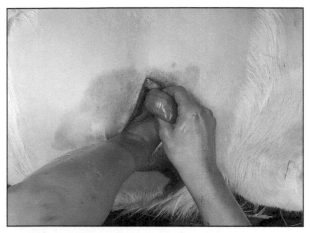

Fig. 3.22 A leg is grasped through the wall of the uterine horn and brought into the incision. (Image courtesy Adelle Isaacs.)

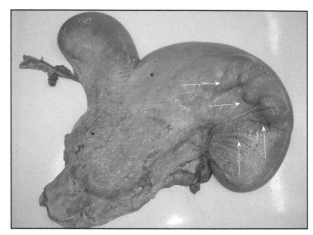

Fig. 3.23 To avoid unnecessary blood loss, the uterine incision is made along the greater curvature where vessels (some highlighted with arrows) are smallest.

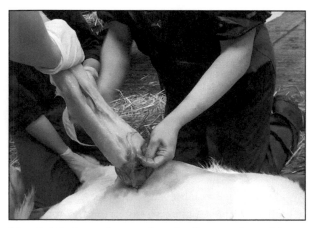

Fig. 3.24 An assistant takes the fetus and provides first care and resuscitation. The surgeon holds the uterus to stop it falling into the abdominal cavity. (Image courtesy Adelle Isaacs.)

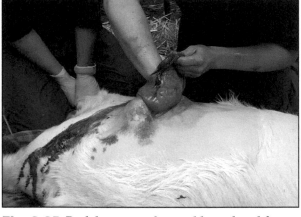

Fig. 3.25 Both horns are thoroughly explored for additional fetuses. (Image courtesy Adelle Isaacs.)

the same incision. Occasionally, this is not possible and a second uterine incision has to be made.

The fetus is removed and passed to an assistant for further care (**Fig. 3.24**). Both horns are thoroughly explored for further kids (**Fig. 3.25**). The placenta is only removed if it comes away easily. Otherwise, any protruding parts are resected, with the bulk left in place.

The uterus is sutured with a continuous inverting pattern (e.g. Lembert or Cushing) through the serosa and muscular layer, using absorbable material, ideally on a swaged needle to reduce tissue trauma. Catgut is a good choice, with less tearing of tissue and less

persistence that may lead to scarring compared with synthetic suture materials. However, synthetic materials, such as polyglactin 910, offer more consistent material strength and better knot and handling qualities. Great care must be taken to avoid including the fetal membranes. The knots should be buried.

After uterine closure, the uterus is lavaged with warm sterile fluid, paying particular attention to removing any blood clots around the ovaries. Prior to routine closure of the abdominal wall (**Fig. 3.26**), the surgeon may wish to instil intra-abdominal antibiotics (soluble and non-irritant, for example benzylpenicillin sodium). If the doe was tied-out

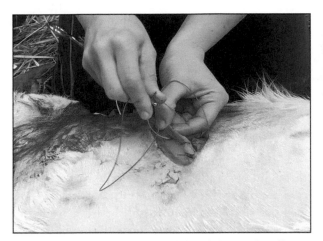

Fig. 3.26 **Routine closure of the abdominal wall. A continuous pattern may be used for both musculature and skin. However, in case of seroma formation, it is good practice to place 1 or 2 simple interrupted sutures at the ventral end of the skin suture.**

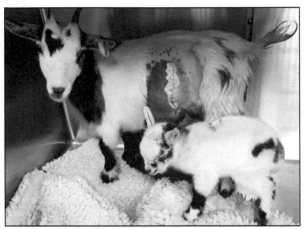

Fig. 3.27 **Depending on the time of year, fly repellent ointment is applied to the wound. (Image courtesy Emily Reeves.)**

during surgery, abdominal wall closure is aided by releasing the leg ties.

Aftercare

The flank and udder are cleaned thoroughly. Postoperative medication includes analgesia, oxytocin to aid involution and fly control where applicable (**Fig. 3.27**). Any hypothermia in the doe is addressed, and any concurrent disease treated. Bonding and colostrum intake is monitored (**Fig. 3.28**).

Complications

Reported kid survival rates range from 40% to 65%. Stage 2 labour of more than 6 hours prior to intervention carries a poor prognosis for kid survival. Doe survival rates of >90% are achievable.

Common complications include RFM, metritis, endometritis, wound breakdown or seroma formation, subcutaneous emphysema and peritonitis (which typically presents clinically within 72–96 hours postoperatively). Good surgical technique is paramount, including asepsis, generous incisions, suture techniques that achieve a good seal and reduce dead space without being overly tight and avoid incorporation of fetal membranes, clean surgical environment, clean preoperative vaginal examination and routine antibiosis.

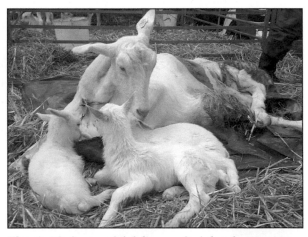

Fig. 3.28 **Successful delivery of triplets by caesarean section. The newborn kids are placed near the doe's head to encourage bonding. (Image courtesy Adelle Isaacs.)**

Fetotomy
Indication
Fetotomy may be considered in cases of fetal maldisposition, feto-maternal disproportion, partial fetal delivery (for example 'hiplock') or when dealing with fetal monsters. It may be of particular benefit where fetal death occurred some time ago and autolysis has set in, and therefore a caesarean section carries a high risk of peritoneal contamination.

An absolute requirement for a fetotomy is that the fetus is dead and that there is sufficient cervical dilation both for carrying out the procedure and retrieving fetal parts. Because of the space constraints and the relative fragility of the uterus, a complete fetotomy is seldom performed in small ruminants. Partial fetotomy, however, has its place.

Contraindications include: fetus still alive (although euthanasia *in utero* may be considered), insufficient dilation of the birth canal and in particular the cervix, fractured pelvis, severe trauma of the birth canal or uterine tears, compromised dam (e.g. septicaemic).

Restraint and position

The doe may be standing or in lateral recumbency (with the fetal limb to be removed lying uppermost), under mild sedation if necessary. A sacrococcygeal epidural (1 ml/45 kg 2% lidocaine HCl) and clenbuterol are administered. Obstetrical lubrication and water and mild disinfectant are prepared.

Technique – front leg removal

This is a relatively easy and quick to perform partial fetotomy that often enables vaginal delivery afterwards. The aim is to remove one (or both) front legs via a subcutaneous method.

Using a scalpel blade, a circular cut is made through the skin just above the fetal carpus, taking care not to sever any tendons (**Fig. 3.29a**). A 2–3 cm long cut along the long-axis of the leg is made in a proximal direction, connecting with the circular cut at its distal end. Using digital pressure and probing, the skin is lifted off the leg's soft tissue (**Fig. 3.29b**). Tension is maintained on the lower limb to aid breaking down of muscular attachments, especially of the shoulder blade (**Fig. 3.29c**). The freed 'skinned' leg is removed (**Fig. 3.29d**).

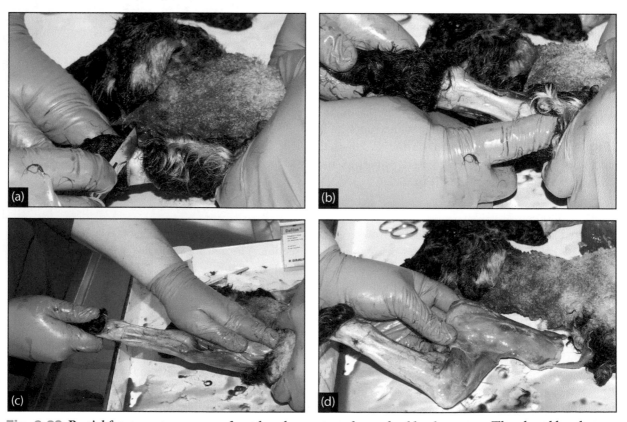

Fig. 3.29 Partial fetotomy to remove a front leg, demonstrated on a dead lamb *ex utero*. The gloved hands on the right mimic the vulva of the dam. A circular incision is made just above the carpus (a) followed by an incision at right-angle to this along the long axis of the limb. Soft tissue attachments are broken down with fingers (b), while maintaining tension on the lower limb (c). The removed, de-gloved limb (d).

Aftercare

It is important to ensure that all fetal parts have been removed. In cases of severe autolysis, uterine lavage with saline may be indicated. Medication consists of antibiosis, NSAIDs and analgesia. Oxytocin is advisable, especially if clenbuterol was used. The doe is monitored for pyrexia, metritis and inappetence over the next several days.

POST-PARTURIENT PROBLEMS

Haemorrhage
Overview
Internal or external post-partum haemorrhage is possible.

Aetiology
Trauma to the soft tissues of the birth canal, especially the vagina and cervix and their associated vessels, in particular the vaginal artery. Internal blood loss may arise from uterine trauma, including placentomes accidentally incised during a caesarean section, and bleeding into the broad ligament.

Clinical presentation
External haemorrhage is apparent at the vulva.

A uterine bleeding point does not usually result in large quantities of blood externally, but the animal will show systemic signs of blood loss. Bleeding into the broad ligament may present as acute or chronic blood loss.

Diagnosis
Careful examination, if necessary with the aid of a speculum, is required to locate the source. The vaginal arteries are located roughly at the 3 and 9 o'clock positions in the vagina and should be inspected for integrity. Blood accumulation in the peritoneal cavity may be confirmed via abdominocentesis or ultrasonography.

Differential diagnosis
Temporary bleeding from the umbilical stump can appear as severe external haemorrhage, but will not deplete the dam's circulatory volume (**Fig. 3.30**). For internal haemorrhage, any other causes of acute or chronic blood loss (see Chapter 7).

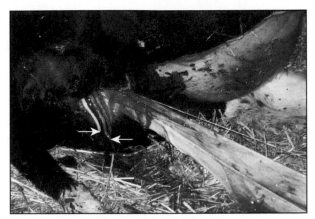

Fig. 3.30 Bleeding from the umbilical stump (arrows; shown here in a cow in left lateral recumbency).

Treatment/management/control
For cervical or vaginal haemorrhage, pressure is applied by packing the birth canal: a stockinette (or freshly laundered sock as first aid) is placed into the vagina and filled with gauze swabs or cotton wool to its maximum capacity. It is left in place for at least 72 hours. The stockinette may be soaked with 1% alum or 1:1,000 adrenaline. If the origin is a vessel and this is accessible, it may be clamped using a pair of haemostats, which are secured to the dam's tail. Ligation can be attempted, but often results in more tissue trauma. Oxytocin is useful to support involution.

For internal haemorrhage, treatment consists of sedation or enforced rest, blood transfusion, antiobiosis, and possibly a laparotomy to find the source of the haemorrhage.

Laceration of the cervix
Overview
Uncommon, but can affect future fertility. Scar tissue may compromise the cervical seal or dilation at subsequent gestation and parturition.

Aetiology
Trauma at parturition, especially if delivery attempted while cervix not fully dilated. The weakest point is dorsally (12 o'clock position).

Clinical presentation
Detected at post-partum or infertility examination, with the aid of a speculum.

Treatment/management/control

Surgery is possible, but access typically proves difficult. Culling is advised if cervical seal fails.

Laceration of the vagina

Overview

A relatively common complication, causing considerable discomfort and being potentially fatal if positioned very cranially.

Aetiology

Spontaneous tearing may result from vigorous contractions forcing a fetal foot through the vaginal wall. More common, however, is excessive force during correction of a malposture. Contributing factors in other species include an overconditioned dam, lack of lubrication and premature or too aggressive interference.

Clinical presentation

Laceration is only detectable on vaginal examination. Care must be taken during exploration to avoid turning a shallow tear into a deeper defect. Most are positioned retroperitoneally, but if full thickness and cranial enough to connect to the peritoneal cavity, signs of peritonitis develop 24–96 hours after kidding.

For treatment and prognosis, categorisation as follows is useful: grade 1 = mucosa only affected; grade 2 = submucosa also involved; grade 3 = full thickness, with prolapse of pelvic fat or able to feel serosal surface of uterus or intestines, depending on location.

Treatment/management/control

- Grade 1: the mucosa normally heals rapidly without treatment.
- Grades 2 or 3: if discovered when fresh, best repaired surgically. A sacrococcygeal epidural is given and stay sutures placed into the vulval lips to aid visual and manual access (held open by an assistant). Commencing at the cranial end of the tear, a continuous absorbable suture is placed incorporating the submucosal and mucosal layers. Systemic antibiosis and NSAIDs are given.

Recto-vaginal fistula

Trauma to the roof of the vagina and vestibulum may lead to loss of the tissue plane that separates these structures from the rectum (**Fig. 3.31**). Where only the vaginal roof is involved, there may be no outward sign. However, the presence of faecal material in the vagina should prompt investigation.

If the case is presented promptly (<12 hours after injury), there is a reasonable prognosis for achieving healing by first intention. Otherwise, surgical repair should be delayed for at least 6 weeks to allow for local swelling to subside and remodelling of granulation tissue to occur. Surgery is carried out in the standing animal under epidural anaesthesia. The rectum is evacuated, the perineal area thoroughly cleaned, and stay-sutures placed into the vulval lips, which are held open by an assistant. In brief, the technique involves freeing a plane of vaginal mucosa (including edges), folding such created flaps ventrally into the lumen, and suturing the dorsal vaginal submucosa in a series of interrupted sutures from cranial to caudal to form a new vaginal roof.

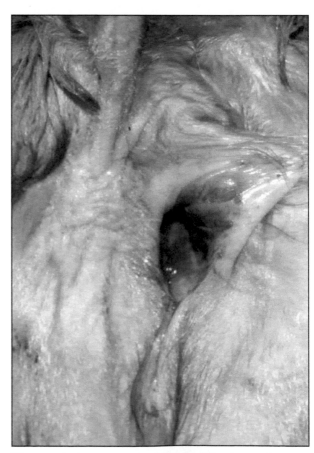

Fig. 3.31 A recto-vaginal fistula. The tissue plane between rectum and vagina has been lost.

Prevention is by early consideration of an episiotomy or delivery by caesarean section.

Vaginal prolapse – post-parturient
Overview
Vaginal prolapse may be a standalone problem or recurrence of a preparturient prolapse. It is sometimes accompanied by rectal prolapse.

Treatment/management/control
As for prepartum prolapse (see earlier). Prognosis is better than in prepartum cases.

Uterine rupture
Overview
Ruminants appear more prone to uterine rupture than other species.

Aetiology
Typically caused by trauma during assistance such as correction of maldisposition, repulsion of fetus or prolonged attempt at delivery. Rarely spontaneous due to contractile forces. Cases with uterine torsion or fetal autolysis are especially vulnerable because of uterine wall compromise.

The weakest point in the wall is dorsally, but damage may occur at any location where undue pressure has been exerted (e.g. near the pelvic brim during correction of a breech presentation).

Clinical presentation
If the defect is caudal enough, it will be obvious on palpation during the routine post-partum check. Loops of intestine may prolapse through the defect and must be confirmed as belonging to the doe rather than to another fetus (if not delivered yet). If the defect is out of reach, signs of peritonitis will develop within 72–96 hours of parturition.

Treatment/management/control
For a small defect, where parturition was without excessive contamination and the fetus is alive, oxytocin to cause uterine contraction is sufficient.

For a small defect, but involving a dead fetus or contamination, oxytocin, antibiosis and NSAIDs are given.

A large defect should be repaired as best as possible, either per vaginam or via a laparotomy. Another approach involves creating a uterine prolapse after administration of adrenaline (does not work if an epidural was used), repairing any defects then replacing the uterus. High-dose antibiosis, NSAIDs and oxytocin are given. If repair proves difficult, euthanasia should be considered.

Uterine prolapse
Overview
Uterine prolapse appears to be less common in the doe compared with the ewe or cow. Typically a sporadic condition, but occasionally 'storms' may be observed.

Aetiology
Suggested contributing factors include: poor uterine tone (e.g. caused by hypocalcaemia); increased post-partum straining because of pain or discomfort secondary to reproductive tract trauma; increased intra-abdominal pressure (e.g. caused by rumen tympany or recumbency); or excessive traction. Possible other factors include high oestrogen content of diet, overconditioned dam and excessive weight of fetal membranes.

Clinical presentation
Most cases present within 24 hours of parturition. One or both uterine horns are prolapsed, exposing the mucosal surface with the caruncles visible (**Fig. 3.32**). The fetal membranes are often still attached. The dam may be in any state from standing and systemically well, to recumbent and in circulatory or toxic shock. The uterus is contaminated, engorged and oedematous, and often traumatised with tears. Initially warm, the uterus increasingly becomes cold to the touch and discoloured.

Differential diagnosis
Owners may be uncertain whether they are presented with fetal membranes or a uterine prolapse.

Treatment/management/control
First aid includes restraining and separating the dam (e.g. with the use of hurdles or bales of straw).

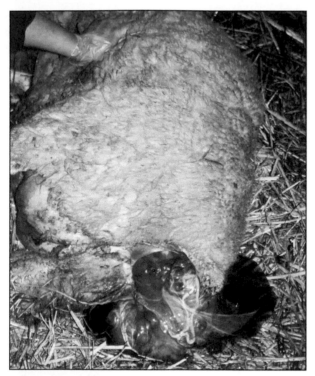

Fig. 3.32 A uterine prolapse (in a ewe). The mucosa is exposed and caruncles visible. Fetal membranes are still partially attached.

If possible, a moist wrap made from a clean sheet or towel is placed around the uterus.

The doe's general condition is assessed, and a decision made as to whether treatment is feasible. A sacrococcygeal epidural is given (see Chapter 18). The doe is placed in either lateral or sternal recumbency with her hindquarters moderately raised (e.g. over a bale of straw), taking care not to cause respiratory compromise. Alternatively, she may be placed in the 'New Zealand' position – in sternal recumbency with both hind legs pulled backwards; this results in the cranial part of the pelvis tilting downwards, thereby aiding the uterus to resume its normal position (**Fig. 3.33**).

The uterus is thoroughly but gently cleaned using a mild disinfectant solution (e.g. 0.1% iodine). Fetal membranes are removed if they come away easily. Any tears are sutured. Using the flat of one's fingers or a fist, the uterus is gradually inverted while pushing it back through the doe's pelvic canal. An assistant parting the vulval lips is of great help. Once replaced, palpatory examination ensures the uterus

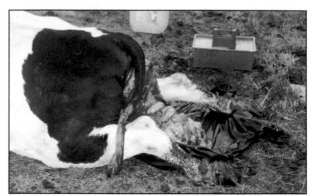

Fig. 3.33 A cow in the 'New Zealand' position for replacing a prolapses uterus. The animal is in sternal recumbency and both hind legs are pulled backwards, resulting in the pelvis tilting forward.

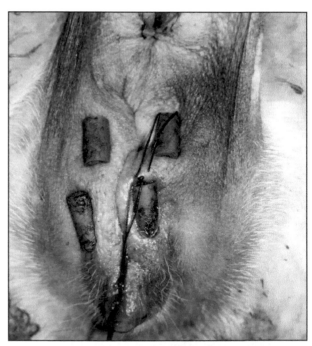

Fig. 3.34 Suturing of the vulval lips is typically not required. However, if performed, the suture is fed through buttons or lengths of tubing to reduce the risk of cutting into the soft tissues.

is fully inverted. Vulval suturing is typically not necessary, but if desired, a Bühner or horizontal mattress suture may be placed. For the latter, the suture is fed through buttons or short lengths of tubing (e.g. a giving set or flutter valve) to reduce the risk of it cutting into the tissue (**Fig. 3.34**).

Medication consists of antibiosis, NSAIDs and oxytocin. Subcutaneous calcium borogluconate (50–100 ml of 20% solution) should be considered.

Uterine prolapse tends to be a one-off event in any particular doe. The female can, therefore, be retained for future breeding, although there is a risk of infertility due to endometritis.

Amputation of the uterus may be considered as a salvage procedure if the prolapsed organ has become devitalised or too fragile to replace. This may enable survival of a pet goat or completion of the lactation in a commercial goat. The technique involves placing a ligature using thick material (e.g. a Penrose drain or Foley catheter) tightly around the uterine body just cranial to the cervix. The uterus is dissected 2–3 cm from the ligature, any bleeding vessels are ligated and the stump oversown, before inverting the reproductive tract remnant.

Retained fetal membranes
Overview
RFM is defined as stage 3 not completed and the membranes not detached and passed by 12 hours post partum (**Fig. 3.35**). Retention is relatively rare in the doe, but impaired fertility and reduced milk yield are likely sequelae in affected females. In small ruminants, there is also the risk of secondary infection with life-threatening clostridial pathogens such as tetanus or malignant oedema (*Clostridium septicum*, *Clostridium perfringens* type A).

Aetiology
The separation process starts well before parturition. Various pathological processes can disrupt this complicated event, such as immaturity of placentomes, oedema or necrosis of chorionic villi, placentitis or metritis, and uterine atony. Postulated risk factors include:

- Physiological: litters >3 kids, induction, shortened or prolonged gestation, dystocia, increasing age of dam.
- Infectious: e.g. abortive agents and also generalised disease.
- Nutritional: deficiency in retinol (vitamin A), tocopherol (vitamin E)/selenium, beta-carotene, calcium, copper, iodine; high BCS, fatty liver.
- Hormonal: lack of $PGF_{2\alpha}$, low progesterone/ high oestradiol.
- Environmental: heat, season, previous RFM, breed.

Clinical presentation
The fetal membranes often protrude from the vulva. Otherwise, a malodorous haemomucoid discharge may be obvious on the tail and perineal area (**Fig. 3.36**). In dairy goats, the malodour may be noticed in the milking parlour.

A good proportion of does are systemically affected, so as a minimum the vital signs should be established.

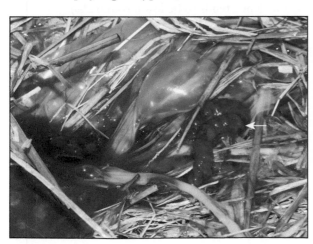

Fig. 3.35 Fetal membranes passed in the normal time frame of 3–4 hours post partum. The brown material (arrow) is meconium.

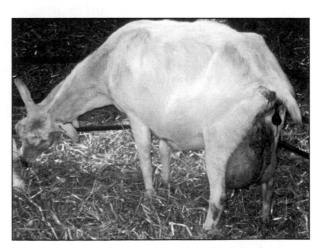

Fig. 3.36 Partial protrusion of retained fetal membranes and staining of the perineal area and caudal aspect of the udder.

Diagnosis
Vaginal examination using a speculum if membranes are not protruding.

Differential diagnosis
Retained fetus, metritis.

Treatment/management/control
Antibiosis
Antibiosis may lead to reduced phagocytosis, antibody response and T-cell function, and delay in the necrotic process necessary to cause separation. Therefore, it is best reserved for systemically affected does. Various factors limit the choice: aminoglycosides have reduced activity in the low-oxygen, acidic environment of the uterus; trimethoprim/sulphonamide combinations are inhibited by the organic debris; the commonly involved *Trueperella pyogenes* is resistant to streptomycin; anaerobes and *Streptococcus* spp. are resistant to enrofloxacin; penicillinase producing bacteria are often present in the first 5 weeks post partum. This leaves tetracycline (≥10 mg/kg), potentiated penicillin and cephalosporin as the main groups.

Systemic administration ensures even tissue concentrations throughout the reproductive tract. Inflammation may reduce drug absorption into uterine tissue, therefore high dose rates should be used. Intrauterine administration is not useful; organic debris inactivates drugs quickly, distribution is haphazard, straining may expel the drug and some drugs are irritating to the endometrium in direct contact.

Hormonal treatment
Hormonal treatment has shown equivocal results in cattle. $PGF_{2\alpha}$ appears beneficial in some females and should be used immediately post partum (i.e. in females considered at risk of RFM). Oxytocin receptors are lost within a few hours post partum in ruminants, and oxytocin may only be beneficial in the few females where hypomotility is a problem. It may be used as a slow i/v infusion or 2 IU every 20 minutes for the first 3 hours post partum; resulting uterine contraction may lead to marked discomfort. Carbetocin is an oxytocin analogue, but possibly with better distribution and longer effect;

the authors have no experience with its use in goats. Oestrogens have a direct uterotonic effect and increase the effect of prostaglandin and oxytocin, but beneficial effects in cases of RFM have not been proven so far, and their use may increase the absorption of toxins.

Other agents
Two not yet commercialised agents are collagenase (to aid breakdown of collagen binding in placentomes) and relaxin (to loosen connective tissue).

Manual removal
Manual removal is no longer advocated, with good evidence that the trauma caused by the manipulation leads to reduced fertility. It should never be used in a septicaemic animal, as toxin release is triggered by the manipulation. At the most, gentle traction for up to 1 minute, and grasping the membranes outside the vulva only, may be tried.

Metritis
Overview
Metritis is acute to peracute inflammation of the endometrium and myometrium soon after kidding. Outbreaks are occasionally encountered in herds where hygiene has deteriorated throughout the kidding period, or where tight batch kidding is practiced. Metritis is one of the main differential diagnoses for depression in a post-partum doe, but its incidence tends to be low (around 2%).

Aetiology
Post-partum uterine infection occurs in all females, but some do not resolve or bacterial growth becomes overwhelming. Commonly involved pathogens include *Trueperella pyogenes* (potentially acting synergistically with *Fusobacterium* spp. and *Bacteroides* spp.), and *Escherichia coli*, *Staphylococcus* spp. and *Streptococcus* spp., plus occasionally clostridial pathogens. Metritis and salpingitis are reported as part of the disease picture of caprine contagious agalactia (see Chapter 12).

Risk factors include abnormal parturition, unhygienic kidding environment, excessive manipulation during assisted delivery, concurrent disease or stress in the doe and high BCS.

Clinical presentation

Metritis commonly results in systemic illness with pyrexia, toxaemia, septicaemia, dehydration, reduced rumen activity, diarrhoea and inappetence. A fetid, haemopurulent uterine discharge (**Fig. 3.37**) is either outright apparent or signs are found on the tail and perineum.

Diagnosis

Vaginal examination using a speculum.

Differential diagnosis

Retained fetus or fetal membranes for this type of vaginal discharge. Other causes of systemic illness (e.g. mastitis). Not to be confused with normal lochia: reddish-brown, non-malodourous discharge for up to 3 weeks post partum (**Fig. 3.38**).

Treatment/management/control

Systemically affected does are treated aggressively with antibiosis (see RFM regarding choice of antimicrobial), NSAIDs and fluids, supported by good nursing care. I/v fluids are ideal (used judiciously to avoid pulmonary oedema), with oral fluids often effective providing some rumen activity is still present. Treatment of mild to moderate cases may be beneficial in terms of future milk yield and fertility.

Uterine irrigation is detrimental in most cases, with a risk of causing rupture of the fragile uterus, delaying involution, irritation of the endometrium by some solutions (e.g. iodine) and lowering the natural defence mechanism of the uterus. Lavage with sterile saline may be considered, as an exception, in cases with large amounts of fetid fluid to dilute toxins present. As much of the lavage fluid should be siphoned off as possible.

Prevention and control involve attention to hygienic kidding environment, sound kidding assistance (degree of manipulation, timing, implements used, hygiene), avoiding dystocia (breed, metabolic disease, body condition), preventing concurrent disease (in particular metabolic disease, which may impair neutrophil function) and adequate nutrition (body condition, deficiencies such as retinol [mucous membrane function] or ascorbic acid [modulates disease resistance]).

Where clostridial pathogens are implicated, a vaccination programme should be instigated. Prophylactic use of intrauterine antibiotics has failed to show a

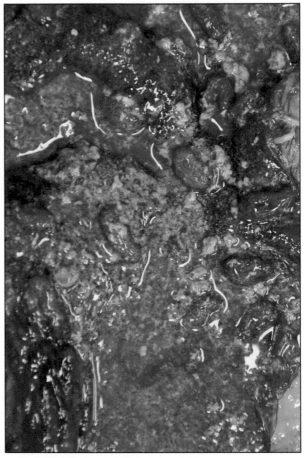

Fig. 3.37 Fetid, haemopurulent discharge typical of metritis. (Image courtesy Ann Courtenay.)

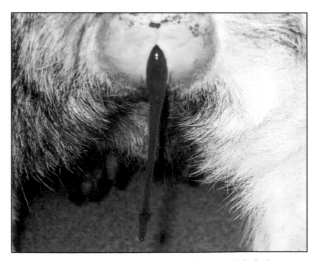

Fig. 3.38 Normal lochial secretions: reddish-brown, and without purulent material or malodour (may have a faint smell of fresh fish or chocolate).

positive effect and may be detrimental to fertility. In at-risk does, antibiotics should be used systemically.

Necrotic vaginitis

Overview
Necrotic vaginitis is an occasional complication of dystocia managed by vaginal delivery, leading to severe discomfort.

Aetiology
Pressure insult of vaginal wall, either by oversized fetus or obstetrician's manipulation.

Clinical presentation
Foul vaginal discharge, signs of discomfort including straining, moderate depression of appetite and milk yield. The vaginal mucosa is inflamed, hard and painful to the touch. Green-coloured plaques may be present on the mucosa. Typically no pyrexia, unless concurrent uterine infection.

Diagnosis
Manual examination of the vagina should be avoided, using a speculum instead.

Treatment/management/control
Emollient cream (e.g. udder cream, Dermisol®), antibiosis, NSAIDs.

Bladder eversion or herniation

Overview
Bladder eversion or herniation is an uncommon, but life-threatening, malposition of the urinary bladder.

Clinical presentation
The bladder either everts through the urethra or herniates through a vaginal tear. It is found within the vagina and may protrude from the vulva. The bladder mucosa is exposed in a case of eversion, whereas the serosa is exposed in a case of herniation.

Treatment/management/control
For eversion, the bladder is manually replaced under epidural anaesthesia by pushing it back down through the urethra. For herniation, the bladder is emptied, replaced and the vaginal tear repaired. A Foley catheter (14–16 Fg) is inserted via the urethra for 48 hours to prevent filling. Antibiosis and NSAIDs are given.

CHAPTER 4

NEONATOLOGY

INTRODUCTION

Whether born naturally, delivered manually or by caesarean section, once the cord has broken the newborn kid must rapidly become a viable unit and adapt to life *ex utero*. The fetal membranes are removed from around its mouth and if obviously viable, the kid is best placed next to the dam's head to facilitate quick bonding.

First movements should be evident within 1–2 minutes of being born, with sternal recumbency being achieved by 5–15 minutes. 'Time to sternal' is a good indicator of vigour. Most kids will be standing within 60 minutes post partum. A kid whose coat is stained with meconium likely has suffered a stressful delivery, and should receive extra care and attention.

WEAK NEWBORN KIDS

There are a number of possible reasons why vigour and normal adaptation may be suboptimal in a newborn kid:

- Injuries and trauma related to the kidding process (e.g. ribcage trauma associated with compression during delivery).
- Anoxia associated with a prolonged birth or premature placental separation.
- Swollen head and tongue associated with prolonged birth.
- Environmental conditions leading to hypo- or hyperthermia or preventing normal adapation.
- Poor *in-utero* development (e.g. caused by abortive agents or nutrition-related poor placenta formation).
- Prematurity, potentially linked to infectious causes of abortion (e.g. *Toxoplasma* spp., *Chlamydia* spp., *Coxiella* spp.).

Congenital abnormalities

Although relatively uncommon, all newborn kids should be examined for congenital abnormalities and these will vary in their influence on survivability. However, not all are apparent immediately, and some may not manifest for months or even years after birth.

Some of these conditions will be covered in more detail in this and other chapters.

Genetic abnormalities

Genetic abnormalities occasionally encountered across all breeds include:

- Cleft palate.
- Undershot/overshot jaw.
- Atresia ani or coli.
- Rectovaginal fistula.
- Penile abnormalities such as hypospadias.
- Cryptorchidism.
- Teat abnormalities such as 'fish-tail' and supernumerary teats.
- Entropion.
- Umbilical hernia.
- Skeletal malformations.
- Spastic paresis.

Developmental insult abnormalities

Abnormalities associated with developmental insult by teratogenic infections during pregnancy include:

- Arthrogryposis and other leg abnormalities (Orthobunyavirus infection such as Schmallenberg or Akabane virus)
- Neurological abnormalities including cerebellar and cerebral hypoplasia/aplasia (border disease and Orthobunyavirus infection).

Mineral shortfall abnormalities

Abnormalities associated with specific mineral shortfalls during critical stages of fetal development include:

• Congenital swayback.

Known heritable abnormalities

Abnormalities associated with known heritability include:

• Beta-mannosidosis, an inherited lysosomal disease of Nubian goats.
• Intersex associated with polledness.

RESPIRATION

Normal adaptation

Lung alveoli form pre-partum and surfactant, which enables the lungs to expand and retain air without individual alveoli collapsing, is produced in late gestation.

The physiological stimulus for the first breath comes from a mix of hypoxia, hypercapnia and respiratory acidosis. Physical stimuli include reduced ambient temperature, tactile stimulus and possibly gravity. The hypoxic stimulus is often reduced in kids delivered by caesarean section, therefore extra attention to respiratory function must be paid in these neonates. They may also suffer from the sedative effects of the anaesthetic agent used (or if delivered after barbiturate euthanasia of the dam).

The kid needs to generate substantial negative pressure to inflate its lungs (each lobe independently), and in part achieves this by gasping against a closed glottis. The ribcage is pliable in newborns, therefore active inspiration and expiration is required.

The amniotic fluid produced in the fetal lungs is physically removed by external pressure on the thorax during the passage through the birth canal, and by absorption via the lymphatics and pulmonary capillaries after lung inflation. The process is completed within a few breaths in a normal neonate.

Asphyxia

Overview

Asphyxia is severe oxygen deprivation.

Aetiology

Dystocia-induced hypoxia and acidosis may diminish the kid's ability to initiate ventilation. Partial or complete failure of the lungs to inflate (atelectasis) may be caused by ineffective gasping or an obstruction (fetal membranes, aspiration of fluid or meconium). Trauma to the ribcage (**Fig. 4.1**) may lead to pain-induced failure of the first deep breath or, if a lung is punctured or with diaphragmatic rupture, failure of sufficient negative pressure to build up.

Clinical presentation

The kid may be in any of the following stages of acute asphyxia:

1 Shallow breaths.
2 Primary apnoea of 1–2 minutes duration, but responsive to external stimuli. Perfusion and body tone are still good and heart rate is normal to elevated. Mucous membrane colour may be cyanotic.
3 Period of gasping.
4 Terminal apnoea unresponsive to stimulation. Perfusion and body tone are poor, and marked bradycardia is present. Mucous membranes appear very pale.
5 Cardiac arrest.

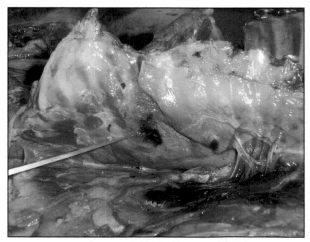

Fig. 4.1 The metal stilet points to bruising on the inside surface of the ribcage caused by a fractured rib. Trauma such as this may lead to failure of the neonate to take an effective first breath to inflate its lungs.

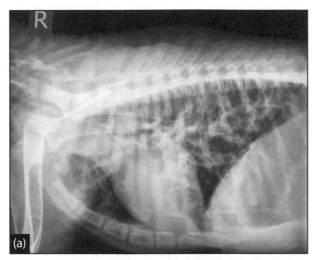

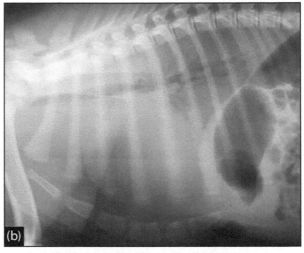

Fig. 4.2 Radiographs showing severe atelectasis in a 2-day-old neonate (a) and lack of lung aeration in a neonate with a ventricular septal defect (b) – the lungs almost appear like solid soft tissue. In both cases, the affected kids appeared normal for the first 2 days post partum.

Signs of atelectasis, in the form of respiratory distress and cyanosis, may not become clinically apparent until day 2 or 3 post partum (**Figs. 4.2**). Similarly, signs of periparturient anoxia or hypoxia may take a few days to become apparent. The kid initially appears normal, then 'crashes' at 2–4 days old.

Treatment/management/control
Clearing airways
Remove membranes and amniotic fluid from upper airways by manual removal or suction. The kid's hindquarters may be raised briefly (<10 seconds; caution: pressure on diaphragm hinders inflation). Handling must be delicate because of the pliable rib cage.

Induction of respiration
- For mild asphyxia. External stimulation by rubbing (**Fig. 4.3**), irritating the nasal mucosa with straw, pinching the tongue or nasal septum or interdigital space, or using hot or cold stimuli.
- Acupuncture. Insertion of a 25 gauge 1.5 cm (5/8 in) needle into the nasal philtrum at right angle to the skin.
- For primary apnoea (respiratory centre still responsive). Analeptics (e.g. doxapram hydrochloride) can be tried. Increases ventilation

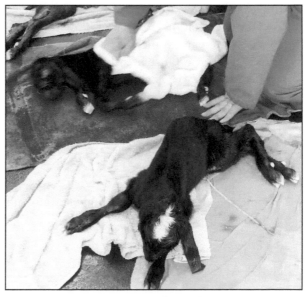

Fig. 4.3 Rubbing (kid on red towel) is one of the physical stimuli that can be tried to stimulate breathing. The lower kid has been placed into sternal recumbency to aid lung inflation.

but does not aid opening of collapsed airways or alveoli. Oxygen requirement is increased.
- Artificial respiration and inflation. Application of intermittent chest compression or movement of the ribcage (hold by humerus and last rib) may help lung expansion, but will not aid

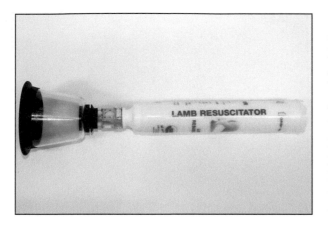

Fig. 4.4 Simple resuscitators, such as the one shown using atmospheric air, are effective in causing lung inflation. The lamb size is suitable for kids. Alternatives include the Ambu-Bag or Breath of Life. With the kid in lateral recumbency, the head and neck are extended fully, the face mask placed over the nose and mouth and the cylinder pulled out and pushed in 4–5 times about every 4 seconds. The kid is placed onto its opposite site, and the same repeated. If available, an assistant can clasp their fingers around the cervical oesophagus to prevent air entering the forestomachs.

initial inflation, and care must be taken not to cause trauma to the ribcage or internal organs. Resuscitators, utilising atmospheric oxygen, are easy to use and quite effective (**Fig. 4.4**). Placing an endotracheal tube (size 5) and exhaling into it is also effective. Positive pressure ventilation (PPV) is ideal, with a rate of 15–25 bpm and sufficient tidal volume to inflate the chest. Once breathing is established and if available, oxygen delivery via a face mask or nasal tube for 1–2 hours at 5 litres/minute is useful, in particular in kids delivered by caesarean section. (**Note:** Mouth-to-mouth respiration is ineffective and carries zoonotic risks.)

Placing the kid into sternal recumbency also aids lung inflation (**Fig. 4.3**).

CARDIAC FUNCTION AND CIRCULATION

Normal adaptation

Closure of the foramen ovale is in response to an increase in lung circulation, leading to increased pressure in the left atrium. Initially consisting of only a thin septum, full-thickness closure happens quite a while post partum. The ductus arteriosus Botalli closure is a reflex response to oxygenated blood, and is typically complete by 24 hours post partum. The umbilical vein collapses in response to absent blood flow, and the umbilical arteries contract when the cord ruptures.

Absent heartbeat

An apex beat should be visible or palpable (**Fig. 4.5**). If not present, external cardiac massage or intra-cardiac adrenaline combined with intubation and PPV, and i/v atropine (0.01–0.03 mg/kg) and adrenaline (0.1–0.2 ml/kg of 1:10,000 IU solution) may be tried, but success rates are poor.

Cardiovascular defects

Cardiovascular defects typically do not become apparent until the kid is several days old and its increased activity accentuates circulatory and oxygenation problems, unless a severe defect is present such as tetralogy of Fallot. (See Chapter 7.)

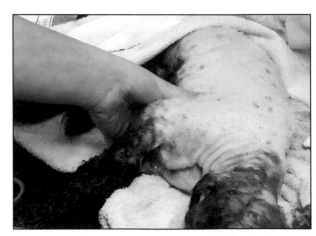

Fig. 4.5 Palpation for apex beat in a newborn, with fingers and thumb placed either side of the ribcage close to the elbow. If present, the beat is easily detected (and may be visible, as well).

THERMOREGULATION

Normal adaptation

The neonatal kid can employ shivering and non-shivering thermogenesis, the latter utilising brown fat for the first few hours of life.

Hypothermia

Overview

Hypothermia is a common condition and fatal if untreated, but almost entirely preventable. Usually in neonates less than 24 hours of age, but can occur at any age.

Aetiology

Risk of excessive heat loss is increased with exposure to an inclement environment, especially the combination of wetness and wind. Failure of the kid to become mobile or dry-off (e.g. in a weak kid) or caused by mismothering (which in turn may be due to dam illness or inexperience, reducing interest in later born kids in a large litter, or disturbance during the bonding process). Low birth weights resulting in both weakness and increased surface to body mass ratio. In general, the relatively little subcutaneous fat deposits and modest insulation characteristics of goat fibre increase the risk of hypothermia.

Clinical presentation

The kid becomes increasingly depressed and eventually comatose. Oxygen consumption increases if cold (i.e. any hypoxia may worsen).

Diagnosis

Easily established by measuring rectal temperature.

Differential diagnosis

Hypothermia secondary to septicaemic or toxaemic shock must be ruled out, and concurrent hypoglycaemia should be considered. Severe parturition trauma or some congenital defects may cause increasing lethargy.

Treatment/management/control

The sequence of treatment steps for marked hypothermia depends on the age of the kid (if brown fat is depleted, alternative energy must be provided prior to warming up to avoid increased metabolism-induced hypoglycaemia) and the degree of depression of the kid (indicating degree of gastrointestinal [GI] atony). **Fig. 4.6** gives the options for treatment, management and control of hypothermia.

Heat lamps should be avoided for warming up, as they cause peripheral vasodilation without increasing core temperature. Suitable methods include

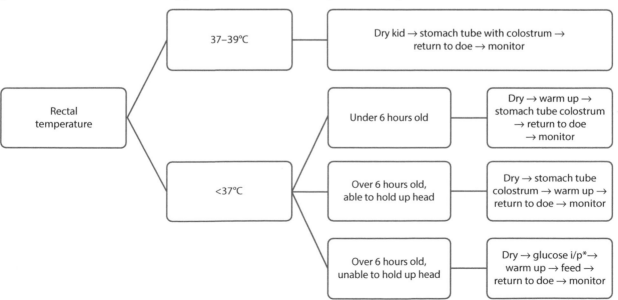

* The dose rate for i/p glucose is 10 ml/kg of 20% bodywarm solution (see Chapter 1 for injection technique).

Fig. 4.6 **Flow chart for the management of hypothermia.**

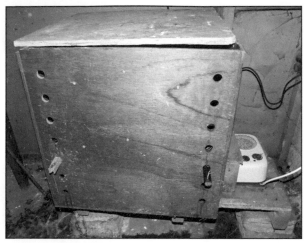

Fig. 4.7 A simple but effective 'hot-box': a household fan heater is used as a heat source and partially inserted into a hole at the bottom of the box. A grid is positioned about one-third up in the box to place the kid onto. (Note: If a metal grid is used, towels are placed underneath the kid.) In this example, the grid is placed onto removable rods to aid cleaning of the box. The box has several vent holes in the walls.

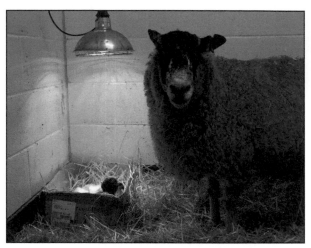

Fig. 4.8 A straw nest is easily manufactured from a cardboard box, and creates a good transitional environment on return of a resuscitated hypothermic kid to the doe. The dam has access to her offspring, and the kid can climb out of the box to nurse.

a heat box (**Fig. 4.7**), hot water bottles (or 'hot hands' – see **Fig. 18.2**, p. 335) placed in the axilla and inguinal region, heat blankets or a Bair Hugger™. The kid is monitored every 30 minutes for response and overheating. Any hyperthermia (indicated by panting and rectal temperature exceeding 41°C) is addressed by dousing with lukewarm water, drying off and returning to the doe.

A 'nest box' (e.g. made from a cardboard box and straw; **Fig. 4.8**), heat lamp and coat are useful on return to the doe. The kid is monitored every hour for a period to check for relapse and for milk intake.

Prevention involves adequate nutrition of the dam, especially during the first 6 weeks (placenta formation) and last 4 weeks of pregnancy (milk yield), providing shelter, preventing mismothering and prompt intervention in dystocia.

IMMUNE SYSTEM

Normal adaptation

Typical for ungulates, the kid is essentially born agammaglobulinaemic and relies on adequate colostrum intake for initial immunoglobulin (Ig) levels. Little specific data is available for kids, but extrapolating from lambs and calves, own-produced Ig first appears at a few days old for IgA and IgM, about 1 week old for IgG_1, and about 1 month old for IgG_2. Intestinal Ig appears from about 1 week old (first IgM, then IgA), but is short-lived unless continuously stimulated.

Non-immune effector cells (neutrophils, macrophages, basophils) are present at birth, but reach full capabilities only after birth. Noteworthy for haematology interpretation is the higher neutrophil count in neonates compared with adults. The complement system is present from the second trimester of gestation, but activity at birth may be close to 0%, reaching 50% at about 2 months of age and full capacity after several months.

Cell-mediated immunity (T cells) is present at birth. B lymphocytes are present at about one-third adult levels at birth, reaching adult concentrations at around 3 weeks of age. They are reduced by steroids, including the endogenously produced ones during parturition, which may persist for up to 2 weeks post partum.

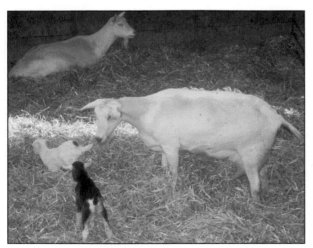

Fig. 4.9 Kids should be standing by 2 hours post partum, and bonding must not be disturbed to facilitate good colostrum intake. The black kid in the foreground demonstrates the wide-based stance that neonates commonly adopt in the first few days of life.

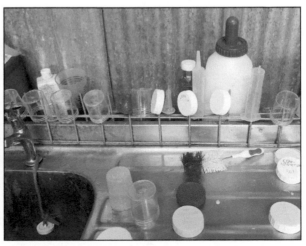

Fig. 4.10 Equipment used to store and feed colostrum must be scrupulously clean to maintain colostrum quality with limited spoilage and reduce the pathogen load in the kid.

The neonatal kid is capable of responding to soluble protein antigens at birth and viral, protozoal and bacterial antigens from about 14–30 days old. However, response is often not 100%, in particular memory capacity. These aspects need to be taken into account for vaccination regimes.

Failure of passive transfer
Overview
Failure of passive transfer is a common and largely preventable condition.

Aetiology
The causes can be grouped into three main categories:

- Intake of inadequate volume of colostrum. Weak kid, recumbent dam or mismothering (**Fig. 4.9**), large litter. Target intake is 10% of birth weight in the first 6 hours post partum, plus another 10% in the following 12 hours.
- Inadequate colostrum quality. Malnutrition and illness in dam including mastitis, delay in harvest post partum, poor storage conditions, dirty feeding equipment (if artificial feeding is used; **Fig. 4.10**).
- Reduced absorption of colostral Ig. Common where the neonate is acidotic or where intake is delayed (absorption ceases at around 24 hours of age). (**Note:** First contact with colostrum appears to trigger gut closure, so once some colostrum has been given, the full dose must follow promptly.)

Clinical presentation
Kids are at higher risk of neonatal disease, in particular septicaemia, umbilical infection (and sequelae such as joint ill) and clostridial diseases.

Diagnosis
If suspected, or for routine monitoring in a herd, blood is taken from kids at least 24 hours old (to allow time for absorption) but less than 1 week of age (when production of own Ig begins).

Total protein (TP) is easy to establish in practice using a capillary tube and refractometer, but hydration status must be taken into account: 55 g/l indicates adequate transfer. Acute phase proteins may artificially increase TP concentrations, which can be addressed by using globulin levels instead (>20 g/l shows good transfer).

The zinc sulphate turbidity test may be used with either qualitative (adequate transfer if it is impossible to read newspaper print through test tube), or quantitative (level >20 OD units is adequate) interpretation.

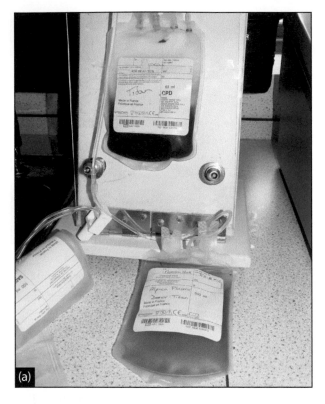

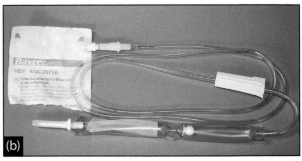

Fig. 4.11 **Plasma transfusion is the best option to address failure of passive transfer. After centrifugation, the plasma is separated with the aid of a homemade 'vice-board'. A human medicine collection set containing the anti-coagulant CPD has been used here (a). A blood transfusion i/v set must be used to filter out any impurities (b).**

Radioimmune diffusion is very accurate, but kits tend to be expensive and processing takes 6–24 hours.

Gamma-glutamyl transferase. Normal levels in the colostrum-deprived newborn are low. A level >44 IU indicates good transfer.

Treatment/management/control

Plasma transfusion is the best option, and despite there being several blood groups in the goat, cross-reactions are rare during transfusions. Harvest requires a blood centrifuge (**Fig. 4.11a**). Plasma will keep at –20°C for up to 12 months, providing temperature fluctuations are kept to a minimum (e.g. by using a dedicated freezer). 30–40 ml/kg of plasma are given i/v through a blood transfusion kit at a rate of 20–40 ml/hour (**Fig. 4.11b**). The kid is monitored for signs of hypersensitivity, which include facial swelling, erythema, dyspnoea and bronchoconstriction. Treatment for acute hypersensitivity type I reaction includes: dexamethasone at 0.1–4.0 mg/kg i/v, adrenaline 1:1,000 at 0.01 mg/kg i/v, or diphenhydramine at 2–4 mg/kg i/m or s/c. Other potential complications include volume overload, hypothermia (if plasma not warmed),

bacterial contamination, air embolism and citrate poisoning.

Other options, used with varying success and lacking supporting studies, include continued colostrum administration (to provide local IgA in the intestinal tract), prophylactic antibiosis (risk of influencing GI tract microflora and potentially supporting fungal infections) or stimulating the non-specific immune-response (for example administering a killed vaccine or foreign protein, or immune-modulators such as levamisole, ascorbic acid (vitamin C), tocopherol (vitamin E) or selenium).

Each herd should have a colostrum bank (**Fig. 4.12**), ideally harvested within 6 hours of birth. Using own does (e.g. those with singletons) avoids any biosecurity risks and ensures antibodies against farm-specific pathogens are present. Sourcing bovine or ovine colostrum from high health status herds is an alternative. Fresh colostrum will keep for several days at ambient temperature. Alternatively, colostrum may be kept frozen at –20°C for up to 1 year. Thawing has to be done gently to avoid denaturing of proteins (i.e. in warm

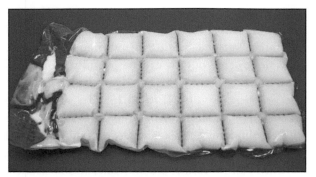

Fig. 4.12 Ice-cube bags are useful to portion colostrum for freezing. They must be thawed gently to avoid denaturing of proteins.

water of 60°C maximum with regular agitation or in a microwave on the lowest setting with periodic removal of any thawed liquid).

Routine procedures such as castration should be delayed until the kid is at least 24 hours old to ensure good colostrum uptake.

Neonatal septicaemia (syn. sepsis)
Overview
Neonatal septicaemia generally means an overwhelming infection in the first week of life. It is often accompanied by a (entero-)toxaemia and bacteraemia. One of the most common causes of mortality in neonates.

Aetiology
Commonly involved pathogens include *Escherichia coli* and other Enterobacteriacaea, *Streptococcus* spp. (in particular Lancefield group B and C) and *Clostridium perfringens*. *In-utero* infection, leading to the birth of an already septicaemic neonate, is occasionally seen with pathogens such as *Salmonella* spp. Otherwise, pathogens most commonly enter via the umbilical or oral route, with subsequent haematogenous spread (**Fig. 4.13**).

Clinical presentation
Initial signs are often vague, with owners reporting the kid being less lively, nursing less and possibly spending more time recumbent. This progresses to signs of septic shock: congested mucous membranes, dehydration, cold extremities, increased capillary refill time, tachycardia, loss of suck reflex and increasing unresponsiveness. Rectal temperature may be elevated, normal or subnormal.

Death results rapidly in peracute cases. In less severe cases, additional signs linked to bacteraemic infiltration may be seen, such as meningitis, endocarditis, kidney and liver abscessation or septic arthritis.

Diagnosis
The sepsis score used in foals can give an indication of septicaemia, but has not been validated in kids.

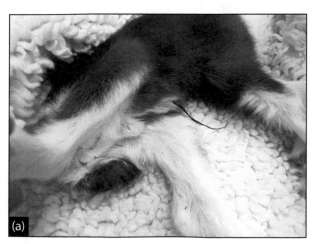
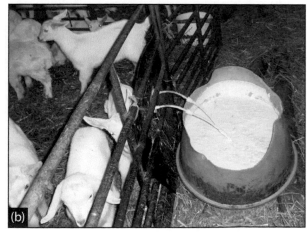

Fig. 4.13 (a) The dried navel in this septicaemic kid suggests that infection did not occur via the common umbilical route. (b) Substandard hygiene levels of feeding equipment contribute to a high pathogen load that may potentially lead to neonatal septicaemia via the oral route.

Blood culture is immensely useful, both for diagnosis and to establish whether a gram-negative or gram-positive pathogen is involved. However, sensitivity of blood culture is not 100%, and clinical impression remains important.

A marked neutrophilia or neutropenia is indicative.

For treatment and prognosis, liver and kidney function biochemistry is useful, as are blood acid–base balance and lactate levels.

Arthrocentesis or limb radiography, ultrasonography of the heart, kidney, and liver, and a cerebrospinal fluid tap are used to detect involvement of organ systems.

Passive transfer is established using one of the tests discussed previously.

Differential diagnosis

Includes hypothermia, hypoglycaemia, uroperitoneum, severe congenital defect and immaturity.

Treatment/management/control

Placing an i/v catheter is invaluable (the jugular, cephalic or saphenous vein are suitable). In an on-farm situation, a large cardboard box, straw bales or hurdles are used to restrain the kid, while allowing the doe to stay in contact if desired (**Fig. 4.14**).

Hypovolaemia is addressed with a sterile crystalloid solution (e.g. Hartmann's or lactated Ringer's).

A fluid rate of up to 40 ml/kg/hour may be necessary initially, but the kid must be monitored for fluid overload leading to pulmonary oedema. Sufficient urine output can be usefully monitored with the aid of a baby nappy (diaper) strapped over the prepuce or vulva (**Fig. 4.15**). To address the likely hypoglycaemia, either glucose is added to the chosen fluid or 2.5–5% dextrose is administered simultaneously.

Until culture results are available, antibiosis must be broad spectrum (including anaerobes). Useful antimicrobials include trimethoprim/sulphonamide (data sheet dose, given i/v q8h) and third-generation cephalosporins (e.g. ceftiofur sodium or hydrochloride at 2 mg/kg q12h). Where aminoglycosides (e.g. amikacin, kanamycin, neomycin, gentamicin) are available for food producing animals, these may be combined with high-dose benzylpenicillin sodium (25,000–30,000 IU/kg q6–8h), bearing in mind the increased risk of nephrotoxicity in a hypovolaemic animal.

Flunixin meglumine (or other NSAID) is useful against toxaemia, providing kidney perfusion is good. After a loading dose of 2 mg/kg, 0.7 mg/kg q6–8h may be sufficient. Failure of passive transfer, if present, is addressed as discussed earlier.

Once a weak suck reflex has returned, the kid is fed milk in frequent small doses. A prognosis of about 50% can be expected with intensive care.

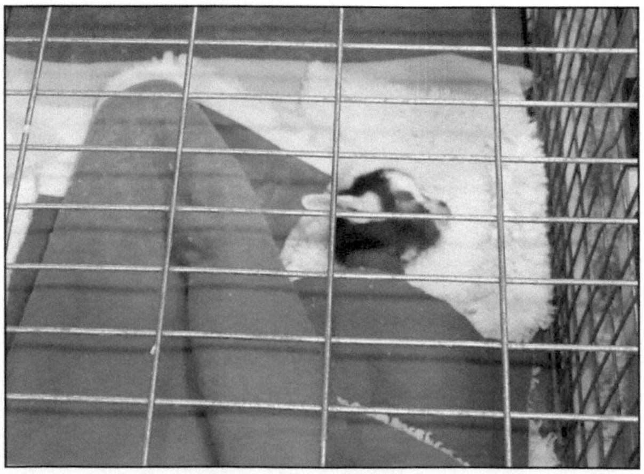

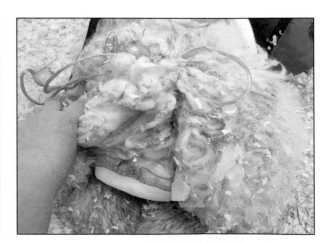

Fig. 4.14 This septicaemic kid requiring i/v fluid therapy was temporarily placed into a dog crate that was available on farm. Equally, a pen can be created from hurdles, straw bales or a large cardboard box.

Fig. 4.15 A baby nappy (here used in a female alpaca cria) is a useful tool to monitor urine output during fluid therapy.

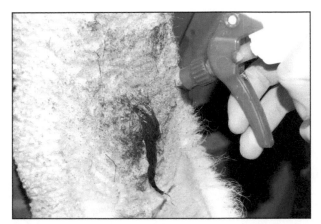

Fig. 4.16 For navel disinfection, spray application keeps the reservoir solution cleaner compared with a dip-cup, but care must be taken to cover the navel all the way round. Strong iodine has the advantage over oxytetracycline solution that it dries out the navel quicker.

Prevention is based on adequate passive transfer, high kidding environment hygiene and good navel care (spray or dip with 7% tincture of iodine or tetracycline spray within 30 minutes of birth, repeated once or twice over the next 12 hours; **Fig. 4.16**).

GASTROINTESTINAL TRACT

Normal adaptation

Hormones, neuropeptides and enzymes have a trophic effect on gut development, causing a major growth spurt. Oral uptake of bacteria during the birthing process and from the kidding environment starts the colonisation of the GI tract, with the intestinal flora comparable to adults after several weeks.

The liver changes from its fetal function as a blood-forming organ to its metabolic function.

Hypoglycaemia
Overview
Kids up to 24 hours old are at highest risk, but older ones may be affected, particularly if the doe develops mastitis or they are exposed to inclement weather.

Aetiology
Starvation may be caused by milk supply problems (e.g. mastitis, teat disorders, mismothering), weak kids unwilling to suckle (e.g. congenital defects,

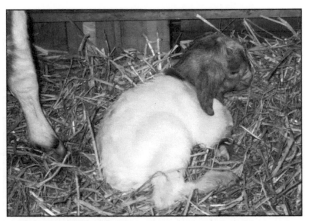

Fig. 4.17 The main differential diagnoses for a neonate that is increasingly dull and unresponsive are hypothermia, hypoglycaemia, septicaemia and marked congenital defect.

swayback, abortive agents), problems interfering with the kid's locomotion (e.g. contracted tendons, fractures) and exposure to inclement environment increasing energy demands.

Clinical presentation
Initially normal at birth, the kid becomes increasingly weak, incoordinated and unresponsive over 12–24 hours (**Fig. 4.17**). Suckle reflex is absent, and dehydration may be evident. Hypothermia is commonly present. Eventually the kid becomes recumbent and comatose, with death within 24–36 hours.

Diagnosis
A tentative diagnosis can be made in the field, supported by blood glucose levels (for example using a hand-held glucosemeter).

Differential diagnosis
Hypothermia, neonatal septicaemia, life-threatening congenital abnormality.

Treatment/management/control
If the kid is able to hold its head up or has a suck reflex, 150–200 ml of colostrum or milk are given by stomach tube. Otherwise, glucose is administered i/v, i/p (see Hypothermia for dose rate; see Chapter 1 for technique) or as a rectal suppository. Steps to prevent or address hypothermia are taken.

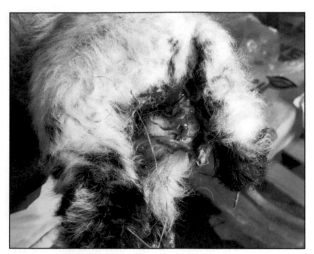

Fig. 4.18 Meconium retention (shown here in a lamb) is easily addressed with an enema.

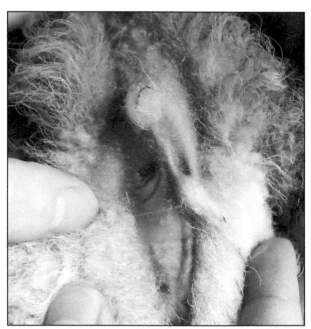

Fig. 4.19 Atresia ani in a newborn male lamb. Because the condition was detected early, no 'bulging' is apparent yet.

The cause is addressed and the kid continued to be supplemented if necessary.

Triplets and quads remaining on the doe should always be monitored for sufficient milk intake and, if lacking, supplemented or fostered on.

Meconium retention
Overview
The meconium should be passed within 24 hours of birth, aided by the laxative effects of colostrum (**Fig. 4.18**).

Treatment/management/control
An enema is gently applied, using either a commercial product (such as Micralax®) or 20 ml of warm soapy water (with a catheter-tipped syringe).

Atresia ani, recti or coli
Overview
A congenital defect where a section of the lower intestinal tract is missing (**Fig. 4.19**). Appears to be rare (around 3 of 1,000 kids born).

Aetiology
Remains unclear, but may have a genetic component.

Clinical presentation
The kid is normal immediately after birth, but develops increasing lethargy and abdominal distension over the first week of life. Mild colic may be present. A high proportion of affected kids also have defects in other body systems, which may cause clinical signs and necessitate a thorough examination to determine prognosis and viability of treatment attempts.

Diagnosis
Absence of an anal opening is obvious on examination, often with outward bulging of the skin in that area from pent up faeces. Ultrasonography or (contrast) radiography are required to diagnose atresia at a more proximal point.

Differential diagnosis
For abdominal swelling: uroperitoneum, abomasitis, peritonitis.

Treatment/management/control
Atresia ani can often be addressed by making an incision over the most prominent point of the bulging in the perineal area, either under topical anaesthetic gel, infiltration anaesthesia or sacrococcygeal epidural. Wound ointment is applied and the tip of

a finger gently inserted, 2–3 times daily for several days.

Surgical treatment of atresia recti may be attempted under sacrococcygeal epidural, but it is often difficult to find the blind end. If it can be located, the rectal serosa is freed from surrounding soft tissue, pulled towards the anus and secured to the rectal sphincter with a series of interrupted sutures.

Prognosis for atresia coli is poor. In pet animals, marsupilisation of the intestine to the abdominal wall can be attempted. However, aftercare is difficult, in particular maintaining skin health and hygiene and fly control.

Cleft palate (syn. palatoschisis)
Overview
Cleft palate is a rare, but typically life-ending, congenital defect in the oral palate. Both the soft and hard palate may be involved.

Aetiology
A genetic component has been considered. It has also been reported as part of congenital skeletal malformations induced by ingestion by the pregnant dam of plants containing piperidine alkaloid toxin (e.g. lupine, poison hemlock, tree tobacco).

Clinical presentation
Milk (and later solid feed) will be visible at the nostrils. The kid may cough or snort while nursing. Suckling is not very efficient, leading to poor growth rate and a potentially distended udder in the doe. Aspiration pneumonia is a commons sequela, with dyspnoea, pyrexia and septicaemia.

Diagnosis
Examination of the roof of the oral cavity will show the defect.

Treatment/management/control
Surgical repair of a small defect in the soft palate may be attempted. Treatment of larger defects, or those involving the hard palate, is unrewarding. If attempted, access is gained by cutting the mandibular symphysis.

URINARY FUNCTION

Normal adaptation
The kidneys are fully formed and functional in the second half of gestation. Post partum, the urachus closes. In response to increased arterial pressure, the glomerular filtration rate increases which, combined with high levels of renin and aldosterone, results in production of a large volume of hypotonic urine in the neonate.

Urine retention
Overview
First urine should be passed within 18 hours of birth.

Aetiology
Possible causes include agenesis or atresia of any part of the urinary tract, vulval fusion (**Fig. 4.20**), uroperitoneum secondary to a ruptured bladder, or severe dehydration. Urination in female kids with a

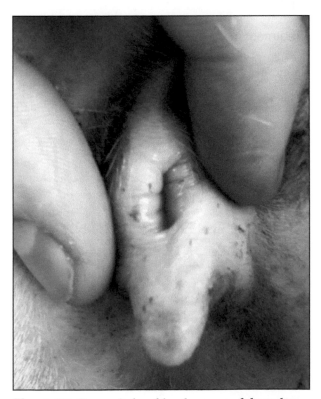

Fig. 4.20 Congenital maldevelopment of the vulva may take the form of complete fusion of the vulval lips, leading to urinary retention (image shows hypoplasia).

patent urachus or male kids with hypospadias may be unobserved.

Clinical presentation

The kid probably appears normal in the first few days of life. As azotaemia worsens, lethargy increases. Bulging becomes obvious in females with vulval fusion.

Diagnosis

Intravenous urograms are the most straightforward method to detect agenesis or atresia of the urinary tract. Ultrasonography will highlight free fluid in the abdominal cavity and aid aspiration to confirm the presence of a uroperitoneum. Haematology and biochemistry are used to establish levels of dehydration and azotaemia.

Differential diagnosis

Other causes of lethargy in the neonate (see Neonatal septicaemia).

Treatment/management/control

Vulval fusion is usually easy to treat: topical anaesthetic gel is applied to the vulval lips and a vertical incision made at the fusion point of the two lips. Wound ointment is applied, and the lips manually parted, 2–3 times daily for several days.

Treatment of a ruptured bladder is covered in Chapter 10 (Urolithiasis).

Unilateral nephrectomy may be considered in cases of unilateral agenesis of the ureter.

MUSCULOSKELETAL FUNCTION

Normal adaptation

The fetus displays leg movements from midgestation, and the bones are generally well ossified at birth. The newborn may display a moderate degree of tendon and ligament laxity, a wide-based stance (**Fig. 4.9**) and an exaggerated gait for a few days.

Contracted tendons
Overview

A congenital defect, typically bilateral and almost exclusively involving the fore legs.

Aetiology

Remains unclear. Postulated are a hereditary component, position *in utero* and manganese deficiency of the pregnant dam.

Clinical presentation

The flexor tendons of the fetlock, plus sometimes the carpus, are contracted, and a plantigrade stance cannot be achieved. In addition, the leg cannot be straightened fully by manipulation.

Diagnosis

The defect is readily detected on clinical examination. However, concurrent congenital defects are common and a thorough and full examination must be conducted.

The kid should also be checked for failure of passive transfer, which is common because of its impaired mobility.

Differential diagnosis

Arthrogryposis may present similarly, but more commonly involves joints in the upper limb or hind leg, as well. Radiography is required to demonstrate joint malformation. Limb joint fixation can also be a feature of Schmallenberg virus infection.

Treatment/management/control

Conservative treatment is sufficient where the leg can be manually extended to achieve a tiptoe stance (**Fig. 4.21a**). After liberal padding, either a splint is secured onto the palmar aspect or the limb is placed in a cast (**Fig. 4.21b**), in both cases from the toe to the proximal metacarpus. The splint or cast is removed after 10–14 days to check for skin integrity and degree of correction. If further support is necessary, the cast can be re-used as a half-cast.

Tendonectomy is indicated if the contracture is too severe to achieve a tiptoe stance. It can be performed under general anaesthesia, sedation and intravenous regional anaesthesia, or local infiltration of both skin and tendon sheaths. A 3 cm skin incision is made on the palmar aspect of the mid-metacarpus. The superficial flexor tendon is cut across followed, if necessary, by cutting the deep flexor tendon and suspensory ligament (**Fig. 4.22a**). The skin is sutured

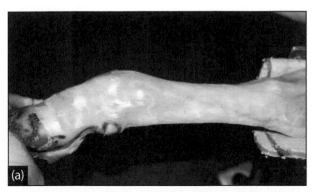
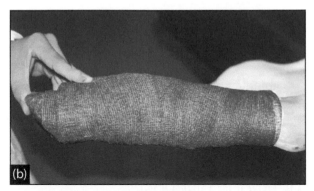

Fig. 4.21 In this calf with contracted tendons, the leg could be manually extended to achieve a tip-toe stance (a); therefore, application of a splint was a suitable treatment option (b).

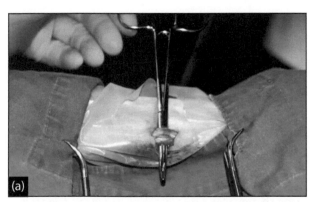
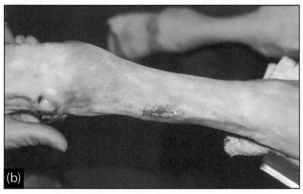

Fig. 4.22 A tendonectomy to address contracted tendons. Both superficial and deep flexor tendons and the suspensory ligament may have to be cut in severe cases (a). The small incision on the palmar aspect of the mid-metacarpus was closed with skin staples in this bovine case (b).

or stapled (**Fig. 4.22b**), and the leg placed into a cast or splinted for 2–4 weeks.

The kid will require aid in standing up and nursing for the first few days. Administration of high-dose oxytetracycline as a treatment is controversial: no effect has been proven in ruminants, and the high dose may induce toxic nephrosis.

Flexor tendon laxity
Overview
Flexor tendon laxity is commonly linked to prematurity, and carries a good prognosis.

Treatment/management/control
Exercise on a hard surface several times a day is helpful. It is also possible to extend the heel with a glued-on wooden block, for example.

Arthrogryposis
Overview
Congenital joint contracture, typically involving multiple joints and often leading to dystocia.

Aetiology
Orthobunyavirus infections, such as Schmallenberg and Akabane virus, may cause this, as may toxins including plant toxins.

Clinical presentation
The kid shows abnormal angulation of the legs and is unable to stand. Also, a normal straight posture cannot be achieved with manipulation.

Diagnosis
Radiography shows abnormal joint formation.

CHAPTER 4

Differential diagnosis
Contracted tendons, fractures, beta mannosidosis (see below).

Treatment/management/control
There are no viable options.

White muscle disease
See Chapter 14.

METABOLIC DISORDERS

Because of their clinical presentation, metabolic disorders are important differential diagnoses for apparent neurological disorders.

Neonatal acidosis
Overview
Acidosis in the neonate is usually a combination of respiratory and metabolic acidosis.

Aetiology
Prolonged parturition or post-partum apnoea are common causes.

Clinical presentation
Often no specific sign, but the newborn may show reduced vigour. Meconium staining of the newborn indicates that the kid experienced *in-utero* stress and is at higher risk of acidosis.

Diagnosis
Definitive diagnosis is based on blood gas analysis.

Treatment/management/control
Intravenous administration of sodium bicarbonate will address the metabolic component. The dose rate is either based on a deficit calculation (body weight × 0.5 × base excess) if blood gas analysis is available, or an empiric dose of 20 mmol i/v is given, in each case slowly over 10 minutes. Adequate lung ventilation must be ensured to enable removal of the carbon dioxide produced by the conversion of bicarbonate.

Colostral Ig uptake is reduced in acidotic neonates, therefore a larger volume is required and the kid should be tested for failure of passive transfer once over 24 hours old.

Prevention relies on reducing the risk of dystocia and prompt intervention when it does occur.

Floppy-kid syndrome
Overview
Floppy-kid syndrome is a metabolic acidosis, without diarrhoea or dehydration, affecting kids typically between 7 and 14 days of life (range 3 days to 4 weeks). Herd morbidity of between 30 and 50% is most commonly reported, although in outbreaks described in North America morbidity approached 100%. Mortality in unrecognised and untreated outbreaks can be high.

Aetiology/pathophysiology
Remains unknown. In some outbreaks, the biggest and healthiest kids are affected, and sometimes only one out of a litter. Both kids nursing their dams and those being artificially reared (on fresh or pasteurised milk) are at risk, with a possible link to recent increase in milk intake. The condition has been recognised in dairy, meat and fibre kids and also in kids reared indoors and outdoors.

The current hypothesis is that bacterial overgrowth may play a role (e.g. *Escherichia coli*, *Clostridium botulinum*). However, kids born to does vaccinated against clostridial pathogens (e.g. *C. perfringens*) appear at equal risk.

Some herds report the problem to be contained to the middle period of the kidding season, with early or late season kids unaffected. Herds affected in one or several consecutive years may then not see the problem for a number of years despite unchanged management.

Clinical presentation
Kids are invariably born healthy, consume sufficient colostrum and suckle well either on natural milk or milk replacer. Early signs include profound muscle weakness and incoordination, giving the impression of ataxia, with affected kids appearing intoxicated. Muscle control is lost across various body systems; for example, tongue paralysis leading to difficulty feeding, dyspnoea and GI tract stasis.

Rectal temperature is normal to slightly elevated. Diarrhoea is absent, but abdominal distension is sometimes seen.

Diagnosis

Diagnosis is often based on elimination of other possible causes. Blood gas analysis will confirm metabolic acidosis, typically with an increased anion gap. Hypokalaemia may be present. Hydration status is normal, as is kidney function. There are no characteristic post-mortem examination findings.

Differential diagnosis

Main differentials include neonatal septicaemia, enterotoxaemia, peracute enteritis, abomasitis or abomasal bloat, meningitis, cervical spinal cord lesion, disbudding injury and swayback.

Treatment/management/control

First aid consists of repeated oral administration of half a teaspoon of baking soda in some water, or frequent oral doses of commercial oral rehydration solution. Bismuth subsalicylate may also be beneficial. Good response is seen to i/v $NaCHO_3$ over 1–3 hours, with the dose calculated based on deficit using base excess (body weight × 0.5 × base excess), or an empiric dose of 50 mmol. Potentiated penicillin may be considered, given the possible bacterial involvement. Until full suckling function has returned, force feeding may be necessary. (**Note:** For i/v use, chemical grade sodium bicarbonate or a commercial $NaCHO_3$ solution must be used, not baking soda, which contains anti-caking agents.)

Once recovered, relapses are rare and kids develop normally. Recovery rates are about 80% with prompt treatment and nursing care.

Control is problematic as the cause is incompletely understood. In outbreaks, *ad-libitum* access to milk or milk replacer should be stopped, and strict feeding hygiene maintained at all times to prevent pathogen build-up in or on milk utensils.

Beta-mannosidosis

Overview

Beta-mannosidosis is an inherited lysosomal disease of Anglo-Nubian goats, leading to oligosaccharide accumulation in brain and kidney because of a deficiency in beta-mannosidase.

Clinical presentation

Signs are evident from birth and include inability to rise, intention tremors, nystagmus-like eye movements, deafness, Horner's syndrome, a mix of joint contractures and hyperextension, and often a dome-shaped skull. Kids are typically unable to suckle.

Differential diagnosis

Swayback, other severe congenital disorders, dystocia-induced trauma and hypoxia.

Treatment/management/control

No treatment is available. Euthanasia is indicated. The site of mutation for beta-mannosidosis has been identified.

Iodine deficiency (congenital hyperplastic goitre)

Affected kids are typically stillborn or born weak and premature. Blindness has occasionally been reported, as has coat thinning (see Chapter 15).

NEUROLOGICAL FUNCTION

Normal adaptation

In principle, all functions necessary for survival are well developed at birth. Spinal reflexes develop early *in utero*; in particular the withdrawal and righting (into sternal) reflexes are well developed at birth. Skin sensation is well developed, including response to warmth or coldness. Responses to auditory and tactile stimuli are possibly exaggerated. All reflexes connected with suckling are present within minutes of birth.

Of note for the neurological examination in neonates are the following: the pupillary light reflex is present at birth, but the menace reflex is a learned response and develops over the first week of life. Mentation and senses adjust within 24 hours post partum, and behaviour within 2–7 days. For gait and posture abnormalities it should be remembered that jerky movements and mild hypermetria are normal in the first few days, as is a mild wide-based stance (**Fig. 4.9**). The normal dominant extensor strength may lead to hyperreflexia. Tendon hyperextension or contraction is a common problem without a neurological basis. In a 'neurological' neonate, basic disorders such as hypothermia, hypoglycaemia and septicaemia must always be ruled out.

Congenital central nervous system abnormalities
Overview
Hypoplasia or aplasia of the cerebrum or cerebellum may be observed with certain infectious diseases (e.g. border disease virus and Orthobunyavirus [see Chapter 2]). The age at onset of clinical signs can vary from a few days to several weeks old.

Congenital swayback
Overview
Congenital swayback is one of the more common abnormalities associated with specific mineral short-falls during critical stages of fetal development.

Aetiology
Copper deficiency in the pregnant dam results in spinal cord demyelination in the fetus from the fourth month of gestation onwards. This results in a progressive ascending paralysis. Recognised forms are congenital and (acute) delayed swayback.

Clinical presentation
Ataxia when driven, muscle incoordination and inability to stand. Prognosis is poor in neonatal animals.

Diagnosis
In the dam, liver copper levels are the only reliable indication of copper status, although serum or plasma levels may be reduced in deficient animals.

Treatment/management/control
Copper supplementation of affected kids is unrewarding.

Prevention consists of adequate copper supplementation of the dam. High soil molybdenum ('teart' pastures) or high soil or water sulphur levels will interfere with copper uptake. Definitive diagnosis of copper deficiency needs to be obtained, however, to avoid copper toxicity. (See also Chapter 15.)

MISCELLANEOUS

Neonatal maladjustment syndrome (syn. 'dummy kid')
Overview
Maladjustment syndrome is a potentially fatal condition, but with good response to nursing care.

Aetiology
Potentially linked to milder forms of intrauterine growth retardation. Kids are full term and parturition is usually without complications.

Clinical presentation
The kid appears strong and achieves standing and walking within the normal time frame post partum. However, it demonstrates altered behaviour and appears to lack first instincts such as successfully seeking and finding the udder. The kid may drift towards any dark corner and even when aided to latch on, fails to initiate suckling. Righting reflexes may be compromised. Some kids may suffer myoclonic seizures.

If not detected and treated, secondary problems ensue such as hypothermia and hypoglycaemia.

Diagnosis
No specific cause is apparent, and no concurrent conditions are evident on clinical and laboratory examination.

Differential diagnosis
Hypoxia, acidosis, hypoglycaemia, congenital defects, neonatal septicaemia and meningitis. Blood and CSF analysis to rule out.

Treatment/management/control
Nursing care is the mainstay, in particular colostrum administration followed by regular milk feeding. Respiratory function may be compromised and, if available, can be addressed by nasal oxygen. Thermoregulation may also be poor, and use of coats and increased ambient temperature is useful. The kid should be in a low-stimulant environment. Anticonvulsive therapy may be necessary in some kids. It may take several days for the kid to adopt normal behaviour.

Prematurity

Overview

Prematurity is fairly commonly encountered, with reasonable prognosis with good nursing care.

Aetiology

Multiple causes may lead to premature live births, including infectious causes of abortion (e.g. *Toxoplasma* spp., *Chlamydia* spp., *Coxiella* spp.), plant toxins, mineral deficiency (e.g. iodine), iatrogenic (PGF$_{2\alpha}$, corticosteroids), placental insufficiency and illness in the dam.

Clinical presentation

Several signs may indicate prematurity, but none are specific: incisors not erupted (**Fig. 4.23**), silky thin coat, floppy ears and tendon laxity. Abortions may be evident in the herd.

The kid may struggle to stand and maintain normal body temperature and demonstrate dyspnoea. It may appear normal for the first few hours post partum before markedly deteriorating.

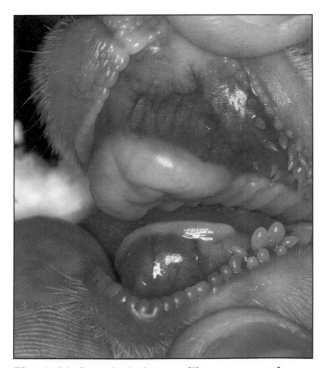

Fig. 4.23 Some body features like non-erupted incisors may indicate prematurity in the neonate, but they are not pathognomonic.

Diagnosis

In herds with good breeding dates, diagnosis is often straightforward based on calculation of pregnancy length. Otherwise, a tentative diagnosis can be made only based on clinical signs.

Treatment/management/control

Kids more than 4–5 days premature are generally not viable and euthanasia should be considered.

The two main aspects to address are lung function and thermoregulation. Surfactant is often not fully developed: a resuscitator will aid inflation and bronchodilators may help (e.g. aminophylline). Thermoregulation is supported by a warm, draught-free environment, use of a coat and ensuring energy intake.

The kid will require help to stand and suckle, and force-feeding colostrum is often indicated, because lactogenesis may not have commenced yet in the dam or because of the kid's inability to stand and suckle. With regard to passive transfer, the premature gut is fully capable of absorbing immunoglobulins.

Joint laxity will gradually disappear with exercise. In the meantime, the kid is aided in standing and walking (e.g. with a belly sling).

Low birth weights

Overview

A major cause of loss within the first 48–72 hours post partum. In the Angora breed, survival is less than 20% for birth weights <1.5 kg, reaching 60% for birth weights of 2 kg. Peak survival is for birth weights of 4 kg, after which the higher risk of dystocia reduces survival rates again (**Fig. 4.24**).

Aetiology

There are two main causes: (1) the doe's nutrition status during placenta formation (roughly first 6 weeks of pregnancy); it must stay level or be slightly increasing; a decreasing level leads to a reduction in both size and number of placentomes formed; and (2) abortive agents.

Treatment/management/control

Nursing care, in particular thermoregulation and colostrum/milk intake, may increase survival chances.

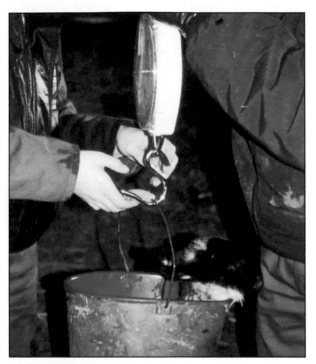

Fig. 4.24 Birth weights are easily established using a spring-loaded or hook scale and suitable container or sling to hold the neonate. Routine monitoring is very useful. As a minimum, they should be checked if a herd experiences high neonatal mortality.

Control of abortive agents is via vaccination and biosecurity. Nutritional cause is addressed by use of a suitable ration in early pregnancy. The risk of large litters versus the benefits of oestrus synchronisation must be weighed up.

Sticky kid disease

Overview
Sticky kid disease is a hereditary condition of mainly Golden Guernsey goats. Male kids seem to be more susceptible than females, and it may affect just one of a litter.

Clinical presentation
Affected kids do not dry off after birth and become susceptible to other diseases (enteritis, pneumonia). Excess sebum secretion is evident in skin biopsies.

Treatment/management/control
Treatment with medicated shampoos is not effective. Kids can be successfully reared with lots of nursing,

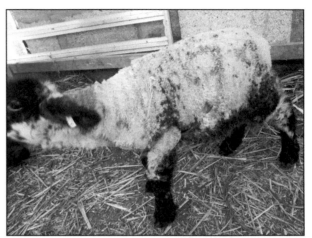

Fig. 4.25 Just as in lambs, the skin of a dead neonate may be placed onto another kid to facilitate fostering. However, this technique is not without disease risk.

but often succumb to secondary disease and, therefore, are probably best culled.

ARTIFICIAL REARING

Fostering
In herds where kids stay on does until weaning, fostering of an orphaned or underfed kid may be tried. Practices that may increase the chance of acceptance of the foster kid include placing the skin of the doe's own dead kid on the foster one (**Fig. 4.25**) or smearing the kid with strong smelling or tasty fluids (e.g. amniotic fluid, aniseed, molasses). The doe is manually restrained every 2–3 hours initially to allow the kid to suckle, with monitoring in between for bullying. Foster crates are an option, but can compromise the doe's welfare.

Supplementing
Where a doe provides some, but not sufficient, milk for her kids, finding the right level of supplementation can be difficult. If the kid is oversupplemented, it may stop seeking the doe's udder and, in turn, stimulation of milk production ceases.

A reasonably successful approach is to estimate the kid's 24-hour requirement, based on 15% of its body weight. Then initially feed one-third of this requirement divided over multiple feeds, while monitoring for sufficient weight gain. If weight gain is suboptimal, increase the supplemented amount to one-half of total requirement for a few days, monitor weight gain and adjust as necessary.

Routine artificial rearing

Advantages of taking kids off does include more saleable milk in dairy herds, having more control over growth rates, breaking disease cycles (e.g. Johne's disease) and dealing with large litters or orphans.

Feeding considerations

Either whole milk or milk replacer may be used, the latter with 24–26% protein, 14–22% fat and 12–16% dry matter (DM) (e.g. 15% DM equates to 1 part milk powder by weight mixed with 5.7 parts water by weight; **Fig. 4.26**). High levels of starch or plant protein in the milk replacer should be avoided.

For just a handful of kids, lamb or human baby bottles placed in a rack work well (**Fig. 4.27**). Bottles should not be hand held when feeding male kids, to reduce the risk of kids developing 'berserk male syndrome'. Where larger number of kids require feeding, a self-feed milk reservoir with multiple teats is more efficient (**Fig. 4.28**). Starting with bodywarm milk for the first few days, kids can be accustomed to

cool milk readily. Where milk is replenished once a day and the ambient temperature is above 15°C, the milk is chilled prior to being placed into the reservoir, and the reservoir ideally insulated to slow down souring. Ice packs can be placed into the reservoir in very warm weather. The reservoir must have a lid (**Fig. 4.29**) and, if too heavy to be tipped, a drainage hole for emptying and cleaning. A third option is feeding from an open trough; this is suitable where milk is given several times throughout the day, but requires training of the kids. For teat-based systems, the drinking height is 50 cm to start with.

Feeding implements must be kept scrupulously clean (**Fig. 4.30**), using hot water and disinfectant (e.g. sodium hypochlorite [bleach]).

As a rough guideline, the kid should be fed 15–20% of its body weight in each 24-hour period. If not offered *ad libitum*, this amount is spread over at least 4 feeds during the first week of life, then 3 feeds up to 4–6 weeks old and twice daily for the remainder. The amount is halved and the frequency reduced to once a day in the 2 weeks prior to weaning.

An example protocol is: week 1 feed 4 × 300 ml, weeks 2–6 feed 3 × 750 ml, weeks 7 and 8 feed 2 × 1–1.5 litres, week 9 feed 1 × 1–1.5 litres, week 10 feed 1 × 500 ml.

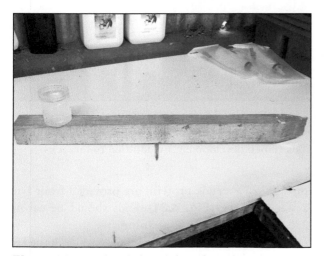

Fig. 4.26 A make-shift weigh scale to measure out milk powder. A timber baton is balanced on a rod. A known quantity of water is placed at one end. A container is placed equidistant at the other end and milk powder added until the baton is in balance again.

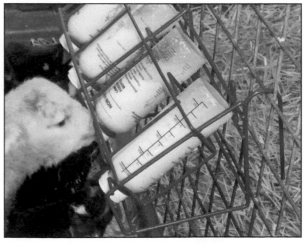

Fig. 4.27 A bottle rack works well for a small number of kids that require milk feeding.

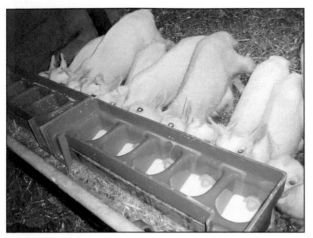

Fig. 4.28 Self-feed teat feeders are a labour efficient way for long-term feeding of larger groups of kids. In the system shown here, where milk is not available *ad libitum*, all kids must have access to a teat at the same time. This type of feeder can be heavy, often resulting in suboptimal infrequent cleaning.

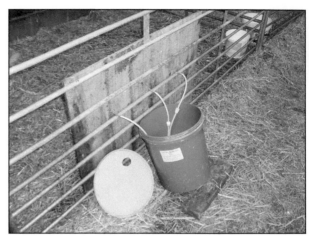

Fig. 4.29 Where milk is replenished to last 12–24 hours, the container must have a lid to preserve milk quality. It should also be insulated and, depending on the climate, cooled.

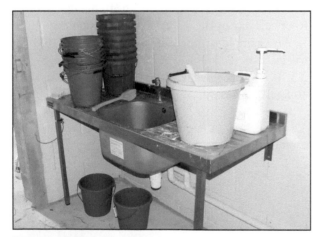

Fig. 4.30 Good practice. An easily accessible cleaning area for feeding buckets, well equipped with brushes, disinfectant and hot water on tap.

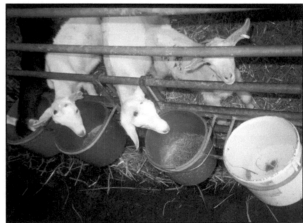

Fig. 4.31 Good access to concentrate, provided from 1–2 weeks of age, as well as to water (white bucket), aids rumen development (in addition to forage).

Where milk is offered *ad libitum*, during the 2 weeks prior to weaning the amount is reduced to half that consumed in the previous week.

Clean drinking water must always be available.

Weaning considerations

To aid rumen development, hay or eating straw and concentrate (kid, lamb or calf pellets or coarse mix; 18–25% crude protein) are provided from 1 to 2 weeks of age (**Fig. 4.31**). Kids should be eating 250 g of concentrates at weaning.

Weaning may be attempted at 6 weeks old if the kid has reached 10 kg body weight. This requires excellent husbandry and a daily live weight gain of 250 g. Often more achievable is weaning at 8–12 weeks old or once they have reached 18 kg body weight.

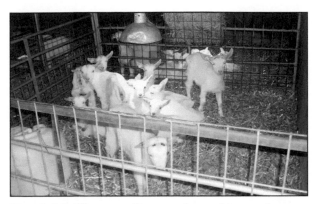

Fig. 4.32 These goatlings are housed in an adequate group size (up to 15 works well, maximum of 25). However, the stocking density is too high and does not fulfil the minimum space allowance of 0.6 m²/kid.

Post-weaning growth rates on good quality pasture range from 100–120 g/day for dairy breeds to 185–245 g/day for Boer kids. Kids on pasture may experience weight stasis in late autumn to early winter, regardless of supplementary feeding.

Housing considerations

Group sizes of 15 work well and should not exceed 25. Minimum space allowance is 0.6 m²/kid (**Fig. 4.32**). Housing must be well ventilated but draught-free, with plenty of clean bedding. Minimum required shed temperature is 5°C, and heat lamps should be considered depending on air space and number of kids. If reared outside, natural or artificial shelter from wind, rain and sun must be available.

CLINICAL EXAMINATION OF THE DIGESTIVE SYSTEM

Oral and dental examination

Examination of the rostral oral cavity is straight-forward; however, the tightness of the goat's mouth means that sedation may be required to allow full examination of the caudal parts (**Fig 5.1**). A pen torch and mouth-gag are invaluable. Integrity of the oral mucosa is of interest. Loss may indicate conditions such as dental disease, drenching gun injury, neoplasia, viral disease or uraemia.

Teeth are checked for absence, malocclusion, loss of anchoring, overgrowth, angulation and discolouration. Halitosis and quidding are signs of dental disease. A rough assessment of cheek teeth alignment can be made by external palpation of the tooth arcades (**Fig. 5.2**).

Abdominal examination
Abdominal contour

The behaviour of fluid (migrating ventrally) and gas (rising dorsally), together with the anatomical location of various structures of the gastrointestinal (GI) tract, allows narrowing down of the likely problem when observing the abdominal contour.

Common origins of bilateral ventral distension are rumen distension (pathological or because of a fibrous, slowly digestible diet), free abdominal fluid (e.g. ruptured viscera or peritonitis) and late pregnancy (**Fig. 5.3**). Bilateral dorsal distension is commonly caused by free abdominal gas (e.g. peritonitis) or severe rumenal tympany. Common causes for distension of an individual abdominal quadrant are: left upper = rumenal tympany; left lower = rumen fluid; right upper = intestine; right lower = abomasum, intestine, late pregnancy.

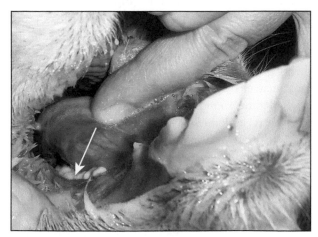

Fig. 5.1 Sedation enabled a thorough examination of the caudal oral cavity (here in an alpaca), and a purulent discharge (arrow) was detected.

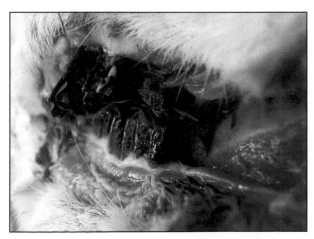

Fig. 5.2 Skyline view (rostral to caudal) of the right cheek teeth, with the lip commissure incised. The abnormal angle of the upper molars could be palpated externally. The animal was quidding and had recurrent feed impaction in the cheek.

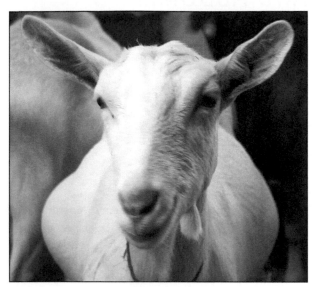

Fig. 5.3 Distension of the right lower abdominal quadrant in a pregnant doe. The abdominal contour should be noted during examination.

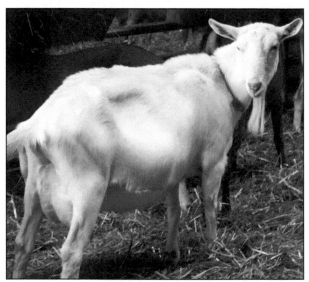

Fig. 5.4 The mildly arched back and backwards stance of the hind legs indicate discomfort in this goat. Origin of pain may be the abdomen, but also the udder, thorax or limbs.

A 'papple' shape (dorsal and ventral distension on left, ventral distension on right) may be seen in vagal indigestion. More discreet swellings can be caused by haematoma, neoplasia or emphysema in the abdominal wall.

Abdominal auscultation and percussion

In addition to the rumen rate (normal: 2–4 contractions in 2 minutes), the character of the contractions is of interest (i.e. whether strong and of normal duration). Quiet sounds mean either reduced rumen function or that the rumen has been displaced away from the left body wall. Rumen fill gives an indication of recent feed intake.

Regular intermittent borborygmi of moderate strength should be audible when auscultating the right flank. Of concern would be excessive or absent borborygmi.

A dull, drum-like resonance on percussion suggests tight distension with gas (e.g. rumen tympany). A high-pitched resonance (like fluid dripping into a metal bucket) indicates a gas–fluid interface, like in a distended abomasum. It is important to be familiar with normal areas of resonance (e.g. a narrow strip just ventral to the lumbar transverse processes associated with the colon).

Pain indicators

Colic signs are often subtle, including general restlessness, shifting weight or lifting a hind leg towards the abdomen. The goat may display grunting or bruxism. However, colic signs are not pathognomonic to the GI tract. Similarly, an arched back may be displayed with pain originating in the abdomen, but also in the thorax, mammary gland or limbs (**Fig. 5.4**). A 'panicked' facial expression may be present. The withers pinch test can be applied in goats; a normal response consists of the goat dipping its back in response to the withers being grasped. If cranial abdominal pain is present, the goat may either grunt on dipping or refuse to dip the second time round. Manual palpation and lifting of the ventral abdominal wall is also useful to detect pain.

The Eric Williams test is used specifically to detect reticular pain. It makes use of the fairly regular cycle of two B-waves (rumen contraction) to one A-wave (reticulum contraction), and involves simultaneous palpation for the rumen waves in the left flank while auscultating the trachea to detect a grunt or catching of breath.

Liver examination

The liver is not readily accessible to physical examination. Protrusion beyond the last rib may be detected, as may be pain on percussion over the right caudal ribcage. Mucous membranes are checked for jaundice. In general, detecting liver pathology involves further diagnostics, such as biochemistry, biopsy and ultrasonography.

Faecal examination

Volume, consistency and abnormal contents (e.g. blood, mucus, membrane casts) are evaluated. Perineal staining indicates diarrhoea. Presence of tenesmus is noted.

Ancillary diagnostics
Ultrasonography

The presence of free abdominal fluid is easy to establish by ultrasonography (**Fig. 5.5**), which may also guide centesis (see later). In the normal goat, only very small pockets of fluid are present, increasing somewhat in a pregnant doe near term.

The gas present in the rumen and abomasum precludes visualisation of changes in the lumen, but the position of the viscus and the integrity and thickness of its wall can be established. Intestines can be visualised through the right flank and typically have a mid-tone echogenicity (**Fig. 5.6**), with regular and obvious peristaltic movements (not to be confused with movement caused by respiration). The loops of the small intestine are irregularly arranged, while the loops of the spiral colon appear more ordered. Of concern are absence of peristalsis or incomplete collapse of a loop during peristalsis, low echogenicity of gut contents, wall oedema or a very different appearance of adjacent loops (**Fig. 5.7**). Intussusception may display the classic 'goggle' appearance (see **Fig. 5.37**).

The liver usually has a homogeneous appearance and the main vessels (e.g. vena cava) and bile ducts can be identified (**Fig. 5.8**). Calcifications within the parenchyma or bile ducts are of interest, as are any masses (e.g. an abscess). The gallbladder may appear enlarged in an inappetent animal.

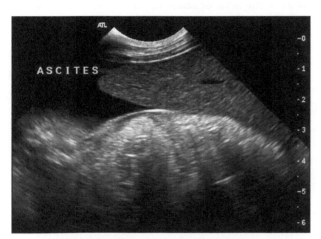

Fig. 5.5 Marked free abdominal fluid (appearing black on ultrasonography) to the left of a liver lobe.

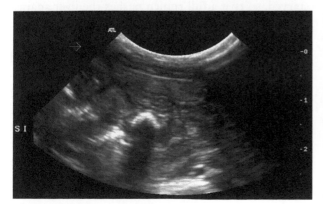

Fig. 5.6 Mid-tone echogenicity of normal intestine. Some bright gas shadows appear in the lower half of the image.

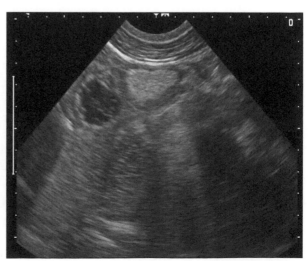

Fig. 5.7 Cross-sections of adjacent intestinal loops showing different ultrasonographic appearance and echogenicity in a case of ileal obstruction.

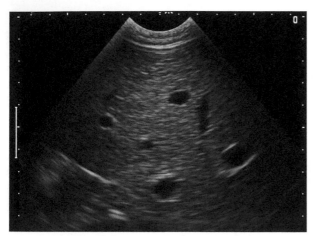

Fig. 5.8 Normal ultrasonographic appearance of the liver. The parenchyma is homogeneous and various cross-sections of vessels and bile ducts can be seen.

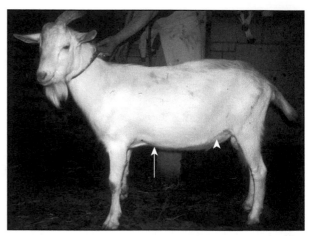

Fig. 5.9 Landmarks for abdominocentesis: either left paramedian about four finger-widths behind the elbow (arrow), or left or right paramedian just in front of the teats in the male or udder in the female (arrowhead).

Computed tomography and magnetic resonance imaging

Computed tomography (CT) and magnetic resonance imaging (MRI) are becoming more accessible and most goats are small enough to fit into a machine used for companion animals. These imaging modalities bypass the limitations of radiography and ultrasonography in ruminants, and reference articles for normal anatomical appearance are becoming more widely available.

Abdominocentesis

Ultrasound guidance, if available, is helpful to perform abdominocentesis. Alternatively, samples may be taken blindly from the following sites: (1) left paramedian, four finger-widths behind the elbow; or (2) left or right paramedian just in front of the udder (or teats in the male; **Fig. 5.9**). The site is clipped and disinfected. An 18–20 gauge hypodermic needle, 3.75 cm (1.5 in) long (5 cm/2 in in overconditioned animals), is inserted at a right angle to the skin and gradually advanced. Fluid may be collected by free-catch or with the aid of a syringe, into both an EDTA and a plain sampling tube.

The omentum is very effective in containing peritonitis, and sampling at various sites and to varying depths may be necessary (also because there may be a substantial amount of intra-abdominal fat).

On farm, the presence of fibrin, ingesta and blood can be established. A subsample is shaken vigorously to check for precipitation of excessive protein. Laboratory analysis includes protein (normal range 20–25 g/l), nucleated cells (normal range $0.2–0.3 \times 10^9/l$) and culture.

Liver biopsy

Liver biopsy is a useful technique to establish pathology in the individual sick goat, but also for routine monitoring of trace element status (in particular copper). The animal is placed into left lateral recumbency, possibly under light sedation. Ideally, it should not be starved, so that a full rumen pushes the liver against the right abdominal wall. An area in the 10th or 11th (penultimate) intercostal space, on a line between the tuber coxae and shoulder joint (**Fig. 5.10**), is clipped and disinfected. After infiltration of skin and intercostal muscles with local anaesthetic, a 1 cm long skin incision is made. A Tru-Cut™ or similar biopsy needle is advanced through the incision, either at right angle to the skin and straight across the body, or aiming towards the left elbow (**Fig. 5.11**). The needle is pushed through the pleura (resistance appreciable, and pain response may be seen) into the thorax. Some centimetres deeper, overcoming resistance indicates that the diaphragm has been penetrated (the needle will move in line with respiration). About 1 cm deeper

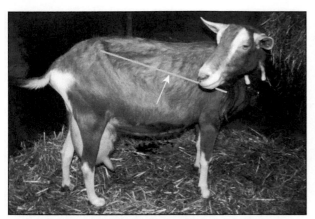

Fig. 5.10 Landmarks for liver biopsy. Needle entry point is in the 10th or 11th intercostal space (arrow) on a line between the tuber coxae and the shoulder joint.

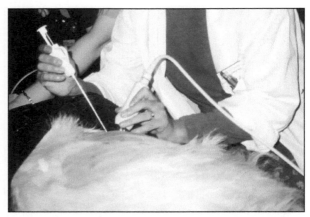

Fig. 5.11 Liver biopsy in a goat (the goat's head is on the left, with its legs towards the operator). Note that the needle is angled this acutely only to gain entry through the stab incision. After that it will be advanced at a right angle to the body wall or pointing towards the opposite elbow. Ultrasound guidance is useful to target a particular lesion, but the procedure can be done blind.

than the diaphragm, and at a total depth of 7–10 cm in the adult goat, renewed resistance indicates the liver capsule. The needle is pushed into the liver tissue for a couple of centimetres (slightly gritty feel to it, like pushing a needle through sand) and the mechanism of the needle is activated to take the sample. A staple or suture is placed into the skin incision

If the sample is taken for copper analysis, as much blood as possible should be washed off with de-ionised sterile water or saline, before placing it into a plain sampling pot. For histology, the sample is placed into 10% formalin.

Ultrasound guidance is useful, in particular to target non-diffuse lesions. Main risk factors include penetration of the gallbladder and haemorrhage from penetrating a large hepatic vessel. Peritonitis is very rare. Animals occasionally exhibit dyspnoea after the procedure due to a pneumothorax. This resolves quickly (within 20 minutes) and, because of the complete mediastinum, does not cause a problem. Ideally, clotting ability is assessed prior to the procedure (e.g. blood drawn into a plain glass vacutainer will clot within 5 minutes in the normal animal).

Rumenocentesis

Rumen fluid analysis is useful to assess subacute rumen acidosis on a herd level or in individual cases with suspected carbohydrate overload or to assess rumen health.

Paracostal collection is carried out in the conscious standing animal, with an optional skin bleb of local anaesthetic. The skin is prepared with surgical spirit. A 3.7–5 cm (1.5–2 in), 14 gauge needle is inserted perpendicular to the skin in the lower half of the left flank close to the last rib and advanced into the rumen. A syringe is attached and the sample collected. Rumen fluid may also be collected by stomach tube, but saliva contamination can artificially increase the pH by 1 to 2 units.

Normal rumen fluid in an animal on a forage-rich diet is green to olive–green in colour and has an aromatic odour. An indifferent smell suggests inactivity, an acid smell and greyish colour suggests low pH, an ammonia smell severe protein overload (e.g. urea toxicity) and a foul smell putrefaction (overgrowth of coliforms and *Proteus* spp.). When the sample is left to stand, sedimentation should take 4–8 minutes. Faster sedimentation, often with absence of floating particles, occurs with inactivity or acute rumen acidosis. Normal rumen pH is 6.5–7.5 on a forage-rich diet, but may be as low as 5.5 about 2–3 hours after a concentrate meal. The normal rumen flora is predominantly gram negative with a wide variety of bacteria (rods, cocci,

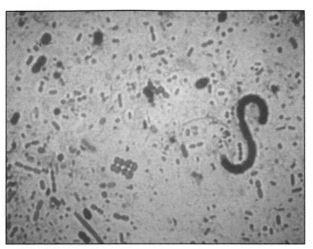

Fig. 5.12 Typical appearance of gram-stained rumen fluid when the ration is forage-rich. Gram-negative bacteria prevail and there is a variety of shapes and sizes.

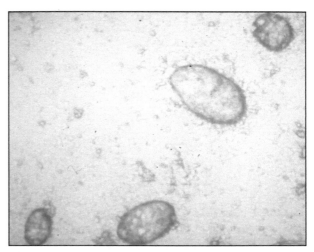

Fig. 5.13 Presence of small, medium and large protozoa suggests a healthy rumen flora. Large protozoa are the first to disappear during flora disturbance and the last to reappear after correction.

singly or in clusters; **Fig. 5.12**) and various sized protozoa (**Fig. 5.13**).

NON-INFECTIOUS DISEASES OF THE DIGESTIVE TRACT AND ABDOMEN

Dental problems

Normal structure and function
Dentition
As is typical for ruminants, the goat has a dental pad in the upper jaw instead of incisors. The dental formula for permanent teeth is:

$$\frac{0I\ 0C\ 3P\ 3M}{3I\ 1C\ 3P\ 3M}$$

The mandibular canine tooth has adopted the position and function of a 4th incisor. Eruption times for deciduous and permanent teeth are shown in *Table 5.1*.

Incisors are used for apprehension of feed. The chewing surfaces of the cheek teeth (premolars and molars) are rough with several ridges. The mandibular arcade is narrower than the maxillary arcade, and each mandibular tooth is offset in a rostrocaudal direction against its corresponding maxillary partner, with the exception of M3. They have a combined serrating function

during cudding. Cheek teeth continue to grow into adulthood.

Dentin is present throughout the length of the tooth, and is covered by enamel in the crown and cement in the root. Enamel cannot repair itself. Secondary dentin can be laid down on the biting surface in response to wear, but needs the right stimulation and good vascular supply and is always of lower quality than the original dentin.

DECIDUOUS TOOTH	ERUPTED BY AGE	PERMANENT TOOTH	CHANGING AT AGE
Incisor 1	Birth	Incisor 1	15 months
Incisor 2	Birth	Incisor 2	19–22 months
Incisor 3	Birth	Incisor 3	21–26 months
Canine	1–3 weeks	Canine	29–36 months
Premolars 2–4	3 weeks	Premolars 2–4	17–20 months
		Molar 1	3–4 months
		Molar 2	8–10 months
		Molar 3	18–24 months

Table 5.1 **Tooth eruption times in the goat.**

Adapted from: Thomé, H (2004) Mundhöhle und Schlundkopf. In: *Nickel, Schummer, Seiferle – Lehrbuch der Anatomie der Haustiere, Band II*, 3rd edn. (eds J Frewein, H Gasse, R Leiser *et al.*) [Oral cavity and pharynx. In: *Textbook of Anatomy of Domestic Animals, Vol. II*, 3rd edn]. Parey Verlag, Stuttgart.

Mandibular brachygnathia and prognathia (syns. underbite/overbite)

Overview

Brachygnathia is a shortened mandible, prognathia a mandible that protrudes beyond the maxilla (**Fig. 5.14**).

Aetiology

Typically congenital, although the extent of the misalignment may alter as the animal grows and matures. A hereditary component is likely and affected animals should be removed from the breeding pool.

Clinical presentation

Teeth alignment and health should always be checked in an animal failing to maintain a satisfactory body condition score. The defect may be obvious visually, but more subtle cases require lifting of the upper and lower lip to check alignment of the mandible in relation to the dental pad. Occasionally, a lateral head radiograph is required to determine whether protruding incisors are due to prognathia or just tooth overgrowth.

Clinical relevance consists of reduced feed intake with an overbite and occasionally broken teeth. An underbite may damage the oral mucosa with secondary infection.

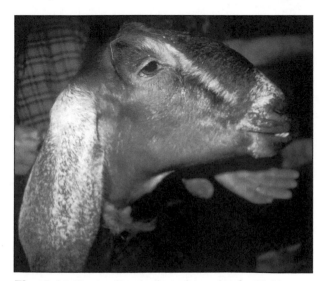

Fig. 5.14 Protruding incisors in an Anglo-Nubian buck. Careful examination, possibly combined with a radiograph, may be required to distinguish true prognathia from tooth overgrowth.

The cheek teeth should always be checked, as they are often also misaligned.

Treatment/management/control

There is no treatment for an underbite. An overbite resulting in clinical problems may be at least partially corrected by trimming the incisors. The goat is lightly sedated. A rolled-up towel or dog tug-of-war rope makes a useful gag to hold the mouth open and the tongue out the way. The teeth may be cut with embryotomy wire or a Dremel rotary tool. Water cooling must be applied to the teeth during the procedure. Great care must be taken not to open the pulp cavities.

Dental disease

Overview

Incisor and cheek tooth pathology are well described in other ruminants and, despite a paucity of literature on the subject, it is likely that the goat is similarly affected with conditions such as malocclusion, tooth loss, periodontal disease and tooth fractures.

Aetiology

Age will cause some inevitable changes, such as uneven wear and formation of diasthemata. Secondary problems to these are trauma to the oral mucosa and food impaction, with periodontal disease.

Occasionally, the eruption of permanent teeth is abnormal with, for example, deciduous teeth not shedding on time or eruption at an abnormal angle.

A high concentrate diet may lead to caries. No information exists on the possible role of retinol, ascorbic acid or calciferol (vitamins A, C and D) and calcium, as implicated in other species.

Tooth root infections may be linked to eruption of permanent teeth or haematogenous infections. Tooth fractures may be the result of trauma to the head or stones or metal in the diet, possibly facilitated by any weakening of the tooth structure.

Clinical presentation

Many affected animals will show no overt signs until dental pathology is well advanced (**Fig. 5.15**). Weight loss or failure to maintain body condition should always trigger a dental examination.

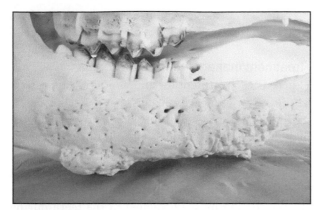

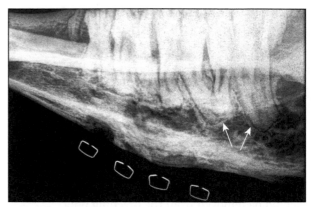

Fig. 5.15 Specimen of severe mandibular bone pathology. The animal (an alpaca) had not shown any obvious signs until 1 week prior to referral, and the owners had performed routine body condition scoring and palpation of the jawline 4 weeks prior. This lateral view shows the rostrocaudal extent of the pathology. Also note the normal offset between mandibular and maxillary teeth.

Fig. 5.16 Radiograph of the mandible showing extensive bone lysis and sclerosis. To determine tooth root involvement, the integrity of the lamina dura is established. Normal appearance can be seen surrounding both roots of M3 and the caudal root of M2: a radiolucent line adjacent to the root, then a radiodense line (arrows). The lamina dura is lost around the cranial root of M2 and the caudal root of M1. The skin staples were placed over the discharging tracts to establish the relative location of the bone lesions. Left dorsal to right ventral oblique view.

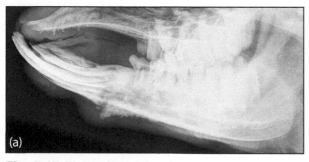

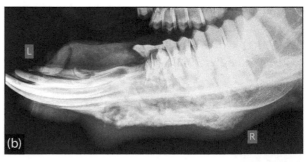

Fig. 5.17 Two radiographs of an alpaca jaw showing the benefit of oblique radiographs. (a) The pathology in the lateral view looks relatively restricted; (b) the oblique view shows the true extent of the pathology.

Incisor tooth pathology may reduce overall intake of forage, leading to weight loss. However, if goats are grazed on varied vegetation, they often compensate by selective feeding.

Cheek tooth pathology will lead to weight loss, but also signs of poor digestion, such as poor rumen fill and undigested fibre in the faeces. Other possible signs include quidding (dropping feed or a cud), feed impaction in the cheek, salivation, bruxism, halitosis, tooth discolouration and taking longer to feed. Where the tooth root is involved, additional signs include jaw swelling, discharging tracts along

the jaw and excessive tear flow (if maxillary tooth affected).

Uneven wear may also lead to changes in the mandibular joint, with associated discomfort.

Diagnosis

Oral examination, with the aid of a pen torch and light sedation, may give an indication of the problem. Diagnosis is aided by radiographs, highlighting involvement of bone structures and tooth roots (**Fig. 5.16**). Lateral, dorsoventral and 30–45-degree oblique views are taken (**Fig. 5.17**), either in the standing goat or in lateral recumbency under sedation. A mouth gag is useful to separate the arcades (e.g. a 20 ml syringe or syringe case, covered in a layer of elastic bandage for grip). Ultrasound is useful to investigate soft tissue changes. MRI or CT is occasionally necessary to identify the specific tooth involved.

Differential diagnosis

A jaw swelling (**Fig. 5.18**) may also be caused by infection of the bone (including actinomycosis, syn. 'lumpy jaw'), a fracture, neoplasia, an abscess (including caseous lymphadenitis [CLA]), a saliva cyst, foreign body reaction (e.g. a blackthorn), cud retention and insect or snake bites.

Treatment/management/control

A loose or malaligned tooth may be removed orally. A 'spike' that has formed in response to malocclusion or a missing tooth can be rasped off. The goat's mouth is rather restricted in its ability to open, but with sedation and using dental floats for miniature ponies the task can usually be achieved. It is

very important to leave some ridges on the biting surface: floating this surface smooth will result in indigestion.

The options for tooth root infections are surgical extraction, surgical curettage (**Fig. 5.19**), medical treatment or a combination of these. Because of the tightness of the goat's mouth, the surgical approach is via the ventral mandible or lateral maxilla. Alternatively, a buccal approach can be used up to molar 2, taking care not to traumatise the parotid duct. General anaesthesia (GA) is advisable, combined with a mandibular and mental block for analgesia (see Chapter 18). Any defect created is plugged postoperatively to reduce saliva loss and contamination (e.g. with gauze swabs or a tampon; **Fig. 5.19**). The plug is replaced, and the wound lavaged daily until granulation tissue is well established. Antibiosis, either as stand-alone treatment or postoperatively, needs to be prolonged (4–6 weeks). A wide variety of pathogens may be involved, including anaerobes. Suitable antimicrobials are florfenicol, penicillin, potentiated penicillin (e.g. with clavulanic acid), tetracycline and ceftiofur.

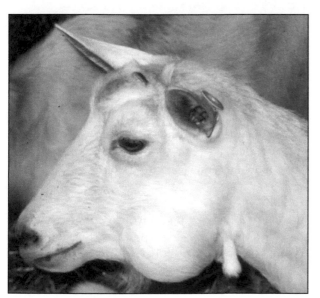

Fig. 5.18 **Marked swelling involving the left mandible. The main differential diagnoses are: bone infection, soft tissue abscess, cud retention, salivary cyst.**

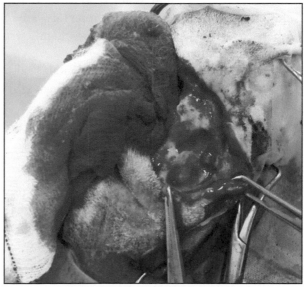

Fig. 5.19 **View onto healthy bone after aggressive curettage to remove any softened and infected bone tissue (animal in dorsal recumbency, with muzzle to bottom of image). A gauze swab is placed into a resulting defect connecting with the oral cavity to act as a postoperative plug.**

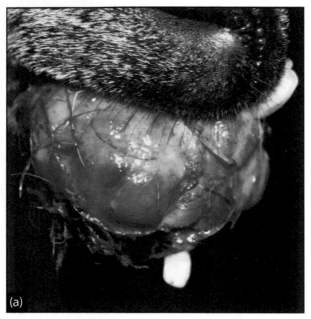
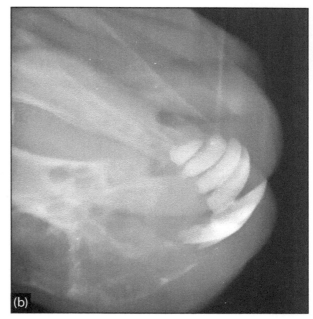

Fig. 5.20 (a) Giant cell tumour in the oral cavity of a mature goat, and (b) associated radiograph showing extensive bone destruction. (Image courtesy Andrew Dobson.)

Cases with extensive bone involvement may benefit from oral potassium iodide (0.5–1.0 g per day for 7–10 days) or i/v sodium iodide (1 g/12 kg as 10% solution, 2–4 times at 7–10 day intervals; an i/v catheter must be used as the solution is highly irritant to perivascular tissue).

Dietary fibre is important for dental health, in particular tooth wear and buffering saliva production.

Oral problems (excluding dental)

Normal structure and function

The tongue has a moderately well developed protuberance in its caudal part, the torus linguae. The oral mucous membranes tend to be relatively pale and, depending on breed, may show heavy pigmentation.

Neoplasia
Overview

Oral tumours occur regularly. Lymphosarcomas may be found in young adults, with other tumours typically affecting middle-aged to older animals. There appears to be no breed predilection.

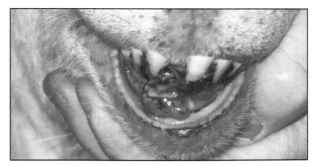

Fig. 5.21 Oral lymphosarcoma in a 7-year-old Anglo-Nubian doe, causing separation of incisors and some food impaction.

Aetiology

Neoplastic changes may involve various tissues of just the oral cavity (e.g. spindle cell or giant cell tumours; **Fig. 5.20**) or be part of a wider spread neoplasia such as lymphosarcoma.

Clinical presentation

Until the mass becomes externally visible, early signs include salivation, bleeding, dysphagia and tooth misalignment (**Fig. 5.21**). Regional lymph nodes may be enlarged, which may contribute to any dysphagia.

Diagnosis

Histology provides a definitive diagnosis. A punch biopsy typically gives a suitable sample. Depending on the site, it is taken under topical anaesthetic gel application, infiltration anaesthesia or regional block. Moderate to profuse haemorrhage should be expected from most oral sampling sites, which can be addressed with direct pressure application.

Differential diagnosis

Bone proliferation may be caused by dental disease or bone infection (e.g. actinomycosis). The main differentials for a soft tissue swelling are abscess, traumatised mucosa with subsequent infection, alveolar food impaction and foreign body reaction. Clinical, ultrasonographic and radiographic examination usually allows a definitive diagnosis.

Treatment/management/control

Prognosis is guarded to poor. It may be possible to surgically remove very discreet masses, possibly followed by radiotherapy. Partial jaw resection is in theory possible; however, the impact on food intake and mastication must be considered. Spread to regional lymph nodes carries a poor prognosis.

Drenching/bolus gun injury

Overview

This is an entirely preventable problem. A large proportion of goats in a herd may be affected, and case mortality rates of around 15% have been reported.

Aetiology

Trauma to the thin mucosa underneath the tongue or near the pharynx is caused by forceful placement or misplacement of a drenching or bolus gun nozzle. Occasionally, the soft palate is traumatised. The mucosal defect is invaded by commensals and opportunistic bacteria, such as *Trueperella pyogenes*. *Clostridium* spp., yeasts and fungi may also be involved. Localised septic cellulitis, tissue necrosis and abscessation result (**Fig. 5.22**).

Clinical presentation

Submandibular or retropharyngeal swelling, often extending along the ventral neck, develops within

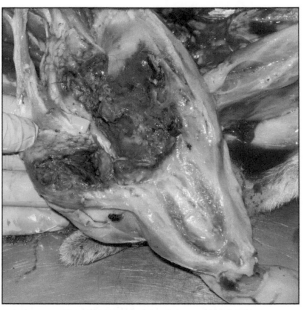

Fig. 5.22 View onto the roof of the oral cavity of a lamb, showing extensive infection and necrosis resulting from trauma caused by a drenching gun. The entry point was small, with the full extent of the lesion only apparent after resection. (© Crown Copyright 2013. Source and kind permission: Animal and Plant Health Agency and Ian Mawhinney.)

a few days of the gun being used. Salivation, dysphagia, halitosis, nasal discharge and enlargement of regional lymph nodes may also be seen. Pain is often displayed in the form of bruxism and inappetence. Abscesses may erode into local vessels, possibly leading to bleeding from the nose and mouth, coughing, collapse and sudden death. Asphyxia can result from misplacement of a bolus. Cases may be peracute, with death within 24 hours.

Occasionally, infection tracks into the cervical spine, with resulting neurological deficits.

Diagnosis

Sudden death is commonly reported, with confirmation on post-mortem examination (PME). In the live animal, sedation may be required to allow thorough inspection of the pharyngeal region. Ultrasonography may aid in identifying the cause of retropharyngeal swellings.

Differential diagnosis

Neoplasia typically affects individual goats only. Caseous lymphadenitis may present as an outbreak, but swellings are typically confined to lymph nodes. Vena cava thrombosis with pulmonary embolism is a differential for haemoptysis, but usually only affects single goats. Dental disease is ruled out during examination.

Treatment/management/control

A misplaced bolus may be surgically removed, but prognosis is guarded to poor. Aggressive antibiosis (broad spectrum, including anaerobes) combined with NSAIDs may be tried. Euthanasia is indicated in severe cases.

Control relies on good drenching technique and training of all staff undertaking drenching. Of particular importance are the following points: taking enough time over the procedure, restraining the animal effectively, taking into account the angulation of the nozzle (especially when an unfamiliar type of gun is used; **Fig. 5.71**) and placing the nozzle on top of the tongue. The minimum body weight of animals to be treated, which most anthelmintic and mineral and vitamin boluses stipulate, must be observed. Guns must be well maintained (no sharp edges) and replaced regularly.

Tongue lesions

Sarcocystosis is common in some countries, although often without significant clinical impact. Also reported are foreign body granuloma, erosions, ulcerative glossitis and fibrosis. Wooden tongue (actinobacillosis) does not appear to be documented in the goat.

Oesophageal problems

Megaoesophagus

Overview

Megaoesophagus is a sporadic and relatively rare disorder involving dilatation and atony of the oesophagus with poor long-term prognosis.

Aetiology

Often idiopathic, but also described secondary to vagal nerve trauma, hiatal hernia, thymoma and oesophagitis caused by choke. May be congenital. The majority of cases appear to affect young adults.

Clinical presentation

Intermittent regurgitation, weight loss, reduced appetite, salivation, coughing related to food or water intake and possibly recurrent bloat. Pyrexia may be present. Where the cervical section is affected, a swelling in the distal neck may be observed, either permanently or during swallowing or cudding (**Fig. 5.23**).

Diagnosis

Fluoroscopy, endoscopy and contrast radiography (**Fig. 5.24**).

Differential diagnosis

Similar clinical signs may be seen with external pressure onto the oesophagus. Other causes of bloat must be ruled out including, in young animals, a persistent aortic arch. Rhododendron poisoning may present with similar signs, but is of acute onset. Oesophageal sarcocystosis is a cause of dysphagia in some countries (not in the UK).

Treatment/management/control

Symptomatic only, including feeding on an incline (e.g. front feet elevated), small meals and highly

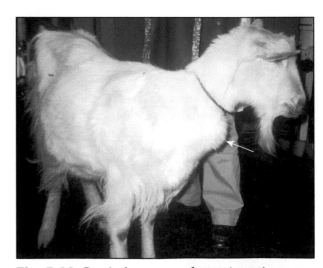

Fig. 5.23 Cervical megaoesophagus (arrow) in a 3-year-old Golden Guernsey presented for weight loss.

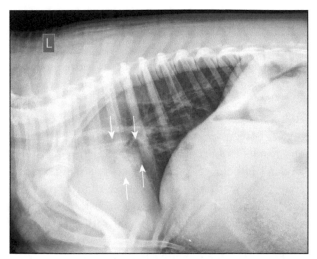

Fig. 5.24 Contrast radiograph outlining the dilated oesophagus (arrows) in the thorax of a 7-month-old Southdown sheep.

digestible feeds. Because of the necessity for cudding in ruminants, long-term control is difficult.

Obstruction (syn. choke)
Overview
Obstruction is occasionally seen, despite the selective feeding behaviour of goats, especially if grazing in orchards.

Aetiology
May result from feeding dry, hygroscopic feeds (such as sugar beet pulp), but more commonly in ruminants when eating large pieces of feed (potatoes, roots, fruit), especially from overhead height (such as picking apples out of a tree). More rarely neurological in origin or caused by external pressure onto the oesophagus.

Clinical presentation
Excessive salivation is seen. Cervical obstructions can often be seen or palpated.

Diagnosis
Inability to pass a stomach tube confirms the diagnosis.

Treatment/management/control
Treatment consists of administering a smooth muscle relaxant (e.g. hyoscine butylbromide [Buscopan®],

alpha-2 agonist, clenbuterol) and retrograde removal of the obstruction (massage, probang), or oesophagotomy if this is not successful (risk of stricture formation).

Forestomach problems

Normal structure and function
The forestomach system consists of reticulum, rumen and omasum. The entry point of the oesophagus into the reticulum is connected to the exit point into the omasum via the oesophageal groove. Its closure is important in unweaned kids to channel milk directly into the abomasum. The caudoventral sac of the rumen is larger than the caudodorsal one in the goat, and extends further caudal in the abdominal cavity. Maximum rumen capacity is around 17 litres. The omasum is about fist-size in the goat, lying at the level of the 8th to 10th ribs.

Rumen tympany (syn. bloat)
Overview
Rumen tympany is a regular problem, with multiple aetiologies that can broadly be categorised as excessive free gas production, formation of stable froth or secondary due to failure to eructate.

Aetiology
Excessive gas production is seen with acute carbohydrate overload or milk fermentation in kids (e.g. following incorrect force feeding of milk or 'rumen drinkers'). Legumes may lead to frothy bloat.

Failure to eructate has several categories of causes: neurological (vagus nerve dysfunction, tetanus), positional (lateral recumbency), physical (external pressure on oesophagus such as neoplasia, lymph node enlargement, persistent aortic arch; or internal obstruction such as choke, proliferative growths), and physiological disturbances (hypocalcaemia, toxicities, inflammation).

Chronic bloat is often a sign of disturbed rumen flora and digestive function, for example in poorly weaned animals or with rumen alkalosis.

Clinical presentation
The left dorsal abdominal quadrant is visibly enlarged, with a dull resonance on percussion.

Dyspnoea, including mouth breathing, may be present in severe cases.

Diagnosis

Passing a stomach tube will detect any oesophageal obstruction and confirm the diagnosis of free-gas bloat. Neck palpation, ultrasonography, endoscopy, thoracic radiography, rumenocentesis and other aids may be necessary to determine the underlying cause.

Suspicion of frothy bloat is based on history and confirmed with trial treatment.

Differential diagnosis

Diffuse peritonitis with gas production may lead to dorsal abdominal distension, but the distension is usually bilateral and the goat will show additional signs of severe discomfort and illness. The causes of secondary tympany, as listed under aetiology, must be considered.

Treatment/management/control

A stomach tube is passed to release free gas. If the animal is in severe respiratory distress, emergency treatment consists of inserting a 12–14 gauge needle or making a stab incision into the rumen. The landmarks for this are on a line from the tuber coxae to the shoulder and close to the last rib. If possible, the area is disinfected first. A stab incision needs to be followed up with surgical wound care. For frothy bloat, the goat is drenched with a surfactant (commercial product such as poloxalene [Bloat-Guard®] or vegetable oil).

In recurrent or chronic cases, either a trocar is used or a rumen fistula created (see Surgery of the rumen).

Supportive treatment consists of transfaunation or drenching with a rumen stimulant, and offering a forage-rich diet for several days. Recently weaned goatlings may benefit from returning to milk feeding for 1–2 weeks.

Control of primary bloat consists of gradual introduction of carbohydrate-rich rations or legumes (and pre-emptive surfactant administration for the latter) and good preweaning management of goatlings to ensure adequate rumen development.

Rumen acidosis (syn. carbohydrate overload)

Overview

Rumen acidosis is recognised in two forms: subacute (syn. SARA) and acute.

Aetiology

SARA is seen in goats on a concentrate-rich ration and results from repeated and extended reduction of rumen pH below 5.5. Dairy goats receiving concentrate feeds just twice daily, rather than as part of a total mixed ration (TMR), are at risk, as are meat goats on a concentrate or cereal ration that is not truly offered *ad libitum*.

The acute form results from carbohydrate overload: animals breaking into a feed store, sudden introduction of a carbohydrate-rich ration or gorging after temporary absence of feed (**Fig. 5.25**).

Clinical presentation

Signs of SARA are often vague, including soft faeces, reduced milk yield and cudding, and erratic feed intake. Secondary effects become apparent some weeks later and include laminitis, liver abscessation, poor body condition score and reduced fertility.

Signs of acute acidosis include rumen atony, inappetence, trembling and diarrhoea. The acidic contents draws water into the rumen, leading to ventral rumen distension and dehydration.

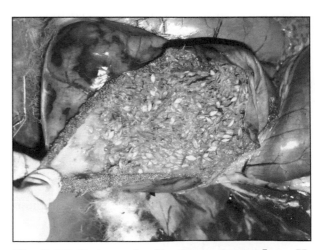

Fig. 5.25 Grain overload in rumen content. Low pH was confirmed.

Diagnosis

A reduction in milk fat (on individual goat samples) reflects suboptimal dietary fibre and gives an indication. Definitive diagnosis relies on rumen fluid pH measurement, with samples taken 2–4 hours after concentrate feeding or, in goats on TMR, 5–8 hours after fresh TMR provision (see earlier for rumenocentesis technique). Ideally, 12 goats are sampled: a rumen fluid pH below 5.5 in more than a quarter sampled indicates SARA.

In acute acidosis, a Gram stain of the rumen fluid will show overgrowth of gram-positive, rod-shaped lactobacilli (**Fig. 5.26**). Blood–gas analysis confirms a metabolic acidosis.

Differential diagnosis

Enteric or toxic causes of diarrhoea and dehydration. Hypomagnesaemia for tremors, but also neurological disorders. Peritonitis for ventral abdominal distension, and forestomach or abomasal outflow problem for rumen distension.

Treatment/management/control

Treatment of acute acidosis consists of increasing rumen pH (1 g/kg sodium bicarbonate orally), correcting dehydration and metabolic acidosis, administering B vitamins (in particular thiamine) and an antimicrobial against *Lactobacillus* spp. (e.g. procaine penicillin or tetracycline), and transfaunation or rumen stimulants. A rumenotomy (see below) or rumen lavage via a large-bore stomach tube to 'wash-out' the feed may be useful if performed within 2 hours of ingestion. Prognosis is guarded overall, and poor in recumbent animals.

In all types of goats, dietary changes must be gradual, with new feeds introduced over 2–3 weeks to allow rumen flora adaptation.

Control of SARA in dairy goats relies on optimal ration formulation, true *ad-libitum* feeding, sufficient trough space and good transition and post-kidding diet management. In particular, neutral detergent fibre levels should be 30% of ration dry matter (DM), with 70–80% from forage (**Fig. 5.27**). Slower fermentable carbohydrates ideally replace some more rapidly fermentable ones. Feeding TMR, rather than twice daily concentrate, is preferable, but care must be taken to mix the TMR well to prevent sorting (while not overmixing, resulting in reduction of effective fibre). However, sorting may not be entirely preventable in goats. Dietary buffers (e.g. sodium bicarbonate) may be added at a rate of 0.75% of ration DM.

Control of SARA in meat goats relies on gradual introduction of the carbohydrate or cereal-rich ration over several weeks, true *ad-libitum* feeding and a clean source of dietary fibre (e.g. straw) being provided separate to bedding.

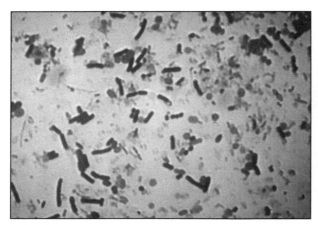

Fig. 5.26 Overgrowth of lactobacilli (gram-positive rods) in rumen fluid during acute acidosis.

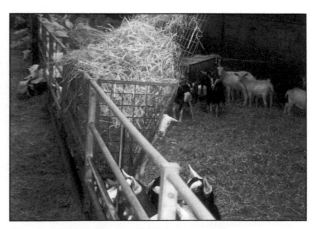

Fig. 5.27 Insufficient SARA control. Straw to increase the fibre level of the ration must be incorporated into the TMR. If offered separately, as in this herd, goats are likely to largely ignore it. Also note that sorting has taken place, and the sparsity of the TMR (i.e. not true *ad-libitum* feeding).

Traumatic reticuloperitonitis
Overview
Traumatic reticuloperitonitis is relatively rare in goats because of their selective feeding behaviour, but odd cases are reported. The aetiology, clinical presentation, treatment and prognosis are similar to cattle.

Surgery of the rumen

Trocarisation
Preparation and equipment
An area in the left craniodorsal sublumbar fossa is clipped and disinfected. A stainless steel cannula with stylet or 'Red Devil' trocar, a scalpel blade and suture material are required.

Restraint
Standing under manual restraint. Local infiltration anaesthesia.

Technical description
A skin incision is made close to the last rib and just below the most prominent point of distension. The trocar is inserted through this incision and advanced into the rumen with a quick stab-like action (or rotating action for 'Red Devil'). The stylet is removed. A stainless steel trocar requires suturing to the skin.

Aftercare
The trocar is left in place for 7–10 days. Prior to removal, the stylet is intermittently inserted for several hours to check whether tympany recurs. Antibiosis may be considered, and petroleum jelly (Vaseline®) applied to protect the skin below the trocar. Fly repellent should be used as necessary.

The skin incision is left to heal by secondary intention after trocar removal.

Potential complications
Peritonitis from leakage around the trocar. A dwell time of 7–10 days ensures some sealing adhesions around the trocar without these becoming too firmly attached.

Rumen fistula
Preparation and equipment
The left craniodorsal sublumbar fossa is clipped, including over the last rib, and disinfected. A small procedure instrument kit and non-absorbable suture material are required.

Restraint
Standing under manual restraint or mild sedation. Local infiltration anaesthesia (inverted L, line or rectangular block).

Technical description
An elliptical piece of skin (3–4 cm long, 2 cm wide) is removed just behind the last rib and over the dorsal gas cap. The abdominal muscles are dissected and the peritoneum incised. The rumen wall is grasped (**Fig. 5.28a**), pulled into the incision and secured to the skin with multiple horizontal mattress sutures. The rumen is incised (**Fig. 5.28b**).

Aftercare
Patency of the fistula is maintained by removing food and inflammatory exudate, and the surrounding skin protected (e.g. with petroleum jelly). Antibiosis may be considered. Fly repellent is used as necessary.

The fistula usually heals over in 3–5 weeks, but a larger incision can be made for a permanent rumenotomy.

Potential complications
Peritonitis is in part avoided by placing the fistula dorsal enough (i.e. above the rumen fluid level). Fly-strike and skin necrosis are potential complications.

Rumenotomy
Indication
Removal of a reticular or ruminal foreign body or toxic plant material, rumen 'washout' in carbohydrate overload, exploratory in chronic rumen tympany.

Preparation and equipment
The left flank is clipped generously and disinfected. Standard surgical kit, stay sutures or pins

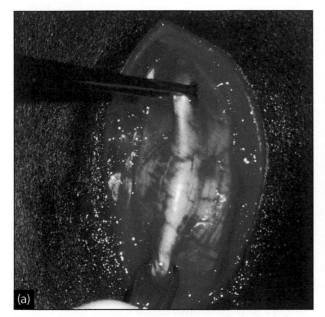
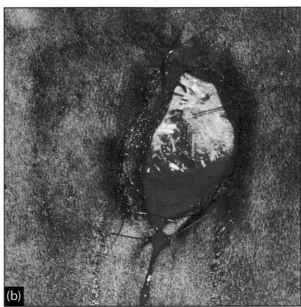

Fig. 5.28 Rumen fistula. An elliptical incision is made through the abdominal wall close to the last rib. (a) The rumen is grasped and pulled into the incision. (b) After suturing the rumen wall to the skin, it is incised.

(for example Steinman pins) and absorbable and non-absorbable suture material are required. In large goats, a Weingart frame can be used.

Restraint
Standing under sedation and regional anaesthesia, or in right-lateral recumbency under GA.

Technical description
A routine laparotomy approach in the dorsocranial flank, with the incision large enough to accommodate the surgeon's hand and forearm. A fold of rumen wall is grasped and pulled into the incision. Prior to incising the rumen, it must be secured tightly to the skin to reduce abdominal contamination. This can be achieved with stay sutures or pins or, in large goats, by use of a Weingart frame. After incising, the rumen and reticulum are explored. If necessary, part of the rumen contents is removed to facilitate exploration.

The rumen incision is closed with a continuous inverting pattern (e.g. Cushing or Lembert) with absorbable sutures. As much contamination as possible is removed, taking care not to wash it into the abdomen. The flank incision is closed in a routine manner.

Aftercare
Routine antibiosis and NSAIDs. Depending on the findings, rumen stimulant or transfaunation. Fly repellent if necessary. Oral or i/v correction of hydration status and, where indicated, metabolic acidosis.

Potential complications
Peritonitis from rumen contents spillage.

Abomasal problems

Normal structure and function
The abomasum is glandular and has a bagpipe-like shape, with a capacity of 1–2 litres. The very acidic content of the abomasum has a pH of 1.5–3. Its cranial end lies midline in the ventral abdomen, then courses towards the right paramedian. Its caudal end rises up along the right caudal ribcage.

Abomasal emptying defect (syns. pyloric stenosis, abomasal impaction, distal vagal indigestion)
Overview
Probably the most common abomasal problem in goats.

Aetiology

Tricho- or phytobezoars and enteroliths may cause physical obstruction of the pylorus (**Fig 5.29**). Functional stenosis can be caused by vagal nerve disturbance, abomasitis and possibly peritonitis. Granulomatous *Actinobacillus lignieresii* lesions can affect the proximal digestive tract, including the pylorus.

Clinical presentation

Affected goats present with abdominal distension, intermittent diarrhoea or reduced faecal output, reduced appetite and gradual weight loss. Heart rate and rectal temperature tend to be within normal limits. Severe abdominal distension causes dyspnoea. The rumen contraction rate can be increased or decreased. Milk yield is reduced.

Diagnosis

Ultrasonography or exploratory laparotomy are useful to confirm the diagnosis. Sometimes the enlarged, doughy abomasum can be palpated in the right lower abdomen. A cranial displacement of the diaphragm may be evident on thoraco-abdominal radiographs.

Moderate elevation of liver enzymes may result from hepatic congestion secondary to increased abdominal pressure. Secondary abomasal ulceration can lead to anaemia.

Impaction of the abomasum is found on PME, with content often more similar to rumen content. Muscular hypertrophy of the abomasal wall may be evident. The reticulum is commonly enlarged.

Differential diagnosis

Duodenal obstruction (enteroliths, bezoars, neoplasia protruding into lumen) or sand impaction of the abomasum. Generalised peritonitis has similar clinical signs, but vital signs are altered and toxaemia or septicaemia is present. Late stage pregnancy involving a large litter, or hydrops uteri, can present similarly.

Treatment/management/control

Surgery to remove obstructive foreign bodies can be attempted. Access should be gained via the abomasum or duodenum rather than the pylorus, if possible, to reduce the risk of postoperative pyloric dysfunction.

Treatment with anti-inflammatories or gastric prokinetic drugs typically does not show any long-term effect.

Abomasal displacement
Overview

Left or right abomasal displacement is only rarely reported in goats.

Aetiology

Too few reports exist to establish whether similar factors as in cattle are involved (such as negative energy balance pre- and post-partum, lack of dietary fibre, post-partum reproductive tract disease).

Left displacement is reported secondary to pyloric obstruction caused by a phytobezoar (**Fig. 5.29**).

Clinical presentation

With left displacement, milk yield is unsatisfactory and appetite may be selective (refusing concentrates but eating forage) or absent. Vital signs are generally normal, including normal rumen contractions, although it may be difficult to auscultate these because of rumen displacement.

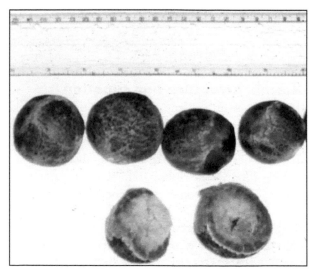

Fig. 5.29 **Phytobezoars removed from an impacted abomasum.**

Simple right displacement presents with similar signs. However, torsion or volvulus on the right leads to rapid deterioration of the animal with abnormal vital signs, dehydration and abdominal discomfort.

Faecal output may be reduced, but malodorous diarrhoea is also possible.

Concurrent disease is often present (e.g. ketosis, mastitis, uterine infection), therefore a full clinical examination is important.

Diagnosis
Simultaneous auscultation and percussion of the left (over or close to last rib) or right flank reveals a high-pitched resonance (like water trickling into a metal bucket). Centesis over this area of resonance reveals acidic fluid (pH 2–3), but carries the risk of peritonitis. Ultrasonographic diagnosis requires some experience.

Differential diagnosis
Peritonitis results in bilateral resonance and a severely compromised animal. Pneumoperitoneum would also be audible bilaterally, with a history of recent surgery.

Abnormal resonance on the left needs to be distinguished from rumen tympany (has a duller sound) and rumen collapse syndrome (resonance more caudal in flank and over larger area). On the right, the main differentials are caecal dilation and volvulus, and the normal gas resonance of the colon.

Treatment/management/control
Surgical correction (via right flank or ventral laparotomy, with abomasopexy or omentopexy) carries a good prognosis for left displacement. Right displacement must be addressed promptly and, because of the more pronounced systemic effect, prognosis for this is guarded. Dehydration is corrected and any ketosis addressed. Concentrates are introduced gradually over 7–10 days. Any concurrent disease is treated as appropriate.

Despite the aetiology not being confirmed in the goat, control measures similar to cattle should be considered. In particular, good transition management, avoiding negative energy balance and providing sufficient dietary fibre.

Abomasal ulceration
Overview
Abomasal ulceration may cause death or clinical disease, but many cases are undetected in the live goat, with incidental finding on PME or at slaughter (**Fig. 5.30**). Particular risk groups may be dairy goats in the first few weeks post partum, and kids of a few weeks of age on milk.

Aetiology
Remains unclear: theories include rapidly fermentable dietary carbohydrates, finely ground feeds, stress, anti-inflammatory drug therapy and secondary to rumen acidosis and abomasal stasis or displacement.

Clinical presentation
Non-specific signs of reduced appetite, rumen activity and milk yield, and abdominal discomfort. Vital signs remain normal unless perforation and peritonitis occur. Mild to moderate anaemia may be present.

Perforation can lead to generalised peritonitis with severe systemic disturbance or localised peritonitis contained in the omental bursa.

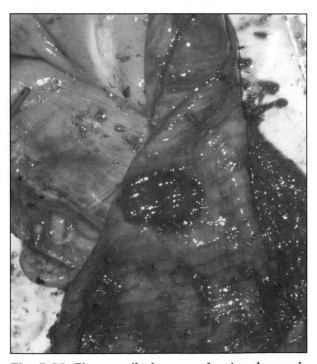

Fig. 5.30 **Circumscribed, non-perforating abomasal ulcer.**

Diagnosis

Deep abdominal palpation may locate the source of any pain to the abomasum. Faecal occult blood is present in some cases. Sampling over several days is advised to increase the detection rate. Ultrasonography of the abomasal wall may show disrupted integrity or thickening, as well as signs of peritonitis in ruptured ulcers (**Fig. 5.31**). For the latter, abdominocentesis is also useful but peritonitis may be contained within the omental bursa.

A moderate inflammatory response and possibly anaemia is evident on haematology.

Differential diagnosis

Other causes of colic and peritonitis. Lymphosarcoma infiltrating the abomasal wall.

Treatment/management/control

Stimulating appetite and feed intake is vital and this may be achieved by offering a choice of palatable feeds and, possibly, administering diazepam (if licensed). A course of antibiotics should be considered, but NSAIDs should be avoided as their role in the aetiology is unclear.

Little information exists on the use of anti-ulcer agents in goats. In general, oral preparations are not useful in ruminants, with the exception of pre-ruminant kids if administered in a way to stimulate the oesophageal groove reflex. Extrapolating from studies in cattle and camelids, the following may be effective: omeprazole at 0.4–1.0 mg/kg i/v q6–8h; pantoprazole at 1 mg/kg i/v or 2 mg/kg s/c, both q24h. The effect of systemic ranitidine or cimetidine appears very short lived.

Blood transfusion may be indicated if bleeding has resulted in severe anaemia.

Surgical repair of a perforated ulcer is often unrewarding because of adhesions and established peritonitis. Localised peritonitis responds reasonably well to conservative treatment, although surgical drainage of the omental bursa may also be considered. Prognosis for generalised peritonitis is poor.

Abomasitis (syn. abomasal bloat)
Overview

Abomasitis is a fatal condition, described in young ruminants including kids of around 10 days to 6 weeks of age. Often only a few out of a group are affected.

Aetiology

Two main pathogen groups are implicated: (1) *Sarcina* spp., a common environmental pathogen present in soil and cereal grain and able to tolerate very low pH levels (**Fig. 5.32**); (2) *Clostridium* spp., in particular *C. sordellii* and *C. perfringens*.

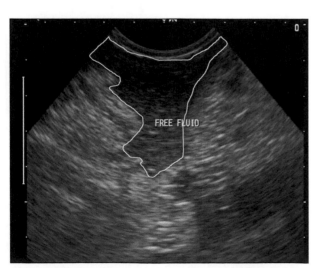

Fig. 5.31 The excessive, hyperechoic free fluid (outlined) in this ultrasonography image is suggestive of peritonitis.

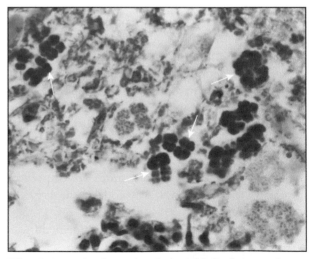

Fig. 5.32 Histology showing multiple clumps of *Sarcina* spp. (arrows) in a case of abomasitis.

The age cut-off is believed to result from increasing carbohydrate digestion in the rumen in older animals, whereby carbohydrates are no longer available to the pathogens in the abomasum.

Clinical presentation

Marked abomasal distension developing over several days and leading to bilateral abdominal distension (**Fig. 5.33**). The kid remains bright, with largely unchanged vital signs, but loses body condition. In herds with infrequent animal observation, many are simply found dead.

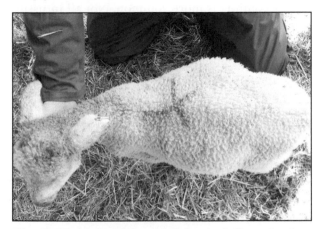

Fig. 5.33 Marked bilateral abdominal distension in a 5-week-old lamb with abomasitis.

Diagnosis

Ultrasonography or radiography shows the dilated abomasum (**Fig. 5.34**). PME shows abomasal haemorrhage, oedema, congestion and emphysema (**Fig. 5.35**). Culture of abomasal fluid is usually negative. Histology shows anaerobic pathogens and, in cases involving *Sarcina* spp., typical packs of eight or more gram-positive bacteria (**Fig. 5.32**).

Differential diagnosis

In rumen tympany caused by milk deposition and fermentation in the rumen (e.g. in 'rumen drinker' or secondary to force feeding), gas can be released by passing a stomach tube. Atresia coli leading to abdominal distension would be evident at a younger age. Intestinal obstruction would present with colic signs and reduced faecal output, and peritonitis with altered vital signs. Congenital malformations or birth trauma may lead to an uroperitoneum, detectable by ultrasonography, biochemistry and abdominocentesis.

Treatment/management/control

Antibiosis with anaerobic spectrum (e.g. penicillin at 25,000–30,000 IU/kg or ceftiofur) can be attempted, but is usually unrewarding.

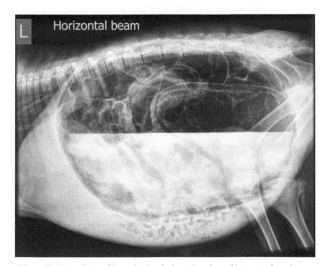

Fig. 5.34 Standing, left abdominal radiograph of a case of abomasitis, showing the extensive abomasal distension and a clear fluid line. Note that fluid does not reach the ventral abdomen or diaphragm, indicating that it is contained within a viscus.

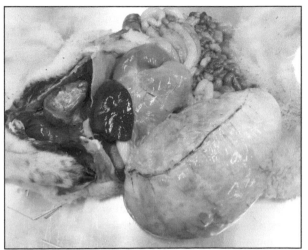

Fig. 5.35 Severe distension and emphysema ('bubble-wrap' appearance) in abomasitis.

Proposed risk factors include unhygienic milk feeding and general poor environmental hygiene.

Intestinal problems

Normal structure and function

Intestine

The pylorus leads into the duodenum (which has a characteristic S-bend), followed by the very long jejunum and then ileum. The jejunum is arranged in curls and folds on a short mesentery and lies in close proximity to, and half encircles, the spiral colon. The ileocolonic junction lies near the most caudal point of the ribcage on the right. The caecum is short, has some fermentation function and points towards the pelvic inlet. The rest of the large intestine consists of the long ascending colon, whose main part is arranged into the spiral colon (in parts on two levels), and the shorter transverse and descending colon, followed by the rectum. Because the stomachs of goats occupy about three-quarters of the abdominal cavity, the intestines are mainly positioned in the right dorsal quadrant. The average length of the intestinal tract is 33 metres.

Water absorption in the hind gut is well developed, leading to formed faecal pellets.

Omentum

The main, simplified clinical and surgical aspects of the omentum are as follows: the greater omentum originates on the left in the horizontal rumen groove, therefore the dorsal rumen is directly accessible during a left-sided laparotomy. It runs ventrally and connects to the greater curvature of the abomasum. On the right, the greater omentum originates high up in the abdomen near the abdominal aorta, and covers most of the abdominal contents. The two layers of the greater omentum form the supraomental process, which is open caudally near the pelvic inlet, thereby allowing surgical access to the intestines via a right flank laparotomy. Embedded in the omentum on the right is the outer wall of the abomasum and the duodenum. The lesser omentum runs from the portal vein to the lesser curvature of the abomasum. A substantial quantity of fat may be present in the omentum of goats in good body condition.

Intussusception

Overview

Intussusception is the invagination of one intestinal segment into an adjacent one.

Aetiology

A history of diarrhoea a few days earlier is common. Young kids may be more affected than adults.

Clinical presentation

May cause acute-onset, severe colic, but a gradual progression with initially only moderate abdominal discomfort is more common. Not all intussusceptions lead to complete obstruction, therefore faecal output may only be moderately reduced rather than completely absent. The degree of dehydration may vary for the same reason. Appetite is typically reduced, with a moderately elevated heart rate.

Diagnosis

In a thin animal, the intussusception may be palpable as an abdominal mass. Ultrasonography is most useful, showing the classic 'goggle' appearance (**Fig. 5.36**).

Differential diagnosis

Functional ileus, low-grade peritonitis, partial pyloric obstruction and other moderately severe GI problems. For a palpable mass, also abdominal neoplasia.

Treatment/management/control

Surgical resection carries a reasonable prognosis if the problem is detected prior to severe systemic compromise or peritonitis. Under GA, a ventral midline or right flank incision is made and the affected part resected, followed by an end-to-end or side-to-side anastomosis (depending on lumen size of the two portions).

Supportive therapy consists of fluid therapy, antibiosis (started preoperatively), analgesia, NSAIDs and gradual reintroduction of the full milk or feed ration over 7–10 days. Complications include narrowing of the lumen, leading to functional obstruction, and peritonitis.

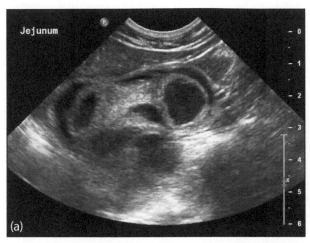
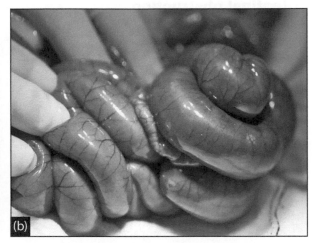

Fig. 5.36 (a) Classic 'goggle' appearance of a jejunal intussusception on abdominal ultrasonography. (b) On laparotomy, the corresponding pathology (on right) with distended loops of jejunum proximal to it (on left).

Torsion of the mesentery or mesenteric root

Overview

Torsion of the mesentery or mesenteric root is possibly more common in kids than adults, and carries a poor prognosis.

Aetiology

Remains unknown. Occasionally, there is a history of diarrhoea or ileus.

Clinical presentation

One of the few causes of violent colic, with acute onset. Vital signs are markedly disturbed, including dehydration. Faecal output is reduced or absent. Rapid deterioration.

Diagnosis

Ultrasonography shows distended intestinal loops (**Fig. 5.37**) and absent peristalsis. Abdominocentesis may show an inflammatory response. Definitive diagnosis is by exploratory laparotomy.

Differential diagnosis

Other causes of colic and 'abdominal catastrophes'.

Treatment/management/control

Surgical correction under GA may be attempted, either through a ventral midline or right flank

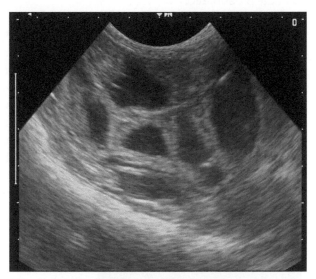

Fig. 5.37 Distended loops of intestine on ultrasonography. The loop in the centre of the image shows wall oedema.

incision. However, the short mesentery often makes it difficult to establish the direction of rotation or, indeed, correct it. Devitalisation occurs rapidly. If surgery is attempted, fluid therapy support, pre-operative antibiosis and postoperative analgesia and NSAIDs are important. Distended loops may be deflated with the aid of a needle. The short mesentery makes 'milking out' of gut contents (either into adjacent unaffected parts or via an enterotomy) difficult.

Intestinal obstruction

Overview

Functional (ileus) or mechanical obstructions occur occasionally.

Aetiology

Ileus can be a sequela to intestinal or abdominal surgery, but also to peritonitis, intestinal inflammation and endotoxaemia. Hypocalcaemia may also play a role.

Enteroliths or phyto- or trichobezoars are common causes of mechanical obstruction. Intestine may become entrapped in a hernia (umbilical or inguinal; **Fig. 5.38**). Spiral colon impaction has been linked to dehydration or reduced milk intake secondary to other events (e.g. disease, transport) in other species.

Clinical presentation

Borborygmi may be increased in the early stage, but are commonly reduced. Faecal output is absent and the animal is inappetent. Mechanical obstruction typically causes discomfort, with associated changes in vital signs. The obstruction may lead to devitalisation of the affected section of intestine, leading to toxic shock and peritonitis. Colic signs are sometimes also present with ileus. Dehydration is common in both functional and mechanical obstruction, and tends to be more marked if the proximal intestine is involved.

Diagnosis

Ultrasonography is the most useful tool; peristalsis is absent and the intestinal wall may appear oedematous. The intestine proximal to the obstruction is markedly distended, with the sections distal to it emptier than normal.

Differential diagnosis

Intussusception, pyloric outflow problem, rumen stasis.

Treatment/management/control

A mechanical obstruction can be corrected by an enterotomy, or by gut resection and anastomosis if devitalisation has occurred. Systemic rehydration may be sufficient in mild to moderate colon impaction.

Prokinetics may be tried for ileus, but little information on these drugs is available in the goat and prognosis is guarded. In horses, lidocaine is used prophylactically either intra- or postoperatively, but can also be used as treatment (loading dose of 1.3 mg/kg i/v followed by CRI of 0.03–0.05 mg/kg/minute). Similarly, metoclopramide may be used prophylactically or as a treatment (0.05 mg/kg i/m q6h). Erythromycin was found to have a positive effect on abomasal tone and emptying in cows, and is used in ileus in horses (2 mg/kg i/v in 100 ml of physiologic solution q12h). Another drug to consider is cisapride.

The risk of postoperative ileus is reduced by gentle tissue handling, keeping exposed intestinal sections moist during surgery, and prompt correction of dehydration.

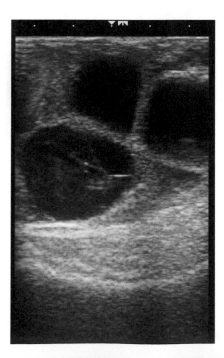

Fig. 5.38 Typical clover leaf appearance of intestinal incarceration in an inguinal hernia.

Rectal prolapse

Overview

Incomplete prolapse involves the mucosal layer only. Eversion of the entire caudal rectum is present in complete prolapse. Depending on the length of prolapsed tissue, mild to severe degrees are distinguished.

Aetiology

Tenesmus caused by rectal inflammation and irritation. Neurological dysfunction is a rare cause.

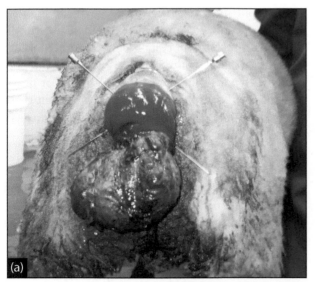

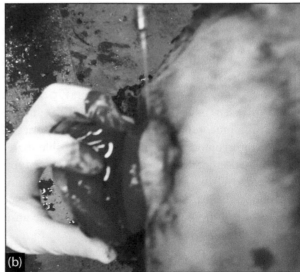

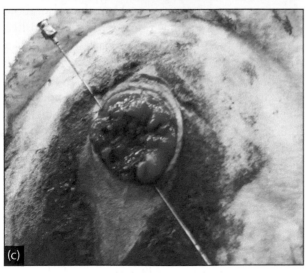

Fig. 5.39 Rectal prolapse in a ram. (a) Substantial tissue eversion exposing the rectal mucosa. Two metal pins (e.g. Steinman) have been placed through the prolapse at the level of the skin for temporary retention during surgery. (b) The prolapsed tissue is resected about 2 cm away from the skin junction. (c) Suturing of mucosa to skin completed and first metal pin removed.

Clinical presentation

Rectal tissue protrudes beyond the anus, with the mucosa exposed (**Fig. 5.39a**). It may be intermittent or permanent.

Diagnosis

Self-evident on clinical examination. For prognosis, the degree and extent of any tissue trauma should be established.

Differential diagnosis

Inexperienced keepers may confuse vaginal and rectal prolapse. Anal or rectal neoplasia may initially appear similar.

Treatment/management/control

Correction is under lumbosacral epidural anaesthesia (see Chapter 18). Addition of xylazine HCl (0.07 mg/kg) to the epidural is useful to prolong its effect. The goat is kept standing or placed into ventral recumbency.

A mild prolapse is replaced after cleaning the exposed tissue, followed by a purse-string suture placed subcutaneously around the anus using nylon tape or monofilament nylon. The suture is tightened to leave a one finger-width opening.

Tissue amputation is required in more severe cases. For a simple, but somewhat crude approach, a 10 ml syringe (or syringe case) open at both ends and with the plunger removed, is placed into the rectum. An elastrator ring is applied over the prolapsed tissue, compressing it onto the syringe. Ischaemic necrosis causes sloughing in a few days. Surgical correction involves placing two Steinman pins through the prolapsed tissue for temporary fixation (**Fig. 5.39a**). The prolapsed tissue is resected (**Fig. 5.39b**), and the remaining mucosa sutured to the skin in a series of simple interrupted sutures, using absorbable material. Digital guidance is used, because vision is typically obscured by mucosal haemorrhage. The pins are removed (**Fig. 5.39c**) and the remaining tissue replaced into the pelvis. NSAIDs and routine antibiosis are given.

The main complication is stricture formation.

Exploratory laparotomy
Indication
Exploratory laparotomy is a useful diagnostic tool to establish the nature of an abdominal problem. In most goats, all parts of the abdominal viscera can be at least palpated, and a large proportion exteriorised. Intraoperative ultrasonography is useful for those parts that cannot be exteriorised. For this, contact gel and the probe are placed into the finger of a sterile glove or sleeve to maintain asepsis.

Preparation and equipment
A compromised patient is stabilised with i/v fluids and any acid–base imbalance corrected (if detected or suspected). Any free rumen gas is released with the aid of a stomach tube to reduce abdominal pressure. The stomach tube may be left in place during surgery.

Standard surgery kit, bowel clamps, sterile solution for lavage, needles and tubing to release gas, suction if available, lap sponges and sterile fluid to keep exposed viscera moist, absorbable and non-absorbable suture material are required. Also euthanasia solution.

Restraint
Unless the goat is too compromised, surgery is best performed under GA for two reasons: (1) findings can be dealt with without time pressure; and (2) optimal surgical analgesia is provided. The latter is important, as handling of inflamed viscera will induce a marked pain response. If performed under local anaesthesia, additional analgesia could be provided with a morphine epidural, pethidine or possibly opioids (butorphanol, buprenorphine), but these drugs are not licensed for food producing animals in most countries.

Technical description
A left flank approach is indicated for suspected rumen problems, and allows rumenotomy and exploration of the reticulum. To reduce spillage of rumen contents, the goat is placed into sternal or 45-degree right lateral recumbency.

A ventral midline approach (**Fig. 5.40**) is indicated for a suspected intestinal problem, but also allows access to the urogenital tract, abomasum and liver (by palpation). A right flank approach gives access to the abomasum, liver (by palpation), urogenital tract and most parts of the intestine.

Regardless of the approach, it is important to explore both lateral and medial to the omentum, reflecting it where necessary. Viscera and tissues must be handled gently, and any exteriorised parts kept moist.

During exploration, the following are noted: amount, character and abnormal constituents of peritoneal fluid (**Fig. 5.41**), adhesions, abnormal location or distension of viscera (**Fig. 5.42**), viability of organs, foreign bodies and masses.

Prior to closure, consideration should be given to thorough lavage with warm sterile fluids, intra-abdominal antibiosis (e.g. benzylpenicillin sodium) and 1% carboxymethylcellulose (to reduce adhesions).

Depending on the findings and their prognosis, intraoperative euthanasia may be indicated.

Aftercare
Antibiosis, NSAIDs and analgesia, continued fluid therapy as necessary. Box rest until wound healed, plus possibly a belly bandage.

Potential complications
Peritonitis, adhesions, wound breakdown or herniation.

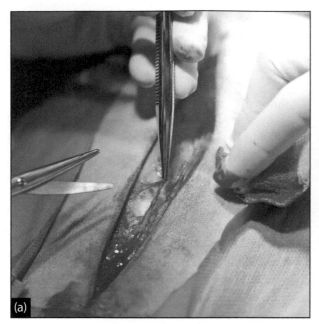 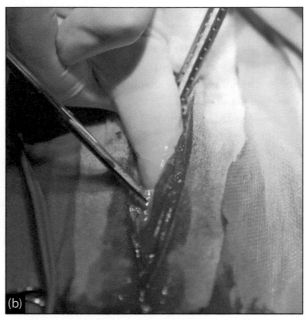

Fig. 5.40 Ventral midline laparotomy. The skin is incised with a scalpel blade; (a) the peritoneum is lifted up with a pair of rat-tooth forceps and cut with scissors; (b) once the incision is large enough, a surgeon's finger is introduced and the incision extended over the finger. This reduces the risk of accidental incision of any underlying structures, especially if they are distended.

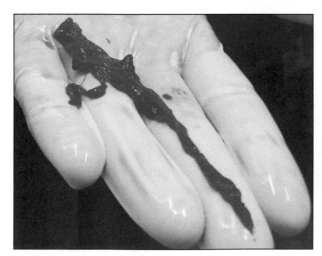 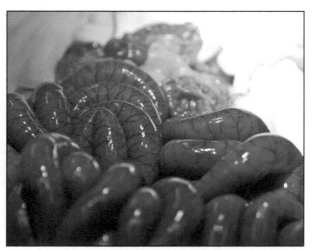

Fig. 5.41 Fibrin or protein clots in the peritoneal fluid indicates an inflammatory reaction.

Fig. 5.42 Distended jejunum proximal to an obstruction. The loops show a change in colour and fluid accumulation in the lumen, and peristalsis was largely absent. Note the healthy pink and collapsed intestinal loops in the background of the image.

Liver and pancreas problems

Normal structure and function

The liver lies encased in the ribcage in the cranial abdomen alongside the diaphragm, extending along the right-hand side. The right and left lobes are not further divided in the goat. The goat has a gallbladder.

The pancreas weighs about 50–70 g, and lies roughly between liver, right kidney and omasum.

Liver abscessation

Overview

Although not always causing overt clinical disease, liver abscessation can lead to substantial financial losses in meat goats because of carcase rejection at slaughter (**Fig. 5.43**), and poor performance in both dairy and meat animals.

Aetiology

Usually dietary, with excessive rapidly ferment-able carbohydrates leading to a ruminitis, followed by either direct migration of pathogens through the compromised rumen wall or dissemination via the portal vein into the liver. Because of the dietary aetiology, a large proportion of goats in a group are affected.

Clinical presentation

Half to two-thirds of liver parenchyma needs to be affected before overt clinical signs become apparent. These include jaundice, abdominal pain originating from the liver region and possibly enlargement of

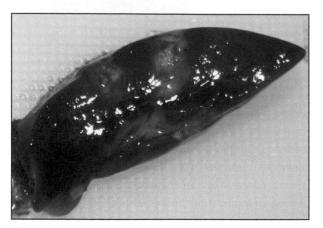

Fig. 5.43 Liver abscessation (in a cross-section). This is often a result of incorrect carbohydrate feeding management.

the liver, with non-specific signs of reduced appetite and milk yield.

An associated manifestation is caudal vena cava thrombosis (see Chapter 7).

Diagnosis

Ultrasonography to confirm abscessation. Blood biochemistry typically shows decreased albumin and elevated bilirubin and liver enzymes (gGT, GLDH, SDH), with a marked inflammatory response on haematology.

Liver abscessation can be detected at slaughter or PME.

Differential diagnosis

Other causes of abdominal pain or peritonitis. For jaundice, causes of acute haemolysis. Hepatic insult, including liver fluke, for elevated liver enzymes.

The ultrasonographic appearance may resemble neoplasia or tuberculosis lesions.

Treatment/management/control

There is no treatment option. Control centres on good management of carbohydrate-rich rations, including gradual introduction of carbohydrates, avoiding engorgement by making feed available truly *ad libitum*, and avoiding infrequent feeding of large amounts of carbohydrate (e.g. twice daily in-parlour feeding).

Hepatic lipidosis (syn. fatty liver necrosis)

See Chapter 14.

Ovine white liver disease

See Cobalt deficiency in Chapter 15.

Metastatic tumours

Malignant tumours may result in metastases in the liver. They may give a similar appearance to liver abscessation on ultrasonography or cursory PME (**Fig. 5.44**).

Pancreatic disorders

The few cases of pancreatic disorders reported include diabetes mellitus type I, insulinoma and congenital cystic disease.

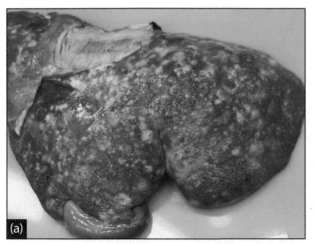
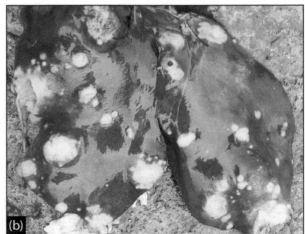

Figs. 5.44a, b Metastatic tumours affecting the liver.

Umbilical disorders

Normal structure and function

In the fetus, the umbilicus consists of the urachus connected to the urinary bladder, the umbilical vein leading to the liver, and two umbilical arteries connecting to the iliac arteries. When the cord is torn at birth, the arteries retract and the urachus and vein close. Normally, the external umbilical remnants dry out and are shed within about 7 days after birth.

Umbilical hernia

Overview

Umbilical hernia is one of the more common congenital defects, and is occasionally life-threatening.

Aetiology

This defect in the abdominal wall may be congenital, with a likely hereditary component, or occur secondary to umbilical infections. Hereditary hernias may jump one generation.

Clinical presentation

A well-circumscribed swelling along the ventral abdominal midline is present. In uncomplicated hernias, vital signs are normal, pain is absent and the hernia is easy to reduce manually. Rarely, either small intestine or abomasal fundus prolapses into the hernial sac, leading to colic signs and making full reduction difficult and inducing pain.

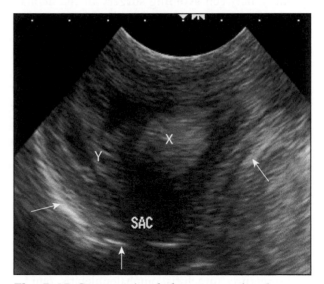

Fig. 5.45 Cross-sectional ultrasonography of an umbilical hernial sac (arrows). The umbilical remnant (X) is surrounded by some omentum (Y).

Other congenital defects may be present, affecting prognosis and treatment economics.

Diagnosis

The defect in the abdominal wall can be easily palpated after reducing the hernia. Ultrasonography is useful to establish whether any viscera have prolapsed into the hernial sac (**Fig. 5.45**).

Differential diagnosis

Similar swellings may be caused by an umbilical abscess, infected umbilical remnant or a haematoma.

A hernia may occur concurrently with other umbilical disorders (see below), and a thorough examination is required.

Treatment/management/control

If congenital, affected males should not be used for breeding. Unless the defect is very large or a visceral prolapse is present, repair is usually not necessary in goats reared for meat.

Females may be reared for milk or fibre production, providing that their offspring are not retained in the herd. Surgical repair (see Umbilical surgery) is advisable as the increased abdominal pressure during pregnancy may lead to problems. Delaying surgery until 2–3 months of age is a good compromise between avoiding surgery in the neonate while still dealing with a relatively small, manageable patient.

Occasionally, applying a belly bandage for a few weeks is sufficient to seal the hernia. Applying a rubber elastrator ring over the hernial sac is not advisable because necrosis and breakdown of the abdominal wall often follow.

Control centres on removing affected animals from the breeding pool.

Umbilical infections

Overview

Umbilical infections are usually chronic in nature. Infection may involve either the external remnant (omphalitis) or tissues (abscess) or the internal umbilical structures (urachitis, omphalophlebitis, omphaloarteritis). A hernia may be present concurrently.

Aetiology

Poor navel and environmental hygiene is the main cause. In group-housed kids, navel sucking may also play a role. A range of opportunistic and environmental pathogens are involved.

Clinical presentation

Infection of external structures presents as obvious swelling in the umbilical region, which is fluctuant in the case of an abscess. The swelling is non-reducible, or partially reducible if a hernia is also present. Occasionally, a draining tract is present. Pain on palpation is typically mild to moderate.

Infection of internal structures similarly presents as a swelling, more commonly accompanied by a discharging tract with pus visible at the point of the umbilicus (**Fig. 5.46**). Omphalophlebitis carries the risk of a bacteraemia. Vital signs may be abnormal and signs indicating infection of other structures may be present, in particular septic arthritis and endocarditis.

Diagnosis

With the goat in lateral recumbency, deep abdominal palpation will reveal thickened internal structures and whether these track cranially (= vein) or caudally (= arteries or urachus). Palpation will also establish the absence or presence of a hernia.

Needle aspiration establishes the presence of pus, taking care not to penetrate a hernial sac or adjacent structures.

Ultrasonography is very useful to establish the extent of infection and structures involved. The probe is initially placed at the junction of the abdominal wall with the external remnant (caudally and cranially, in turn) and then gradually rotated to visualise the abdominal cavity. This will highlight whether the external umbilical structures continue intra-abdominally and whether any internal structures are enlarged (**Fig. 5.47**) and/or filled with pus.

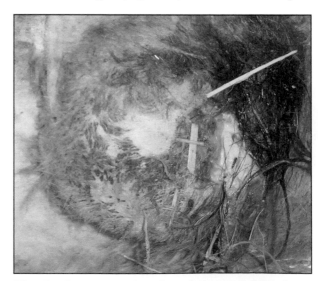

Fig. 5.46 Patent, infected urachus and umbilical hernia in a male calf (lying in lateral recumbency). Note the purulent discharge towards the right of the hernial sac (near the prepuce).

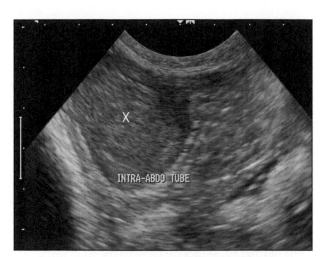

Fig. 5.47 The enlarged umbilical remnant (here in cross-section, labelled X) could be followed all the way from the hernial sac deep into the abdominal cavity on ultrasonography.

Differential diagnosis

A complicated hernia (i.e. one with a visceral prolapse) must be ruled out prior to needle aspiration or lancing.

Treatment/management/control

With the goat in lateral recumbency, an abscess (or identifiable pus-filled pocket in omphalitis cases) is lanced with a scalpel blade, followed by drainage and lavage with saline or a 0.1% iodine solution. Sedation and local anaesthesia are usually not necessary. Lavage is repeated once or twice daily for several days until the infection is resolved. Antibiosis is not required unless a hernia is also present for which surgical repair is planned. Such repair is delayed until the infection is brought under control.

Infected internal structures require surgical removal. If a drainage tract is present, careful lavage and antibiosis for a few days are used to partially control the infection prior to surgery.

Patent urachus
Overview

Patent urachus is a condition that requires surgical treatment to avoid discomfort and chronic inflammation from the resulting cystitis.

Aetiology

The urachus fails to close post partum, leaving a permanent connection with the urinary bladder. Concurrent infection is often present.

Clinical presentation

Urine escapes through the umbilical stump. While quite easy to detect in the female, close observation is required in the male because of the close proximity of the prepuce and umbilicus. Cystitis is a common sequela, causing dysuria, mild abdominal discomfort and abnormal urinalysis.

Diagnosis

Clinical observation is often sufficient, but may be confirmed with ultrasonography. Any concurrent infection of the urachus needs to be established in order to inform the treatment approach.

Treatment/management/control

Surgical removal of the urachus (see Umbilical surgery), with resection and oversewing of the bladder apex. Even in meat animals treatment is advisable, as urine staining of the ventral abdomen may lead to fly strike or rejection at the abattoir.

Umbilical surgery
Indication

Repair of an umbilical hernia or treatment of infected or patent umbilical structures.

Preparation and equipment

If infection is present, lavage and antibiosis are used to at least partially bring the infection under control prior to surgery. Cover against clostridial pathogens needs be considered (either vaccination, maternally derived antibodies or suitable perioperative antibiosis).

A generous area of the ventral abdomen is clipped and prepared. In the male, the preputial opening is covered with a sterile absorbent swab, held in place with a towel clamp.

A laparotomy surgical kit, including bowel clamps if the urachus involved, is required.

Restraint

The goat is placed in dorsal recumbency. GA is the method of choice in anything but a simple hernia to eliminate any time constraints. A simple hernia may be repaired under moderate to deep sedation, and V-shaped local infiltration (with the point of the V towards the sternum, and extending either side of the hernia).

Technical description
Simple hernia
In the female, an elliptical incision is made around the hernia, extending about 1 cm cranially and caudally. In the male, a pear-shaped incision is made with the blunt end just cranial to the prepuce. Care is taken in the male not to dissect too far laterally to avoid trauma to the nerves in the paramedian region that supply the retractor penis muscle. Excessive skin from the hernial sac is removed with the incision (**Fig. 5.48a**).

Closed reduction is preferable, especially for on-farm surgery, as the peritoneal cavity is not entered. For this, the skin over the hernial sac, including as much of the subcutaneous tissue as possible, is removed with a combination of blunt and sharp dissection. Tissues are separated thoroughly down onto the hernial ring. This is facilitated by placing Allis tissue forceps either side of the incision and the centre of the sac, and applying tension. The skin will be tightly attached to the sac near the umbilical scar, and accidental incision of the sac may occur (if it does, the resulting defect is oversewn). Once completely freed from surrounding tissues (**Fig. 5.48b**), the hernial sac is inverted into the abdomen. Suturing is as described below.

Infected internal structures or patent urachus
The skin incision around the hernia (as above) is extended cranially up to the xiphisternum for removal of the umbilical vein or, for removal of the umbilical arteries or urachus, caudally up to the pelvic inlet (midline in the female and just lateral to the prepuce in the male). This cranial/caudal incision is continued through the linea alba (after deflection of the prepuce in the male) into the abdominal cavity. The hernial sac is incised close to the ring, using digital guidance to avoid incision into viscera or omentum (**Fig. 5.49**), and the surplus tissue removed.

The proximal end of the infection is located, gently breaking down any adhesions while taking care not to rupture any abscess. Two pairs of artery forceps are placed across the uninfected, healthy part of the structure, followed by a double ligature using 3.5 metric absorbable suture material between the two pairs of forceps. The structure is transected between the distal pair of forceps and the ligature and removed together with the hernial sac. In cases of a patent urachus, artery forceps are placed across the proximal urachus. A bowel clamp is placed across the bladder apex and, after resection of the urachus, the bladder is closed with an inverting suture pattern.

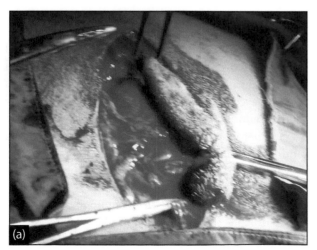
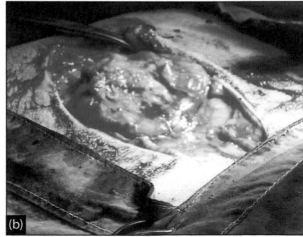

Fig. 5.48 Closed reduction of an umbilical hernia. (a) The elliptical skin incision around the hernia is made in such a way that excessive skin is largely removed. Here, the skin is already partially dissected from the underlying sac. (b) The hernial sac has been freed completely and is ready to be inverted into abdomen.

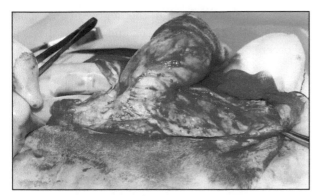

Fig. 5.49 Open reduction (here to remove an umbilical remnant). After making a small opening through the sac, the incision is extended under digital guidance.

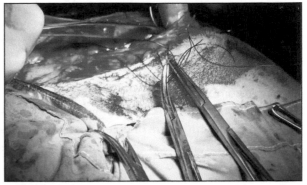

Fig. 5.50 When closing the defect, accurate placement is made easier by first placing all the sutures (securing the ends with artery forceps), then tying them off.

Closure of the defect

A modified Mayo-Mattress suture ('Vest-over-Pants' suture) or simple interrupted sutures are suitable to close the hernial defect, using 4 metric polydioxanone (PDS). Non-absorbable material may be used, but carries a higher risk of fistula formation. Sutures are placed through the outer edge of the hernial ring, using the index finger or the back of a scalpel holder inside the abdomen to push away any abdominal contents and to keep the hernial sac close to the abdominal wall during closed reduction. It is often easier to place all the required sutures first, securing their ends with artery forceps before tying them off (**Fig. 5.50**). The edges of the hernial defect should be overlapped (or pulled together for simple interrupted sutures) as closely as possible. The use of a polypropylene mesh implant is rarely required in a goat and is inadvisable if infection is present.

A simple continuous subcutaneous suture is placed, using 3 metric absorbable suture material and ensuring that the tissue covers the hernia sutures. The skin is closed with simple interrupted or cruciate sutures with 3.5 metric non-absorbable material. A rolled-up gauze swab can be placed over the wound as a stent, held in place with two stay-sutures (**Fig. 5.51**). Alternatively, a belly bandage is used.

Aftercare

NSAIDs are given. Repair of a simple hernia under sterile conditions does not require antimicrobials. Where infection is present, however, antimicrobials

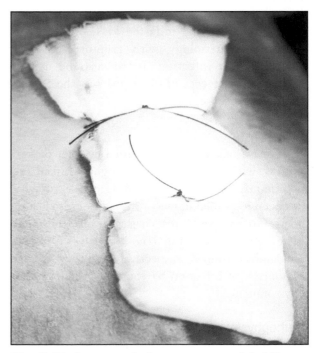

Fig. 5.51 A stent made from a gauze swab held in place with two stay sutures exerts some pressure over the wound and keeps it clean.

are administered for 3–10 days (longer duration where contamination occurred during surgery or if the entire infected structure could not be removed). Clavulanic-acid potentiated penicillin is suitable. The goat should be kept confined in a small pen for 6–8 weeks, with a companion animal to prevent escape attempts.

The stent or bandage is removed after 3 days in a female and 1–2 days in a male (when it becomes soaked with urine). Skin sutures are removed after 12–14 days.

Potential complications
Breakdown of the repair, caused by residual infection or weakness in suture or excessive exercise postoperatively. Peritonitis because of rupture or leakage of an infected structure during removal.

INFECTIOUS DISEASES OF THE DIGESTIVE SYSTEM AND ABDOMEN

Rotavirus
Definition/overview
Rotavirus is associated almost exclusively with diarrhoea in young, milk-fed kids, often as part of a mixed aetiology with cryptosporidia and *Escherichia coli* infection. It can also be demonstrated in the faeces of older goats in the absence of clinical disease.

Aetiology
Rotaviruses are classified within a number of serogroups, with reported disease in goats linked predominantly to groups A and B. Group C rotavirus has been identified in faeces from otherwise healthy goats. Group A and B rotaviruses are also commonly identified as causes of diarrhoea in calves (group A) and lambs (group B), respectively, and these may act as sources of infection to young kids and/or their environment.

Pathophysiology
Rotaviruses replicate in the non-dividing mature enterocytes near the tips of the villi in the small intestine, leading to progressive shortening of villi with villus fusion and thickening of the crypts. The villus surface area reduction leads to malabsorption, with the severity of the diarrhoea linked to the degree of villus damage.

Clinical presentation
Diarrhoea in kids <2 weeks old, most commonly in the first 7 days of life, the severity of which depends on the weight of infection, the degree of any hypogammaglobulinaemia present and the involvement of other concurrent enteric pathogens.

Diagnosis
Laboratory detection of group A and B rotaviruses by polyacrylamide gel electrophoresis (PAGE) or ELISA tests. Many commercially available ELISA kits marketed for detection in calves will detect only group A rotaviruses.

Differential diagnosis
Other causes of neonatal diarrhoea, such as cryptosporidia and *E. coli*, although rotavirus is often involved in mixed infections with these same pathogens. Also non-infectious causes, including dietary.

Treatment/management/control
Treatment is aimed predominantly at reducing the effects of diarrhoea (i.e. dehydration and resulting electrolyte imbalance).

Emphasis must be placed on attention to detail when rearing kids, particularly when they are reared artificially. Good colostrum management is a key factor, and many confirmed rotavirus incidents are linked to failure of passive transfer. Other risk factors include unhygienic kidding environment, overcrowding, unhygienic or haphazard feeding regimes, a cold and damp environment and concurrent disease.

Bovine rotavirus vaccines, given to does in late pregnancy, have been used with varying success. If used, it is important that kids receive colostrum from vaccinated does for 2–4 weeks after birth.

Cryptosporidiosis
Definition/overview
Cryptosporidium spp. infect a wide range of mammals and are highly prevalent in ruminants, particularly young calves, lambs and kids. The parasite is a major cause of severe diarrhoea in kids <4 weeks of age (**Fig. 5.52**), particularly in intensive systems of rearing. They are a significant zoonotic pathogen, being a particular risk to young children coming into contact with infected animal faeces (**Fig. 5.53**).

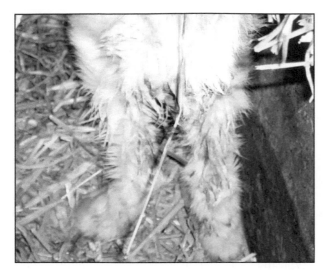

Fig. 5.52 Diarrhoea in a goat kid with confirmed cryptosporidiosis.

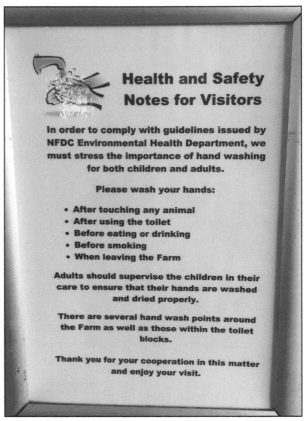

Health and Safety Notes for Visitors

In order to comply with guidelines issued by NFDC Environmental Health Department, we must stress the importance of hand washing for both children and adults.

Please wash your hands:

- After touching any animal
- After using the toilet
- Before eating or drinking
- Before smoking
- When leaving the Farm

Adults should supervise the children in their care to ensure that their hands are washed and dried properly.

There are several hand wash points around the Farm as well as those within the toilet blocks.

Thank you for your cooperation in this matter and enjoy your visit.

Fig. 5.53 Goat kids are popular at open farms. Suitable signs should be clearly visible emphasising the potential risks of zoonotic infections such as cryptosporidia and *E. coli* O157.

Aetiology

Cryptosporidia are small protozoal parasites in the phylum Apicomplexa. Over 150 species of mammals, reptiles, birds, amphibians and fish have been reported as hosts. Molecular techniques for taxonomic classification have identified many different species, a number of which have reportedly affected goats following both natural and experimental infection. While many such infections will be subclinical, disease in goats is almost always associated with *Cryptosporidium parvum*.

The oocyst stage responsible for transmission is ubiquitous in the environment and cryptosporidiosis can be acquired through a number of routes including goat to goat (directly or indirectly), from other ruminants (directly or indirectly) or by ingestion of contaminated food or drinking water.

Oocysts are very resistant in the environment and are able to survive the effects of many disinfectants. Products are available with declared efficacy of reducing environmental contamination.

Pathophysiology

Infection is by the ingestion of infected faecal material from the immediate environment. The severity of infection is linked to the dose of oocysts ingested (and hence degree of environmental contamination), the immune status of the goat (more severe in kids with poor passive transfer) and the presence of concurrent infection such as rotavirus and enteropathogenic *E. coli*.

Once the oocyst is ingested, it excysts and releases sporozoites that then colonise the intestinal enterocytes, followed by an asexual phase of schizogony, resulting in a new wave of infected cells by the release of merozoites. This is then followed by the sexual phase or gametogeny, resulting in further waves of enterocyte invasion and the production of oocysts in faeces and perpetuation of the life cycle. This process leads to progressive destruction of enterocytes and of the intestinal villus architecture, causing malabsorption and maldigestion and resulting in the clinical signs of diarrhoea.

Clinical presentation

Watery diarrhoea in kids usually aged between 5 and 14 days, rapidly leading to dehydration and electrolyte imbalance, dullness and inappetence. Cases will often become more severe and widespread as the kidding season progresses, and the weight of environmental infection increases. Explosive outbreaks of disease can be encountered in intensively reared kids, with up to 100% morbidity and up to 20% mortality (higher in mixed infections).

Diagnosis

Laboratory tests include the detection of oocysts in faecal smears stained with Ziehl–Neelsen (ZN) or Giemsa, faecal flotation, ELISA tests, fluorescent-labelled antibody tests and PCR.

Differential diagnosis

Other causes of neonatal diarrhoea, such as rotavirus and *E. coli*, although rotavirus is often involved in mixed infections with these same pathogens.

Treatment/management/control

Management and control are based on reducing environmental contamination with viable oocysts by:

- Ensuring a clean dry environment for rearing, with clean bedding that is regularly replenished.
- Ensuring kids have received adequate colostrum.
- Ensuring all feeding utensils are scrupulously clean.
- Ensuring that a consistent feeding regime is followed to avoid dietary upsets.
- Practicing an 'all-in-all-out' system, in particular avoiding the temptation to hold back poor performing kids.
- Practicing a thorough pen cleaning routine between batches of kids, removing all visual signs of faecal material, followed by steam cleaning and the use of disinfectants with a declared efficacy against oocysts.

There are no licensed therapeutic or prophylactic products for goats in most countries, but anecdotal evidence suggests that halofuginone lactate at lamb/calf dose rates and frequency may be beneficial in severe cases. Treatment is aimed predominantly at reducing the effects of diarrhoea (i.e. dehydration and resulting electrolyte imbalance).

Coccidiosis

Definition/overview

Coccidiosis is one of the most important and common causes of diarrhoea and ill thrift in young goats worldwide. It is caused by a protozoal parasite of the genus *Eimeria*. Although coccidiosis is a problem in many animals and birds, the causative *Eimeria* spp. are predominantly host specific (e.g. cattle *Eimera* spp. will not affect goats and vice versa). Goats of all ages may shed *Eimeria* spp. in their faeces, but it is only in younger goats that clinical signs will develop (typically between 4 weeks and 5 months old). Disease is more prevalent in goats that are housed or where stocking density on pasture is high, where environmental contamination can rapidly develop. Conversely, it is rarely encountered in extensive management systems.

Aetiology

Up to 20 different *Eimeria* spp. have been recorded in goats, some of which can cause severe disease; others can coexist in the gut with no adverse effect on the host. The most pathogenic species are *E. ninakohlyakimovae*, *E. caprina*, *E. christenseni*, *E. arloingi* and *E. hirci*. Consequently, relying on a coccidial oocyst count alone for diagnosis could give misleading results, since a high count of non-pathogenic oocysts is of no clinical significance whereas a lower count of a pathogenic species is highly significant. Confirming a mixed population of several species of *Eimeria* is not unusual. Identification is based on the size, shape and structure of each oocyst.

The life cycle is direct. Ingested oocysts sporulate and release their sporozoites, which enter the gut cells to produce schizonts. Following a cycle of asexual reproduction, a first generation population of merozoites is produced. These in turn break out from the cells and continue the cycle by further cell invasion in a process referred to as schizogony, of which a number of cycles can occur, thus creating a massive multiplication potential (**Fig. 5.54**). The cycle then moves to a sexual stage whereby male and female gametes are produced, resulting

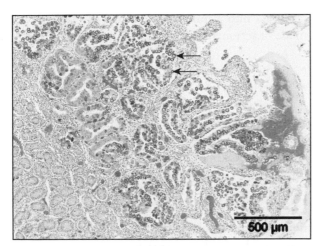

Fig. 5.54 *Eimeria* multiplication in intestinal wall (arrows indicate two examples of the developmental stage).

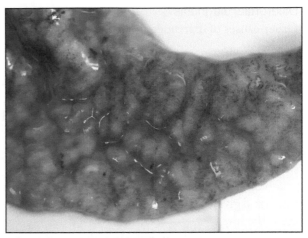

Fig. 5.55 Thickened ileum of a goat with chronic coccidiosis.

in fertilisation and the production of zygotes, further gut cell damage and the eventual release of a final population of oocysts. The ingestion of a single oocyst can result in the eventual excretion of up to one million oocysts.

Pathophysiology

The pathology is associated directly with the damage occurring at gut level as the life cycle progresses. The affected part of the gut may vary slightly depending on the dominant species involved, but the lower jejunum, ileum, caecum and colon can all be affected. There is variable inflammatory damage and haemorrhage at the mucosal level, with compensatory gut wall thickening (**Fig. 5.55**).

Clinical presentation

Clinical signs will usually develop 7–14 days following exposure to oocysts. The pathology results in diarrhoea, with bleeding and blood loss in severe cases. Affected goats may show tenesmus and abdominal pain in the acute phase, and rapidly deteriorate and die if untreated. Subclinical infection may lead to poor growth rates, dull coats and pasty faeces with perineal staining (**Fig. 5.56**). Recovered cases may remain stunted due to chronic gut damage and thickening of the gut wall. These chronic effects often cause the main economic loss in an affected herd.

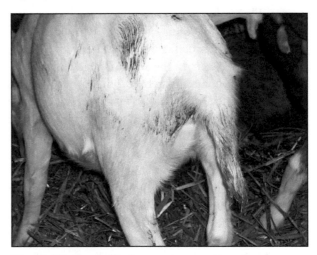

Fig. 5.56 Pot-bellied appearance and perineal staining in a goat with coccidiosis.

Diagnosis

Faecal oocyst counts, accompanied by speciation to assess whether pathogenic species are present. In the prepatent period, clinical signs can precede oocyst excretion. Hypoproteinaemia and hypoalbuminaemia can be marked.

At PME, there is characteristic thickening of the gut, often nodular in appearance (**Fig. 5.55**). Oocysts may be present in faeces or, in acute cases, schizonts may be identified in gut scrapes. Histological examination will show the developmental stages in gut sections with associated inflammatory change.

Differential diagnosis
Other causes of diarrhoea in young goats.

Treatment/management/control
Specific anti-coccidial products for use in sheep and cattle include decoquinate (for in-feed medication), diclazuril and toltrazuril, all of which have been used effectively in goats (off-licence) at sheep dose rates. Other products include ionophores, such as monensin and lasolocid, amprolium and sulphonamides.

Severely affected goats should be isolated, kept warm and given suitable fluid and electrolyte replacement therapy.

Control is based on reducing the oocyst environmental challenge. Ideally, young goats should be exposed to low levels of oocysts to allow immunity to develop, but this is difficult to achieve in practical terms. The problem is greatest on units where successive populations of young goats move through a rearing system, with inadequate cleaning between batches. Oocysts are resistant in the environment, and any faecal material or contaminated bedding from a previous batch of infected kids will provide a heavy challenge for the next batch. Oocysts can survive from one year to the next in contaminated litter. Buildings should be thoroughly cleaned between batches (using disinfectants with known anti-coccidial properties). An all-in-all-out system should be practiced; holding smaller stunted kids back may rapidly start a heavy oocyst challenge if they are chronic coccidiosis cases. Both in housed and in grazing groups, floor feeding should be avoided and feed troughs covered to reduce faecal contamination. Moving feed troughs every few days may also aid control.

Escherichia coli
Definition/overview
Unlike coli-enteritis in calves and lambs, there is very little evidence that *Escherichia coli* is a major problem in goats, but its potential role as a causative agent in neonatal diarrhoea outbreaks has been occasionally reported.

There is a zoonotic risk from the serotype O157.

Aetiology
E. coli is a ubiquitous organism, with many commensal organisms present as part of the background intestinal flora. Disease producing *E. coli* are classified into a number of groups describing their mode of action and virulence, including:

- Enterotoxigenic *E. coli* (ETEC).
- Enteropathogenic *E. coli* (EPEC).
- Enterohaemorrhagic *E. coli* (EHEC).
- Necrotoxigenic *E. coli* (NTEC).

The verotoxin producing EHEC, *E. coli* O157:H7, rarely causes illness in goats or other ruminants, but intestinal gut levels and faecal excretion rates can be high. The organism is an important zoonotic risk, particularly to young children, in which a potentially fatal haemorrhagic colitis and haemolytic uraemic syndrome can develop.

Pathophysiology
Disease producing *E. coli* (particularly ETEC and EPEC) are potent toxin producers, causing local damage to gut enterocytes by effectively adhering to the villi whereby toxins can be readily absorbed.

Clinical presentation
Diarrhoea is the main clinical presenting sign in neonatal kids. Heavy infection, particularly in immunocompromised animals, may result in more serious consequences such as colisepticaemia, with localisation of infection in, for example, joints or brain, or death from overwhelming septicaemia and toxaemia.

Diagnosis
Isolating *E. coli* from intestinal content, faeces or a rectal swab is insufficient evidence due to the ubiquitous nature of the organism and its presence in the gut of healthy goats.

More specific evidence includes the demonstration of specific fimbrial antigens such as F5 or F41, although their exact significance or global prevalence remains unknown. Histological examination of very fresh fixed intestine at PME has been used successfully to demonstrate the adherence capabilities of the bacteria.

Differential diagnosis
Other causes of neonatal diarrhoea such as rotavirus and cryptosporidia, although rotavirus is often involved in mixed infections with these same pathogens.

Treatment/management/control

Oral antibiotics effective against *E. coli*, together with parenteral antibiotic and NSAIDs in septicaemic cases, should accompany fluid therapy.

Attention to detail during kid rearing is key to controlling colibacillosis/colisepticaemia, mirroring the management points highlighted in the section on cryptosporidiosis.

E. coli vaccines are available for use in pregnant cows to boost colostral immunity, but there is limited evidence for their potential use in goats.

Salmonellosis

Definition/overview

Salmonellosis is a worldwide problem in a wide range of livestock systems including ruminants, pigs and poultry. Goats can be affected at any age. *Salmonella* organisms can also be carried asymptomatically by wild birds and vermin, which can readily introduce and spread new infections. The zoonotic risk includes close contact and food-borne infection via contaminated milk and undercooked meat. Salmonellosis is reportable in the UK.

Aetiology

A gram-negative, rod-shaped organism in the family Enterobacteriaceae. Salmonellae are classified according to their serotype or serovar, of which there are >2,000. The most commonly isolated salmonella serotype is *Salmonella typhimurium*, further classified according to its phage type (an important factor in epidemiological investigations). A wide range of other serotypes have been identified as potentially causing clinical signs in goats.

Pathophysiology

Following ingestion, organisms become established in the gut, resulting in an inflammatory enteritis and damage to enterocytes via potent endotoxins, resulting in severe diarrhoea. As gut damage progresses, organisms can gain access to the lymphatic system and hence to the blood stream, resulting in multisystemic infection. Whether carrier status can develop in goats is speculative.

Clinical presentation

Severe diarrhoea in goats of all ages is the most common clinical sign, often accompanied by the passage of blood, mucus and 'shredded' mucous membranes. Affected goats are often dull and pyrexic, and rapidly become dehydrated. If a bacteraemia/septicaemia develops, then a variety of other clinical signs may develop, including abortion in does and meningitis and septic arthritis in kids.

Diagnosis

Isolation of the infective organism from faeces or from gut content at PME. *Salmonella* organisms will grow readily on blood agar and MacConkey agar, but can also be enriched through selenite broth. Confirmation of serotype and phage type requires input from specialist laboratories.

Differential diagnosis

Differentiate from other causes of diarrhoea in goats by laboratory examination, particularly enterotoxaemia.

Treatment/management/control

Any suspect clinical case should be isolated and barrier nursing employed. A faecal sample is taken for laboratory confirmation. Treatment is most effective in the early stages and is based mainly on supportive fluid therapy and NSAIDs. Oral or parenteral antibiotics are widely used in clinical cases, but many serotypes have developed multiple antibiotic resistance profiles, so antibiotic selection should be guided by *in-vitro* sensitivity. Parenteral antibiosis in young goats may prevent other sequelae such as septic arthritis.

Any investigation into an outbreak of salmonellosis needs to be undertaken in depth to identify and hence eliminate the original source. Common routes of infection are:

- A purchased goat.
- Other livestock species in direct contact.
- Rodents or wild birds contaminating feed or water troughs.
- Infected slurry, sewage, bedding or litter (from any livestock species, including poultry, and humans).
- Contaminated feed.
- Boots and clothing of farm personnel and equipment.

Pooled faecal samples are useful to establish morbidity and, together with environmental samples, to monitor successful control.

Strict biosecurity aimed at keeping salmonellosis out of goat units and preventing spread between units is vital.

Salmonellosis vaccines are available for use in other species, with limited data on their effective use in goats.

Suspicion or confirmation of salmonellosis should always trigger an emphasis of the potential zoonotic risks to those working with or handling the goats, or consuming any unpasteurised milk or dairy product. Young children, the elderly and those on immunosuppressive therapy are most at risk. Some dairy herd contracts require the milk buyer to be informed.

Yersiniosis

Definition/overview

Yersiniosis has been reported in goats as a sporadic problem in many countries. It is most commonly associated with enteritis and with internal abscess formation. It has also been linked to abortions and mastitis.

Aetiology

Yersinia spp. are gram-negative, predominantly aerobic bacteria of the family Enterobacteriaceae. They are comparatively slow growing on blood agar, and the resultant small colonies can be overgrown by other colonies and easily overlooked. The two organisms associated with disease in goats are *Y. pseudotuberculosis* and *Y. enterocolitica*. It is a potential zoonotic infection. Wild birds and rodents represent a reservoir of infection, and have been linked to outbreaks of disease via contamination of feed supplies.

Pathophysiology

Both organisms are widely distributed in the environment, affecting a wide range of animals. It is likely that many new infections contracted by goats are eliminated with no evidence of clinical disease. Clinical disease is often linked to exposure to new infection and concurrent stress factors, such as exposure to cold wet weather, transport, overcrowding or excessive handling (particularly in feral goats).

Infection is via the oral route, leading to multiplication in the gut and gut wall colonisation. Local spread to lymphatics leads to the characteristic lymph node enlargement.

Clinical presentation

Although all ages of goat can potentially be infected, most cases occur in goats <12 months old. In the enteric form (as opposed to abortion), diarrhoea is the key feature, often with mucus. Incidents can be transient and self-limiting or progressive, leading to weight loss, particularly when mesenteric lymphatics are involved.

Differential diagnosis

Other causes of enteritis or diarrhoea.

Diagnosis

Diagnosis in the live goat is by isolation of the organism in faeces. Pathological changes include a characteristic enlargement of the mesenteric lymph nodes with marked oedema. Gut changes may be minimal, although focal areas of mucosal necrosis may be evident (**Fig. 5.57**).

Treatment/management/control

Treatment with antibiotics is effective in the early stages, together with supportive fluid therapy.

Control is problematic as the organism is ubiquitous in the environment of many domestic and feral goats and most cases are sporadic. Keeping feed stores bird- and rodent-proof is important, as is the need to keep stress factors such as handling and transport to a minimum, including provision of shelter from inclement weather.

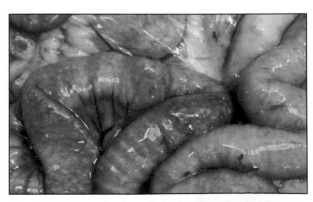

Fig. 5.57 Intestinal yersiniosis. Note the focal areas of mucosal necrosis.

Clostridium perfringens (syn. enterotoxaemia)

Definition/overview

Clostridium perfringens is one of the more important causes of diarrhoea (and death) in goats of all ages, although more prevalent in mature goats.

Aetiology

Caused by *C. perfringens*, an anaerobic, gram-positive, rod-shaped, spore-forming bacterium. It produces a number of potent exotoxins that characterise the specific *C. perfringens* types (*Table 5.2*).

C. perfringens type D is by far the most common cause of the condition referred to as enterotoxaemia. Types A and C have been occasionally linked to clinical disease, but incidents have been reported only sporadically. This section will focus on disease associated with type D.

The organism is a commensal in the intestinal tract of goats and other ruminants, is shed in the faeces and can be found in bedding and soil contaminated with the spores. It possesses the ability to multiply rapidly in gut content when stimulated.

Pathophysiology

Although goats can acquire infection from their environment, most cases result from the sudden multiplication of harmless low levels of bacteria in the gut, overgrowing other bacterial flora and producing high levels of its potent exotoxins.

Cases are more likely to develop in goats that are reared intensively or semi-intensively than those kept extensively, and the condition is rarely encountered in feral goats. The stimulus for overgrowth to occur and outbreaks to develop is most often associated with dietary changes such as:

- Sudden change in dietary constituents.
- Sudden increase in dietary intake.
- Turnout to lush grazing.
- Bringing in freshly cut green forage in zero-grazing systems.
- Accidental access to feed stores and overeating of grain, for example.

A build-up of infection in the environment will undoubtedly occur in outbreaks of disease in housed goats, and this may in turn increase the pathogen load in the gut of susceptible goats, creating a cyclical problem.

Sporadic incidents are often more difficult to explain, but may be linked to ill-defined stress factors such as:

- Parturition and periparturient problems.
- Environmental stresses such as excessive cold or heat.
- Concurrent illness such as severe foot lameness.

The resulting increased level of epsilon toxin appears to damage the gut wall, leading to increased vascular permeability and hence absorption, resulting in a gradually overwhelming toxaemia. The toxin is necrotising and also acts as a potent neurotoxin, causing severe damage to the brain and other vital structures.

Clinical presentation

Peracute cases commonly present as sudden death, particularly in younger goats.

In older goats, there is a sudden acute depression, pyrexia and inappetence, coupled with visible signs of abdominal discomfort such as arching of the back and kicking at the flank. Watery diarrhoea quickly develops, often with blood and shredded mucous membranes (**Fig. 5.58**). There may be ill-defined neurological signs, but affected goats can quickly become comatose as death approaches, all within a 12–24 hour time period.

In acute cases, the signs are less severe, and may progress over 2–4 days. Diarrhoea is persistent and

CLOSTRIDIUM PERFRINGENS TYPE	ALPHA (α)	BETA (β)	EPSILON (ε)
A	+	−	−
B	+	+	+
C	+	+	−
D	+	−	+

Table 5.2 **Exotoxins associated with different *C. perfringens* types.**

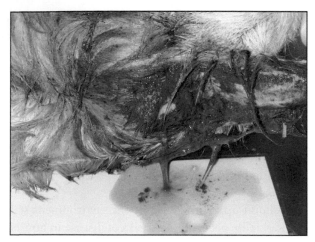

Fig. 5.58 Severe haemorrhagic diarrhoea in a confirmed enterotoxaemia case.

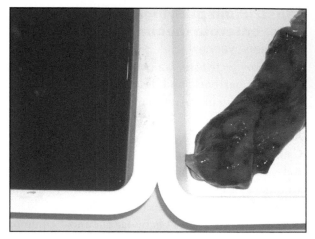

Fig. 5.59 Ileal content (pure blood) and section of colon wall showing ulceration in an enterotoxaemia case.

watery in consistency. Affected goats are often inappetent, but less frequently exhibit signs of abdominal discomfort. As the condition progresses, they become dehydrated and acidotic.

A chronic form has also been described: it is an ill-defined presentation in which affected goats, usually housed intensively, show progressive weight loss, reduced milk yield and soft pasty faeces. It is thought to be related to heavy and constant environmental challenge causing low-grade gut damage due to toxin release in vaccinated goats.

Diagnosis

Diagnosis is based on a combination of clinical signs and recent history. At PME, the most consistent finding is an enterocolitis. In severe cases, the gut wall is intensely congested with pinpoint haemorrhages, ulceration, mucous membrane sloughing and content that may be pure blood (**Fig. 5.59**). In less severe cases, gut wall changes may be fibrinous and gut content often copious and liquid in consistency. Other features include pulmonary and mesenteric lymph node oedema. The hydropericardium associated with pulpy kidney in sheep (also caused by *C. perfringens* type D) is not a feature in goats. Renal tubular necrosis has been described, and this may lead to visible softening of the kidney cortex (in fresh carcases).

Being a commensal, the isolation of *C. perfringens* from gut content or faeces is not confirmatory, but the heavier the growth the more significant the finding. Impression smears of the intestinal mucosa (in fresh carcases) may demonstrate high numbers of gram-positive, rod-like organisms. The most useful test confirms the presence of epsilon toxin in intestinal content or faeces using either an ELISA test or a number of PCR tests – approximately 5 ml of gut content or faeces are submitted. The toxin is labile, however, and rapidly degrades as the carcase autolyses.

Differential diagnosis

Peracute cases need to be differentiated from other causes of sudden death such as plant or chemical poisoning, acute listeriosis, anthrax or abdominal catastrophies. For acute haemorrhagic diarrhoea, salmonellosis is the main differential. Parasitic gastroenteritis (PGE) should be considered for acute, watery diarrhoea.

Treatment/management/control

Treatment success is directly proportional to the severity of the condition. Comatose goats and those passing haemorrhagic diarrhoea carry a poor prognosis. Supportive therapy is important, providing warmth and i/v or oral fluid therapy. Antibiotics may reduce further bacterial proliferation in the gut, and gut active astringents may be helpful, together with NSAIDs. If available, *C. perfringens* epsilon antitoxin may also be of benefit.

Because this is an unpredictable disease that develops when a gut commensal becomes overgrown for a variety of often ill-defined reasons, the universal advice is that all goats (particularly those kept intensively or semi-intensively) should be vaccinated against the condition. It is preferable (unless other clostridial conditions are a known local problem) to use vaccines that contain a minimal number of clostridial antigens, but ensuring that *C. perfringens* type D and *C. tetani* are covered. In most countries, sheep vaccines have to be used in the absence of licensed goat products. The immune response to vaccination is of a shorter duration than in other ruminants, and the recommendation is to boost at least every 4–6 months following the primary course; even then the immunity imparted appears to be variable.

Booster doses should be given strategically 3–4 weeks before perceived risks such as anticipated feed changes or transport. Boosting pregnant does 4–6 weeks prior to kidding will enhance colostral immunity for suckling kids. These should then receive their first dose of vaccine around 4–6 weeks of age, giving three doses for the primary course to account for any immaturity of their immune system and presence of maternally-derived antibodies.

Johne's disease (syn. paratuberculosis)
Definition/overview
Johne's disease is a worldwide problem causing clinical disease in intensively managed ruminants including goats. Many wildlife species including rabbits are able to carry and thus maintain infections locally, and can also spread the organism from unit to unit. It is now recognised that there are specific cattle and sheep isolates, with most goat infections identified as cattle strains. Goats will contract infection from other goats, from cattle (and more rarely sheep) kept in close association or from faecal contamination of their environment.

Aetiology
The main causative organism of Johne's disease in goats is the cattle strain *Mycobacterium avium* subsp. *paratuberculosis* (MAP). Once introduced into a group of goats, uncontrolled infection progressively becomes established and can be very difficult to eradicate.

Infection is mainly transmitted to young kids <6 months old by ingestion of faecally contaminated feed or water supplies and also potentially from contaminated teats and udder while suckling. Contamination of pooled colostrum can readily transmit new infection to a group of susceptible kids. There is also confirmed intrauterine infection of kids, from dams that are heavily infected in late pregnancy. Goats >6 months of age become progressively more resistant to new infection, although lateral spread even in adult goats may occur if the environment becomes heavily infected.

Although susceptible to sunlight and desiccation, MAP organisms can reportedly survive for up to 1 year on pasture (not forgetting potential maintenance in local wildlife).

Pathophysiology
There is an extended incubation period during which infected goats will appear fit and healthy, but may be shedding organisms in their faeces, thus adding to the environmental challenge.

Clinical signs may develop from 12 months of age, but more commonly from around 2.5 years old. The stimulus for infection to become clinical is still poorly understood, but may include stressful incidents such as kidding, transportation, poor nutrition or concurrent disease such as endoparasitism.

After infection, MAP localises in the wall of the ileum, lower jejunum and associated lymph nodes. This in turn stimulates a local macrophage response, resulting in phagocytosis and a progressive thickening of the gut wall and lymph node enlargement. Depending on a number of host-to-pathogen factors, this infection may then be controlled with the goat becoming resistant to infection with no further shedding or clinical disease, or the infection may progress to intermittent shedding and subclinical disease or become clinical with heavy shedding. In an endemically infected herd, it is likely that all three manifestations are present, thus further complicating its control.

Clinical presentation
Initial clinical signs may be subtle, including progressive weight loss and reduction in milk yield, with appetite often unaffected. As the condition develops, anaemia and a lacklustre coat may become apparent together with submandibular oedema as a result of the progressive hypoalbuminaemia. The diarrhoea

associated with the disease in cattle is not a feature of the condition in goats until the terminal stages.

Diagnosis

There is no single reliable test that can be used to confirm infection because of the complex aetiopathogenesis and long period of latent infection in clinically healthy goats. The organism demonstrates typical acid fastness when stained with ZN, either in the faeces of live goats or at PME in the lower bowel content or intestinal scrapes. Growth on culture is very slow, with colonies often not visible for 6 weeks. Serum antibody responses in infected goats prior to the development of clinical signs are poor, becoming stronger as clinical disease develops. Therefore, false-negative results are common with currently available commercial tests such as ELISA during the dormant period, with sensitivity increasing as clinical disease develops. PCR techniques have added to diagnostic tools.

- *Clinically healthy goats:* most available tests are ineffective during this phase of disease; there will be little if any humoral response detectable, and the sporadic shedding of organisms in faeces may be below detectable limits.
- *Infected goats in early clinical phase:* humoral antibody levels and shedding begin to rise, and faecal examination, using ZN stains, culture and PCR techniques, begins to give fewer false-negative results, but overall sensitivity remains low. Goats

may give a positive result on one day, then a negative result when retested – these goats will invariably retest as positive in time.
- *Infected goats in advanced clinical phase:* sensitivity of all available tests increases, as the humoral response becomes stronger and faecal shedding increases.
- *Valuable or pet goats:* laparotomy and histopathological examination of lymph node biopsy tissue has been described.

At PME, the gut wall thickening evident in the lower jejunum and ileum is more subtle (**Fig. 5.60**) than that seen in cattle, in which 'corrugation' and apparent folding of the mucosal surface is evident. This sectional subtle thickening may be palpable when the unopened gut is passed between finger and thumb. On opening, the affected mucosa has a velvet appearance with mucosal fissures. Mesenteric lymph nodes may be grossly enlarged and oedematous, with caseation and even calcification (**Figs. 5.61, 5.62**) being a feature of later stage infections.

Histological examination of affected gut or associated lymph nodes reveals the acid-fast organisms within infected macrophages (**Fig. 5.63**). ZN smears can be undertaken on intestinal mucosal scrapes, content can be cultured or PCR techniques can be undertaken. An ELISA test can be performed on blood taken from fresh carcases.

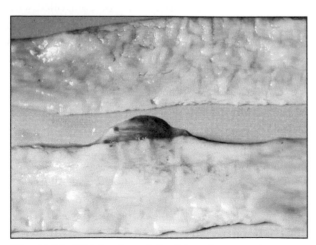

Fig. 5.60 Thickening of the jejunal mucosa in Johne's disease (paratuberculosis).

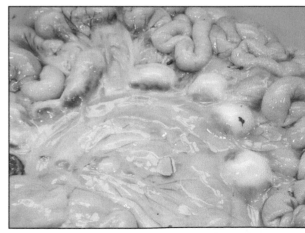

Fig. 5.61 Enlarged mesenteric lymph nodes in Johne's disease (paratuberculosis).

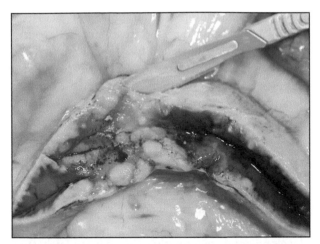

Fig. 5.62 Section of lymph node showing caseation and calcification in Johne's disease (paratuberculosis).

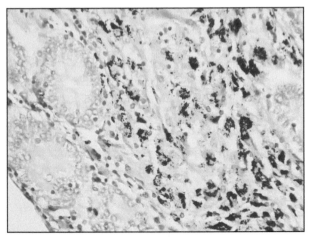

Fig. 5.63 Macrophages stained with ZN showing reddish–purple acid-fast mycobacteria.

Bulk milk monitoring is utilised widely in dairy cattle, and may in time be available when validated for dairy goat herds.

Differential diagnosis

Differential diagnoses for the combined signs of weight loss, reduced milk yield and anaemia in the absence of diarrhoea include fasciolosis and haemonchosis. At PME, lesions may appear similar to tuberculosis.

Treatment/management/control

There is no known treatment for Johne's disease.

Effective control is difficult to achieve, because of the long subclinical incubation period, shedding by these subclinical goats and the low sensitivity of the currently available tests.

Eradication may be achieved over several years, but will need considerable commitment by the herd owner and attending veterinarian. It is based on regular whole herd testing using serology and faecal monitoring, with culling of test-positive goats. Two consecutive negative herd tests are the ultimate aim. An alternative to culling is to separate positive and negative goats into a clean and dirty herd.

Such a control programme must be supported by:

- Prompt identification and removal of clinical cases.
- Minimising faecal contamination of feed and bedding, particularly for young kids.

- Snatching kids at birth and rearing away from adults.
- Feeding colostrum from test-negative dams, possibly combined with pasteurisation, and avoiding the use of pooled colostrum.
- Culling kids born to does developing disease or becoming test positive in late pregnancy (because of the risk of *in-utero* infection).

Control can also be achieved in endemically infected herds by the use of vaccination, widely available and licensed for use in goats in many countries. Vaccination will result in far fewer clinical cases and increased productivity, but will not eradicate infection, effectively allowing a unit to continue in production. Vaccination may influence an animal's response to intradermal tuberculosis testing, and its use must be declared to, or approved by, the animal health organisation in some countries.

Parasitic gastroenteritis

Definition/overview

Abomasal and intestinal nematode infestation is one of the most important diseases of goats worldwide, particularly in those kept outdoors for all or part of the time. Clinical signs may vary from weight loss and reduced milk yield to marked disease and rapid mortality. The biology and life cycle of these parasites is similar to that in other grazing ruminants, but there are a number of important and often subtle differences in goats including:

- An apparent inability to produce age-dependent resistance (possibly because of their evolutionary development as 'browsers' with less pasture exposure than 'grazers', resulting in a poor or defective IgE response).
- A poor understanding of the pharmacokinetics of many of the commonly used anthelmintics.
- A potential need to use anthelmintic dose rates exceeding those recommended for use in sheep and cattle.

Many commercially reared goats such as those in the dairy sector will be housed continuously, thus removing the disease and production risk that exposure to nematodes would pose (**Fig. 5.64**).

Aetiology

The species of nematodes affecting goats are identical to those of both sheep and cattle with some minor exceptions. The parasites that contribute predominantly to clinical disease belong to the genera *Teladorsagia/Ostertagia*, *Cooperia*, *Nematodirus*, *Oesophagostomum*, *Trichostrongylus*, *Strongyloides* and *Trichuris*, and to *Haemonchus contortus*. There is variation between and within countries as to the locally significant nematode population, and the strategic use of laboratory testing enables the establishment of prevalence patterns. This in turn facilitates the development of suitable control programmes.

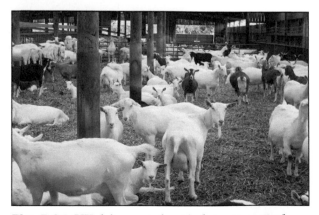

Fig. 5.64 UK dairy goats kept indoors to control parasitic gastroenteritis.

An understanding of the basics of nematode life cycles is important for treatment and control attempts. The superfamily Trichostrongylidae, which includes some of the genera above, has a direct life cycle, with adults in the alimentary tract producing eggs that are voided in faeces, thus contaminating the pasture (so-called 'patent infestation'). Eggs hatch, then pass through two larval stages to the infective third stage larvae (L3), which migrate onto surrounding herbage where they are ingested by the grazing animal. The time period between ingestion of L3 and the appearance of worm eggs in the faeces is typically between 16 and 21 days. The developmental stages within the goat are fairly standard, but those taking place outside the goat can be very variable depending on environmental conditions. Under favourable conditions, hatching of the eggs and development to L3 takes around 7–10 days. However, this can be prolonged (and very unpredictable) in periods of drought or cold weather. Both eggs and larvae are able to survive in pasture from one season to the next.

Pathophysioloy

As with all host–parasite relationships, the pathogenic effects of acquired worm burdens depend on:

- The species of worms and stages of life cycle present.
- The numbers of worms present.
- The predilection site – abomasal worms are generally the more pathogenic.
- The host's age and immunity, which directly affects the worm populations and pathogenicity.

Teladorsagia/Ostertagia nematodes present in the abomasum cause symptoms and pathology similar to those seen in cattle and sheep. Parasitised gastric glands are hyperplastic and contain undifferentiated cells leading to increased abomasal pH and leakage of pepsinogen into the plasma. Macroscopically, infected glands appear as raised nodules which, in heavy infections, coalesce to produce a 'morocco leather' effect, sometimes leading to mucosal necrosis and sloughing with oedema and hyperaemia present. The reduction in functional gastric mucosa leads to impaired digestion and diarrhoea.

Infection with intestinal nematodes produces villous atrophy and crypt hyperplasia. Resultant rapid cellular turnover of immature epithelial cells permits loss of fluid and plasma proteins into the intestinal lumen, causing a protein-losing enteropathy. There is also a deficiency in brush border enzymes that affects nutrient absorption.

H. contortus is a blood sucking nematode (larvae and adults) in the abomasum, causing anaemia.

Clinical presentation

Signs can be encountered in goats of any age, including adults that may have been exposed regularly, because of the poor or variable immunity produced.

Clinical signs will depend on the factors already outlined, together with recent grazing history. With the exception of *H. contortus*, these signs may vary from weight loss/poor weight gain and reduced milk yield, to severe watery diarrhoea leading to hypoalbuminaemia, dehydration and death (**Fig. 5.65**).

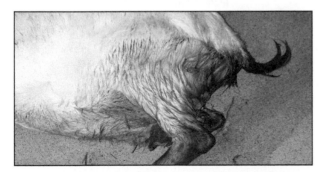

Fig. 5.65 Severe diarrhoea in a case of acute parasitic gastroenteritis.

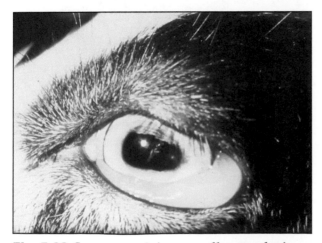

Fig. 5.66 Severe anaemia in a case of haemonchosis.

Progressive faecal staining of the hind end is often present. Heavy burdens of *H. contortus* can produce acute anaemia (**Fig. 5.66**) and death; lighter burdens may produce an iron deficiency anaemia and oedema, which may manifest as submandibular oedema, with faecal consistency unchanged.

Diagnosis

Traditionally based on faecal egg counts (FECs) in live goats (**Fig. 5.67**), although this relies on the presence of a mature, egg-laying (patent) worm burden, and can lead to false-negative results in prepatent burdens. Interpreting the significance of FECs must take account of age of goat and clinical signs present (e.g. there often is poor correlation between FEC and actual worm burden in mature goats). As a general guide, FECs in excess of 2,000 epg are usually clinically relevant. Counts of 500–2,000 epg are suggestive of subclinical parasitism and subsequent reduced production.

In haemonchosis cases, haematology may confirm a clinical suspicion of anaemia coupled with low serum albumin levels. An additional diagnostic aid is the FAMACHA© system developed in South Africa, initially for use in sheep, but also validated for use in goats. It uses a laminated card with five different colour shades representing the varying degrees of anaemia evident in the conjunctival mucous membrane (**Fig. 5.68**, *Table 5.3*).

At PME, pathological changes in the gut are relatively non-specific, although some larger nematodes may be clearly evident in gut content,

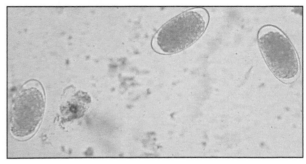

Fig. 5.67 Faecal egg counts are an important part of the development of an anthelmintic control programme.

such as *H. contortus* in the abomasum (**Fig. 5.69**). Investigation is based on identification of nematode burdens in the abomasum and intestinal tract following standard gut washing techniques, supported by FECs.

Differential diagnosis

Other causes of weight loss and diarrhoea such as enterotoxaemia, salmonellosis and coccidiosis. For haemonchosis, include Johne's disease, fasciolosis, other causes of anaemia or dependent oedema (see Chapter 7).

Treatment/management/control

Successful management and control requires a sound knowledge of the life cycle of the parasites and the resultant host response. Several countries disseminate parasite forecasts, highlighting particular risk periods. *Nematodirus battus*, with its mass hatching in spring, is a good example where these forecasts are invaluable, allowing pre-emptive management. Because of the many shared nematodes with grazing sheep and cattle, any control programme on a mixed stock unit must be integrated.

Anthelmintic resistance is becoming a serious issue worldwide, thus anthelmintics must be used appropriately and correctly, and always be combined with pasture management steps to reduce pasture burden. Owners should be encouraged to monitor faecal egg output regularly (**Fig. 5.70**) and only treat where there is clear clinical, FEC or post-mortem evidence of PGE. Criteria to identify goats for targeted selective treatment, based on production efficiency, weight gain and diarrhoea score, are being evaluated. Epidemiological studies in grazing dairy herds show that within a herd, first lactation does and high-yielders are most at risk of high worm burdens, and could be considered for targeted selective treatment.

To prevent introduction of resistant nematodes by incoming stock, the following protocol is recommended: sequentially administer two different classes

Table 5.3 **The FAMACHA© categories and corresponding parameters.**

CATEGORY	CONJUNCTIVAL MEMBRANE COLOUR	PACKED CELL VOLUME (l/l)	TREATMENT RECOMMENDED
1	Red	≥0.28	No
2	Red-pink	0.23–0.27	No
3	Pink	0.18–0.22	Possibly
4	Pink-white	0.13–0.17	Yes
5	White	≤0.12	Yes

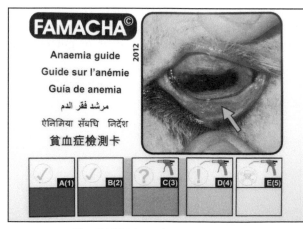

Fig. 5.68 The FAMACHA© chart is a simple tool to check for anaemia based on conjunctival mucous membrane colour. It has proven effective for early detection and selective anthelmintic treatment in the control of haemonchosis.

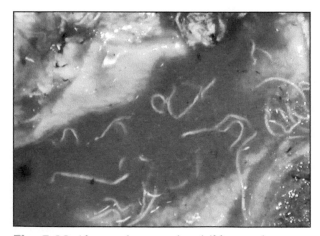

Fig. 5.69 Abomasal nematodes visible grossly.

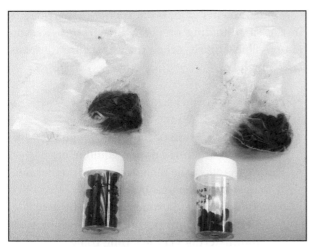

Fig. 5.70 Regular faecal egg monitoring. Screw top containers are preferable to plastic bags for sample submission.

Table 5.4 **Comparison of suggested anthelmintic dose rates in sheep and goats.**		
	SHEEP	**GOATS**
Group 1: benzimidazole	5 mg/kg	10 mg/kg
Group 2: levamisole	7.5 mg/kg	12 mg/kg
Group 3: ivermectin	0.2 mg/kg	0.3–0.4 mg/kg
Group 3: doramectin	0.2 mg/kg	0.2–0.4 mg/kg
Group 3: moxidectin	0.2 mg/kg	0.2–0.4 mg/kg
Group 4: monepantel (see comment in text on its use)	2.5 mg/kg	3.75 mg/kg

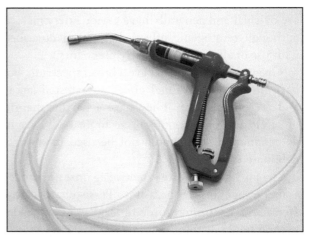

Fig. 5.71 Automatic dosing gun used for anthelmintics. The angulation of the nozzle must be taken into account when placing it into the oral cavity.

of anthelmintic, hold animals in a solid floored pen for 2–3 days, incinerate faeces and any bedding, then turn out onto 'dirty' pasture (i.e. already contaminated with nematode eggs). The two new classes of anthelmintic (see below) may be used for this quarantine drenching.

Management by zero grazing is particularly successful and practised by many large commercial units.

For haemonchosis, an additional control measure is the injectable vaccine Barbervax®. It reduces excretion, thus resulting in lower pasture contamination and reduction in disease, and is reportedly effective against anthelmintic resistant strains. Jointly developed by researchers in the UK and Australia, it is currently being assessed for efficacy in goats.

Identifying the genetic basis for individual goat resilience and resistance is being explored, and may offer selective breeding options in future.

Choice of product and route of administration

There are few, if any goat-specific anthelmintic products worldwide, and in many countries there are no authorised or licenced products available. As a result, in Europe, for example, products are used under the veterinary prescribing cascade.

One problem this lack of goat-specific products has led to is the paucity of information on efficacy, dose rates and pharmacokinetic properties of the main anthelmintic groups in the goat, and it is now recognised that using recommended sheep dose rates may have resulted in underdosing, possibly increasing the resistance risk.

The three most widely available groups of anthelmintics are all effective in goats, but at higher dose rates: *Table 5.4* is based on observations and recommendations cited worldwide. Oral products provide more consistent results than injectable or topical products (**Fig. 5.71**). The benzimidazole group is only available in oral forms. Both s/c and oral levamisole will yield similar good efficacy, since the active ingredient is rapidly absorbed by both routes. However, following s/c administration absorption is extremely rapid, with higher peak plasma concentrations that are more likely to cause toxic reactions. Oral absorption is slower, producing a lower peak and thus greater safety. For macrocyclic lactones the oral route is the most effective since the worm has the greatest contact with the product, even though studies show higher bioavailability after s/c administration. In addition, the period of residual subtherapeutic levels is reduced following oral administration, therefore there is less selection for resistance. Any oral anthelmintic should be administered at the back of the oral cavity to avoid spillage and potentially trigger a stronger oesophageal groove reflex.

Group 1 products are broad spectrum and very effective against arrested hypobiotic larvae. They are ovicidal and generally have a wide safety margin (although teratogenic effects have been described with use of albendazole in early pregnancy).

Group 2 products also have a broad spectrum, but have no or only minimal effect on arrested larvae and are not ovicidal. They have a narrow margin of safety in goats, requiring accurate body weight determination, and should not be used in severely debilitated animals.

Group 3 products are effective against nematodes and a range of ectoparasites. Persistence against *H. contortus* has been recorded as 22 days for moxidectin and 14–25 days for doramectin. Eprinomectin as a pour-on preparation has a product licence in some countries for use in goats. The pharmacokinetics in goats are relatively unknown, and results have often been disappointing with suboptimal nematode kill rates.

Group 4 and 5 are two new classes of anthelmintic, now available as 'prescription only' products in many countries (Group 4 AD: monepantel; Group 5 SI: derquantel). It is important that use of these new classes is kept under control, particularly as isolated cases of nematode resistance to monepantel have arisen in various countries including the Netherlands, New Zealand and Uruguay (associated with a very high frequency of monepantel use on the premises).

Apparent failure of efficacy

Inherent problems of controlling nematodes in goats may contribute to apparent failure, but more common is owner error or inexperience (particularly in the smallholding or pet/hobby sector). Reasons for possible failure, other than anthelmintic resistance, include:

- Dosing with insufficient anthelmintic:
  - Incorrect dose rate.
  - Underestimation of the goat's weight.
  - Poorly maintained dosing equipment.
- Failure to follow the manufacturer's instructions:
  - Not storing the product correctly.
  - Using products beyond their use-by date.
  - Mixing anthelmintics with other products.
  - Administering via the wrong route.
- Rapid reinfection from heavily contaminated pastures.

If anthelmintic resistance is suspected, then post-dosing FEC (drench testing), FEC reduction testing or *in-vitro* larval development and egg hatch assays can be undertaken.

Guidelines to limit anthelmintic resistance

Several countries have developed guidelines because of the concern over rising resistance to anthelmintics in grazing animals. If not checked, this resistance could have a catastrophic impact on animal welfare and economic production worldwide. It is recognised that anthelmintics are a necessary part of nematode control, but their use must be judicious and effective. UK guidelines include SCOPS (sustainable control of parasites in sheep) and COWS (control of worms sustainably). The principles can be applied to goats, and advice points veterinarians can apply include:

Do:

- Encourage the development of farm health planning including worming strategies.
- Establish full grazing management programmes and regular FECs to reduce treatment needs.
- Target the drug used to the parasite (and stage) to be treated.
- Leave proportion of group untreated to preserve susceptible worm population.

- Emphasise and avoid the common reasons for underdosing: underestimation of body weight, maladministration of the product or lack of calibration of the dosing device.
- Depending on the product used, do not move treated animals immediately onto clean pasture.
- Explain and emphasise the importance of quarantining incoming animals and give individual guidance on their treatment.
- Investigate suspected clinical cases of resistance and advise on the selection of alternatives from other classes.
- Report suspected cases of lack of efficacy to the relevant authorities.

Do not:

- Treat unnecessarily or randomly.
- Blanket treat.

(**Note:** The same anthelmintics and principles are applicable to the control of lungworm [see Chapter 6, p. 173].)

Liver fluke (syns. fascioliasis, fasciolosis)

Definition/overview
Liver fluke infection is a widely reported problem around the world. It is a parasite shared with other ruminant species, and can be a major constraint on production.

Aetiology
Disease is caused predominantly by the two trematode parasites, *Fasciola hepatica* and *Fasciola gigantica*. *F. hepatica* has the widest distribution, with *F. gigantica* limited to the more tropical areas of Africa, Asia and the Middle East.

Pathophysiology
The life cycle of both parasites is an indirect one, involving a mud/water snail of the family Lymnaeidae, of which many species have been identified. In the UK, for example, it is *Galba truncatula* that maintains the fluke population in the local environment. The mature flukes inhabit the gallbladder and bile ducts. Eggs voided in faeces pass through

a number of developmental stages involving the intermediate host, before being available again to be ingested with herbage and complete the life cycle. Following ingestion, the immature flukes migrate through the gut wall across the abdominal cavity to the liver, where they penetrate the liver capsule eventually ending up in the biliary system. In large numbers severe parenchymatous damage and capsular haemorrhage can occur, resulting in acute fasciolosis. Mature flukes may survive in the bile ducts and gallbladder for 3–4 years, and during this phase result in chronic fasciolosis.

Clinical presentation
The acute form can be encountered in goats (**Fig. 5.72**), sometimes presenting as sudden death from severe internal haemorrhage. More typically, affected goats show progressive weakness, anorexia and marked pallor of mucous membranes. Respiratory rate may be markedly elevated in response to anaemia. In the chronic form, depending on the degree of damage elicited, early signs include weight loss, anorexia and drop in milk yield. As the condition develops, weight loss can be dramatic, with subcutaneous oedema secondary to hypoalbuminaemia most commonly manifesting as submandibular oedema or 'bottle jaw'. Faeces may be unchanged initially, but in later stages diarrhoea may develop.

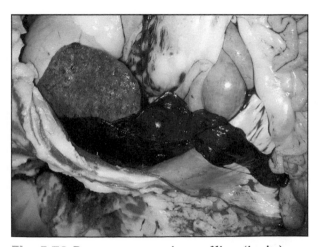

Fig. 5.72 **Post-mortem specimen of liver (*in situ*) showing acute fasciolosis in a lamb.**

Diagnosis

In the live goat FECs, taking the prepatent period into consideration (which can be as long as 8 weeks). Even a single fluke egg found on a FEC is noteworthy. Most acute cases are diagnosed at PME. In early acute cases, local knowledge of the presence of flukes on a unit together with the known seasonality of the condition will lead to a tentative diagnosis, aided by haematology and biochemistry (GLDH, AST) confirming anaemia and liver damage. In chronic cases, serum biochemistry will demonstrate a rise in gGT as a result of biliary damage, and typically hypoalbuminaemia. Fluke serology tests confirming exposure, and PCR tests to identify fluke antigen in faeces, have been developed, but validation for use in goats varies. At PME of chronic cases there is marked accentuation of the biliary tree by fibrosis and, in long-term cases, by calcification. Mature fluke may be identified in the gallbladder and bile ducts (**Fig. 5.73**).

Differential diagnosis

Includes Johne's disease, haemonchosis, other gastro-intestinal nematodes, and other causes of anaemia or dependent oedema (see Chapter 7).

Treatment/management/control

Forecasts are issued in the UK, giving advance warning of the likely risk periods and severity. As the parasite is shared with both sheep and cattle, any control programme should incorporate all co-grazing species.

Management is aimed either at removing the developmental stages of the parasite from the liver of the goat, or at avoiding known parasite–intermediate host interaction in the environment.

Several flukicides are marketed for the treatment and control of flukes. If the product has no licence for use in goats, it is recommended to use the sheep dose (without increasing the dose rate, as for anthelmintics, because of potential toxicity).

Some flukicides can be used in all classes of goat, others should not be used in lactating goats. Depending on the time of year it is to be used, attention must be paid to whether the product is effective in killing immature stages or only mature fluke. Products currently available include clorsulon, closantel, nitroxynil, oxyclozanide and triclabendazole. (**Note:** Resistance reported in the UK.) Albendazole may also be suitable (care in pregnant does).

Where possible, goats should be kept off known snail habitats or these areas should be fenced off. Snail supporting areas do not have to be constantly wet. The area around a leaking water trough or temporary puddles formed after a particularly rainy period can form an excellent snail habitat.

Small liver fluke (syn. lancet fluke)

Dicrocoelium dendriticum is present in many European and other countries, and occasional cases are seen in sheep in the UK. Inside the ruminant host, the parasite migrates up, and lives in, the bile system. Because there is no migration through the gut wall and liver parenchyma, as in fasciolosis, infection is often subclinical and only detected at slaughter or PME.

Sedimentation and McMaster FEC methods tend to be insensitive for this parasite, with flotation using a high specific gravity solution recommended. The life cycle includes land snails and ants, making control via habitat management very difficult. Keeping free-range poultry can reduce snail numbers to a degree, and fencing off ant nests is recommended.

Tapeworms (cestodes)

Definition/overview

Intestinal tapeworms have been identified in goats worldwide, but rarely cause any significant

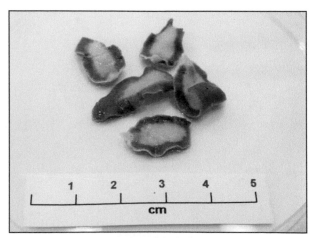

Fig. 5.73 Mature flukes (*Fasciola hepatica*) found in the gallbladder and bile ducts.

clinical disease. Owners may be disturbed by the physical presence of tapeworm segments in faeces.

Aetiology
Moniezia spp. are the most common, and can achieve lengths of several metres, consisting of a head or scolex, and many segments or proglottids. It is the mature egg-containing proglottid that breaks off and appears in the faeces.

Pathophysiology
Light infestations are generally asymptomatic. Very heavy infestations may lead to competition for nutrients in the gut, and can also cause partial or complete intestinal obstruction, or even torsion.

Clinical presentation
If clinical signs do develop, they are usually in younger goats, and can be very vague in nature, including weight loss or poor weight gain. Large burdens resulting in intestinal obstruction or torsion present with colic signs and reduced faecal output.

Diagnosis
Presence of segments in faeces.

Differential diagnosis
Other conditions causing ill thrift in younger goats, including nematodes, coccidiosis, liver fluke and nutritional problems.

Treatment/management/control
Treatment is not usually necessary as the condition is relatively mild, although many anthelmintics are effective against intestinal cestodes.

Metacestode disease
Metacestodes are the intermediate stages in the life cycle of cestodes and can occasionally be found in goats as intermediate hosts (with carnivores the definitive host). The most important species worldwide are hydatid cysts, the intermediate stage of the tapeworm *Echinococcus granulosus*. These cysts can be found mainly in the liver and lungs, often presenting at PME (as an incidental finding) or meat inspection. Clinical signs may be encountered if the cyst enlarges, causing pressure on vital structures such as the bile duct. Control is based on breaking the life cycle, firstly by treating dogs in known endemic areas for tapeworms on a regular basis, and secondly by preventing access to ruminant carcases by scavenging dogs. There is no specific treatment for hydatidosis in infected goats. Hydatidosis can be a significant zoonotic problem. Coenurus cysts (gid) are discussed in Chapter 8.

Peste des petits ruminants (syn. goat plague)
Definition/overview
Peste des petits ruminants (PPR) affects small ruminants so far in almost 70 countries in Africa, the Middle East and parts of Asia. It is a highly contagious disease, which causes massive economic losses each year in regions that are home to over 80% of the world's sheep and goat populations and to more than 330 million of the world's poorest people, many of whom depend on them for their livelihoods. The disease threatens food security and livelihoods, and prevents animal husbandry sectors from achieving their economic potential. Disease has been spreading out from these traditional areas, having been endemic in Turkey since 2000 and now common in North African countries bordering the Mediterranean, both scenarios posing a risk to Southern Europe. Goats appear to be more susceptible than sheep.

PPR is a disease listed under the OIE Terrestrial Animal Health Code and must be reported to the World Organisation for Animal Health. There is currently a global strategy for the eradication of this disease.

Aetiology
PPR is caused by a morbillivirus in the family Paramyxoviridae. In naive herds, the introduction of PPR virus can result in devastatingly high morbidity and mortality figures of up to 100%. Recovered animals produce very strong and lasting immunity. In an endemic area, the adults therefore become naturally immune (or are immune following vaccination) and newborn kids are protected via colostral antibodies. Clinical disease is, therefore, restricted to younger goats between 3 and 12 months of age.

Pathophysiology

The virus is secreted in ocular and nasal discharges, saliva, sputum and faeces. Therefore, disease spread is through close contact between goats and other susceptible species, especially through inhalation of aerosol droplets from coughing and sneezing. Water, feed troughs and bedding can also be contaminated with secretions and become additional sources of infection; however, the virus does not survive for long outside the body of a host animal. Since the virus can be carried and shed before clinical signs develop, PPR can be spread by movement of infected but apparently healthy animals.

After a short incubation period of 2–6 days, the virus localises in the tonsils and pharyngeal and mandibular lymph glands. This rapidly results in viraemia and the virus colonising visceral lymph glands, spleen and bone marrow. Replication also occurs in the mucous membranes of both the respiratory and digestive systems, the latter leading to widespread erosions causing stomatitis and a severe watery diarrhoea. Immunity is compromised as a result of lymphoid tissue damage, and many deaths are hastened by secondary bacterial infections such as pneumonia.

Clinical presentation

Sudden onset pyrexia with severe depression, loss of appetite and initially a clear nasal discharge. The nasal discharge becomes thicker and yellow, often becoming so profuse that it forms a crust that blocks the nostrils, causing respiratory distress. Goats may sneeze persistently in an effort to clear the debris. Ocular involvement includes conjunctivitis, which causes the eyelids to mat together with discharge (**Fig. 5.74**). Gradual epithelial necrosis causes small pinpoint erosions leading to ulcers on the gums, dental pad, palate, lips, inner aspects of the cheeks and dorsal surface of the tongue. These areas increase in number and size, eventually coalescing. In some cases, oral mucous membranes may be completely obscured by thick fibrino-necrotic material covering the erosive changes beneath. Similar changes may also be seen in the mucous membranes of the nose, the vulva and the vagina. The lips tend to swell and crack and become covered with scabs.

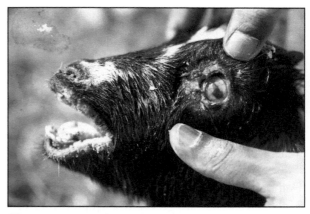

Fig. 5.74 **Peste des petits ruminants case showing severe conjunctivitis and nasal discharge and crusting. (Image courtesy Peter Roeder.)**

Progressive diarrhoea develops, with faeces becoming watery, malodorous and sometimes containing blood and pieces of intestinal tissue, leading to marked dehydration and weight loss. Pneumonia is common in the later stages, and pregnant animals may abort. Clinical progression can be rapid, with death within 5 days from onset, or peracute resulting in sudden death. However, disease can also be mild or non-apparent, and circulate in an area causing little or no illness until susceptible goats are exposed.

Diagnosis

Tentative diagnosis is based on clinical signs. If suspected, PPR is a notifiable disease in those countries in which it is not endemic, and the relevant authorities should be contacted. In the live goat, blood and tissue samples are submitted for virus isolation or antigen detection with PCR. Serum antibody can be detected in more long-standing cases, but is of no value in acute disease.

At PME, the carcass is usually emaciated, the hindquarters soiled with soft or watery faeces, and dehydration is evident. The eyes and nose contain dried-up discharges. The mucosal changes described clinically are evident in the mouth, often extending down the oesophagus. There is often evidence of a secondary bacterial pneumonia. Both small and large intestine show marked congestion of the serosal surface, and congestion and erosive change of the mucosa.

Differential diagnosis

PPR is frequently confused with other diseases that present with pyrexia and grossly similar clinical signs, especially when it is newly introduced. The epidemiological profile, including the often high morbidity and mortality in the herd, is as important as the findings in a single goat or sheep.

Mouth lesions could be confused with foot and mouth disease, bluetongue or contagious pustular dermatitis (orf), the respiratory element with pneumonic pasteurellosis or contagious caprine pleuropneumonia, and the diarrhoea with PGE, enterotoxaemia or coccidiosis. The combination of clinical signs, severity of disease and the geographical location aids in achieving a diagnosis.

Treatment/management/control

In those countries in which PPR is not recognised, management is subject to outbreak measures to control and eradicate the disease.

In countries where the disease is endemic, control is based very heavily on the use of strategic vaccination, aimed most commonly at young goats in their first year of life after colostral antibody has waned. Immunity following vaccination or recovery from natural infection is long-lived. Ring vaccination around endemic areas is used to prevent further spread.

Bluetongue

Signs described include pyrexia, loss of appetite and milk yield with hyperaemia and mild erosive damage to the oral mucosa. On occasion, more severe cases may be encountered in which these oral changes progress to ulcerative and necrotic changes to the tongue, lips and gums, resulting in marked salivation. Diarrhoea may also develop. (See also Chapter 17.)

Miscellaneous conditions

- Adenovirus – adenovirus-associated diarrhoea in young kids has been reported and should be considered if other more common conditions have been eliminated.
- Giardia – this protozoal parasite has been reported as a potential cause of diarrhoea and ill thrift in goats, but can also be found in the faeces of apparently healthy goats, suggesting that its overall pathogenicity may be questionable. Of greater significance is its role as a zoonotic pathogen, and infection in goats may well be identified as part of tracing to identify the source of human infection.
- Caprine herpesvirus – can present as a number of clinical disorders, including diarrhoea in young kids accompanied by pyrexia, weakness, abdominal pain and oral lesions. (See Chapter 2.)

CHAPTER 6

RESPIRATORY SYSTEM

NORMAL STRUCTURE AND FUNCTION

The goat's nasal cavity mirrors the anatomy of other ruminants. Clinically relevant aspects include:

- The ventral meatus, being the widest, carries most of the air flow and allows passage of an endoscope or nasal tube.
- Various recesses and bullae exist, which can only be assessed using advanced imaging techniques.
- Sinuses are connected rather than isolated entities.
- The lateral section of the frontal sinus connects with the horn base.

The cartilages of the tracheal rings are U-shaped in the goat, connected dorsally by a membranous wall. The bifurcation into left and right main bronchus is at the level of the 4th to 6th intercostal space, with an additional bronchus just prior to the main bifurcation into the right cranial lung lobe. On the right, there are two additional smaller lung lobes, in addition to the main lobe. On the left, there is a smaller cranial lobe and the main lobe. The goat has a complete mediastinum.

CLINICAL EXAMINATION OF THE RESPIRATORY SYSTEM

General aspects

Of particular interest for investigation of respiratory tract disease are: season, housing environment (**Figs. 6.1, 6.2**), type of animal (e.g. goatling, first lactation versus adult doe), recent animal movements (regrouping, return from show; **Fig. 6.3**), individual versus group affected, vaccination status, location of pathology (upper versus lower respiratory tract), likely type of pathology based

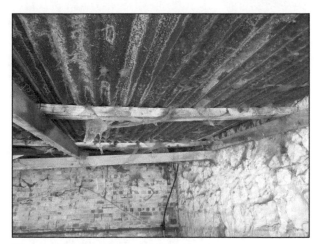

Fig. 6.1 Signs of poor ventilation. Cobwebs indicate poor air circulation; rust on the metal roof and 'tiger-stripes' on the beams indicate frequent condensation.

on auscultation, percussion and observation of other abnormalities (e.g. type of nasal discharge, changes in lung sounds).

It is important to remember that several systemic conditions can alter respiratory tract parameters (e.g. pain, excitement, ambient temperature and humidity, rumen tympany, metabolic alkalosis and acidosis, septicaemia).

Specific observations

The normal respiratory rate is 15–30 bpm in adults and 20–40 bpm in kids, with a moderate abdominal effort to respiration. Nasal discharge is normally clear and non-copious. A mucopurulent discharge indicates inflammation (**Fig. 6.4**); haemorrhagic discharge indicates inflammation, bleeding disorder or mucosal ulceration; and presence of feed or milk indicates a cleft palate, dysphagia or regurgitation.

Air-hunger signs are abducted elbows, extended and lowered head and neck (**Fig. 6.5**) and, in severe cases, mouth breathing.

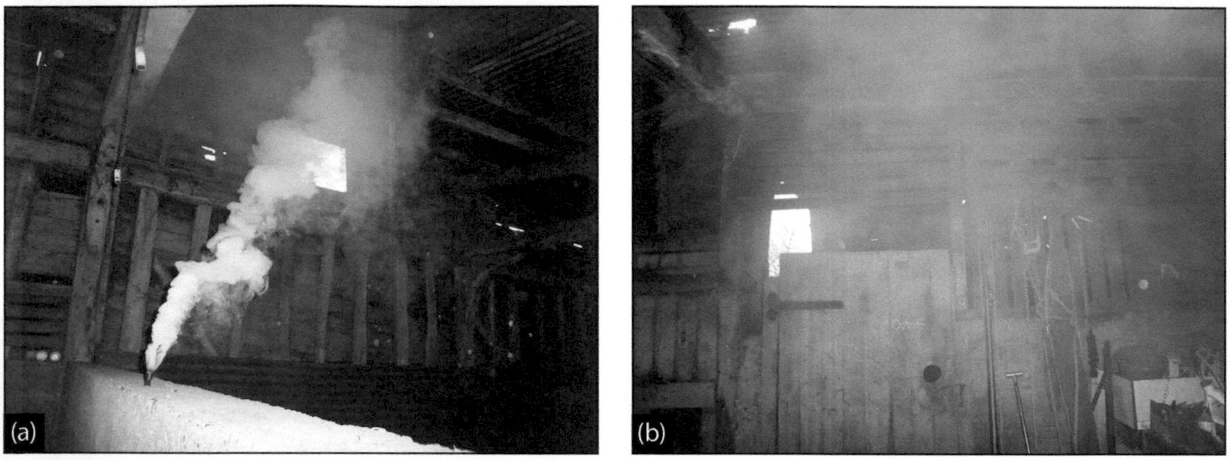

Fig. 6.2 Smoke-bomb test to check ventilation. The smoke rises well initially (a), but then fails to exit the building (b). This suggests reasonable air inlet through the sides, but poor air outlet in the roof.

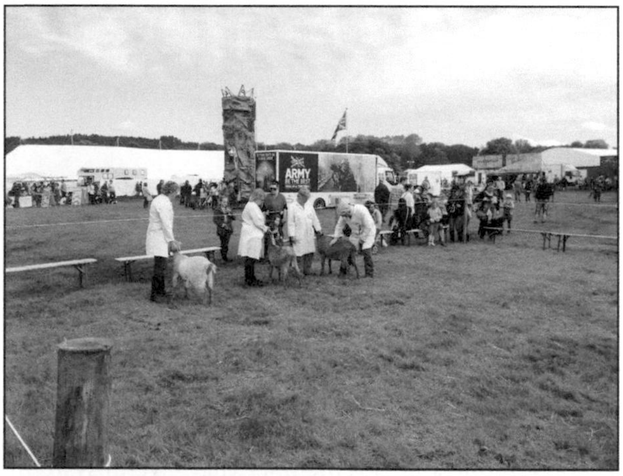

Fig. 6.3 Any recent animal movements are of interest for disease investigation, including goats returning from shows. (Image courtesy Jenny Hull.)

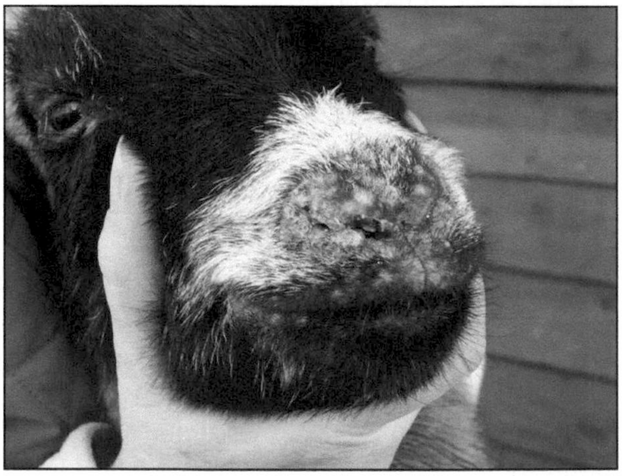

Fig. 6.4 Nasal discharge suggests involvement of the respiratory tract. The mucopurulent nature seen here indicates an inflammatory pathology.

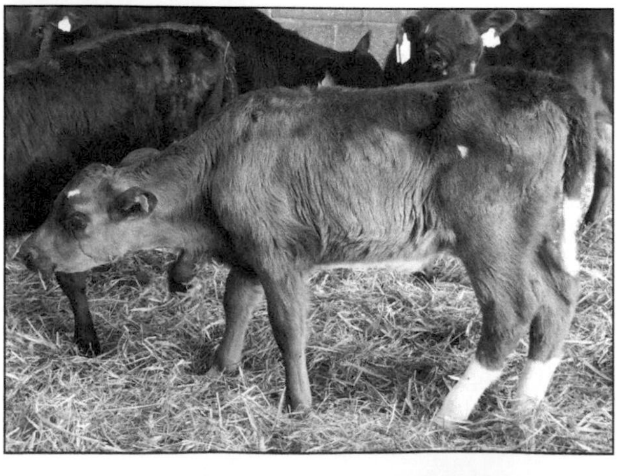

The goat should be observed for spontaneous coughing and whether a cough can be elicited by palpation of the larynx or trachea.

For auscultation, the lung field roughly extends from the penultimate intercostal space in a straight line towards the elbow, becoming inaccessible in the shoulder area. The area around the thoracic inlet is included in the auscultation for the cranial lobes.

Fig. 6.5 Air-hunger signs in a calf. Head and neck are lowered and extended, and elbows abducted. Also note the presence of epiphora: conjunctivitis accompanies several respiratory diseases.

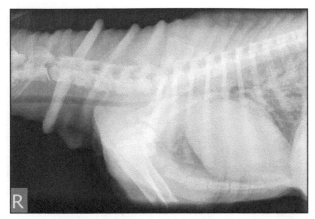

Fig. 6.6 Congenital narrowing of the trachea at the level of the shoulder in a lamb. Adventitious sounds were loudest over the trachea in the distal neck area.

Where adventitious sounds are present, it is important to establish the point of maximum intensity of these sounds. This in part allows differentiation of upper versus lower tract disease (**Fig. 6.6**). Equally, it must be remembered that tracheal sounds may be referred into the thorax.

Ancillary diagnostics

These include endoscopy, tracheal wash or bronchoalveolar lavage for cytology and pathogen isolation, ultrasonography (e.g. to detect pleural effusion or lung tissue consolidation), faecal examination (for parasitic disease such as lungworm) and haematology (to establish eosinophilia in parasitic lung disease or an inflammatory response). Thoracic radiography is of limited value because of the fairly poor correlation between parenchyma pathology and radiographic appearance in ruminants. Lung masses (e.g. neoplasia, tuberculosis nodules; **Fig. 6.7**) need to be at least 5 mm in diameter to become radiographically detectable.

Post-mortem material is invaluable for establishing a definitive diagnosis, especially when a group-affecting disease is suspected.

TREATMENT PRINCIPLES

General treatment principles include: isolation of affected animal(s); anti-inflammatory drugs (NSAIDs or corticosteroids); antibiosis for primary bacterial infections and possibly to control opportunistic secondary pathogens, with the choice ideally based on

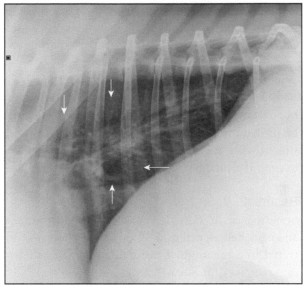

Fig. 6.7 Lateral chest radiograph showing a lung abscess (arrows). Masses have to be at least 5 mm in diameter to be detectable on x-ray. (Image courtesy Jenny Hull.)

culture and sensitivity; ensuring adequate hydration status (to address fluid loss caused by tachypnoea and ensure optimum cilial function); well-ventilated but draught-free environment (pasture with shelter may be best); and maintaining feed intake.

Antimicrobials with good penetration of lung tissue include: trimethoprim-sulphonamides, tetracyclines, macrolides and florfenicol. Moderate concentrations are achieved with the penicillin group (ideally potentiated, e.g. amoxicillin and clavulanic acid) and cephalosporin.

Chronic pathology precludes complete cure and return to normal production. Where fibrous tissue reaction is suspected, iodides may be beneficial (see Chapter 5, Dental problems).

Tracheotomy
Indication
Severe respiratory distress caused by obstruction of the nasal passageways or larynx. Also to provide rest to an inflamed and oedematous larynx.

Preparation and equipment
The ventral neck is clipped and surgically prepared. Equipment includes an uncuffed tracheotomy tube

(e.g. Portex®; inner diameter of 5 mm for kid, 8 mm for yearling, 10 mm for adult) and a small procedures kit, ideally including a pair of Allis tissue forceps. The distal end of a stomach tube can be used in an emergency.

Where dyspnoea has led to cyanosis and severe hypoxaemia, a 14–16 gauge hypodermic needle may be placed into the distal trachea as an interim measure while the surgery is carried out (connected to oxygen if available).

Restraint

Standing or in sternal recumbency, with the head and neck held in extension. Local anaesthetic is infiltrated in a rectangular fashion around, or as a line over, the incision site.

Technical description

A 3 cm long, vertical skin incision is made in the midline of the ventral neck, one-third to one-half the way down. Blunt dissection is used to separate the left- and right-hand side muscle bundles. The trachea is manually pushed towards the incision and fixed either manually or with the aid of Allis tissue forceps, taking care not to cause too much compression.

Using a scalpel blade, the annular ligament between two rings is cut over one-third to half of its length/circumference (**Fig. 6.8**). In adults, it may be possible to remove a crescent-shaped piece of cartilage out of the two adjacent rings. However, this must not be done too aggressively, otherwise the trachea may collapse once the tube is removed.

The tracheotomy tube is inserted and secured with the supplied tapes around the neck (taking care that the tape is not across the opening of the tube; **Fig. 6.9**).

Aftercare

Prophylactic antibiosis and anti-inflammatory medication. The tube is changed twice a day and thoroughly cleaned each time (physical removal of debris, followed by chlorhexidine then thorough rinsing with tap water). Once the primary problem is deemed to have resolved, the tube is removed for trial periods of several hours.

The skin incision is allowed to heal by secondary intention.

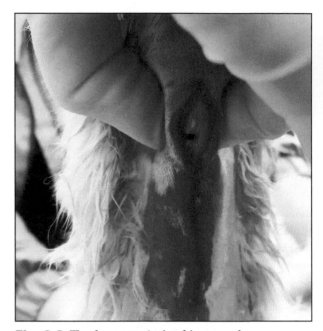

Fig. 6.8 Tracheotomy (animal in sternal recumbency). A vertical skin incision and blunt dissection of the muscles expose the trachea, here manually pushed towards the incision. The annular ligament has been cut and a small section of cartilage removed out of each of the two adjacent tracheal rings to create a circular opening.

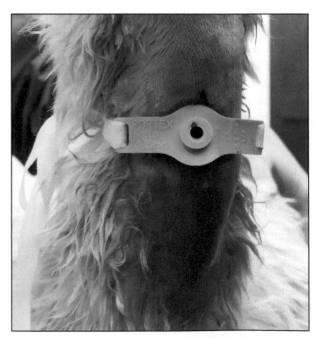

Fig. 6.9 Tracheotomy tube (Portex®) in place and secured with tapes around the neck.

Potential complications
Pneumonia, wound infection, fly strike.

NON-INFECTIOUS DISEASES OF THE RESPIRATORY SYSTEM

Conditions affecting the nasal passages and sinuses
Overview
Various conditions may lead to narrowing of the nasal passageways, resulting in dyspnoea.

Aetiology
Obstruction of the nasal passages may be caused by trauma, neoplasia, foreign bodies or infection of the nostrils, turbinate bones or sinuses. *Actinobacillus lignierisi* infection occasionally occurs in the nasal mucosa, producing granulomatous lesions. Other infections include opportunist pathogens such as *Trueperella pyogenes* that gain entry following trauma or exposure of the frontal sinuses after dehorning. The sheep (*Oestrus ovis*) or deer bot fly can lead to nasal myiasis. Sinusitis may occur secondary to maxillary tooth abscessation.

Clinical presentation
Often noticeable are an abnormal nasal discharge, reduced or absent air flow through one or both nostrils, stertorous breathing in cases of partial obstruction, unpleasant smell of exhaled breath and pain and dull resonance on percussion of the frontal or maxillary sinuses.

Diagnosis
Direct inspection is only possible in the most rostral section. Useful imaging modalities are endoscopy, radiography, CT and MRI. Culture and biopsy are used to establish the aetiology.

Differential diagnosis
Nasal discharge is also seen with some ocular abnormalities and with pathogens causing primarily tracheitis and pneumonia. Stertor may be caused by laryngeal disorders.

Treatment/management/control
Anti-inflammatory therapy is indicated for most conditions. For infectious causes, prolonged antibiosis is used, possibly combined with iodides where actinobacillosis is suspected. For fungal infections, drugs from the azole group (e.g. itraconazole) may be considered. With the patient under GA, the drug is instilled into the nose and left *in situ* for 1 hour.

Sinusitis is addressed by surgical drainage (and tooth removal if involved in the aetiology) and repeated flushing, with concurrent antibiosis.

Laryngeal problems
Overview
Laryngeal problems are occasionally seen in both adults and kids, typically affecting individuals only.

Aetiology
Damage to the laryngeal mucosa allows opportunistic pathogens such as *Fusobacterium necrophorum* to establish a necrotic laryngitis or abscess (**Fig. 6.10**). Drenching gun injury (see Chapter 5) is an example of such trauma and should be considered if several animals are affected. An equivalent to the distinct disease of calf diphtheria is seldom recognised in goats. A genetic predisposition to narrow upper airways, as in some cattle and sheep breeds, has not been reported in goats.

The laryngeal infection is often complicated by local oedema, which is self-perpetuating by forced respiratory movements. Paralysis of the vocal folds may also occur.

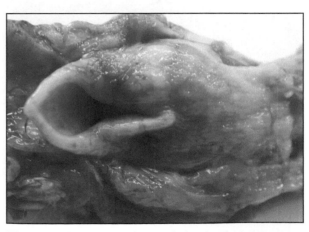

Fig. 6.10 Unilateral laryngeal abscess (post-mortem specimen, 2-week-old alpaca).

Clinical presentation

An inspiratory stertor is evident and the goat commonly adopts an air-hunger position. Astute owners may report a change in the goat's bleating.

Diagnosis

Examination of the oropharynx by laryngoscope, speculum or endoscopy shows oedema and infectious plaques of the arytenoid cartilages (**Fig. 6.11**).

Differential diagnosis

Enlarged retropharyngeal lymph nodes, partial nasal obstruction or external pressure onto the trachea (e.g. thymoma) cause a similar stertor. Ultrasonography is useful to confirm these conditions.

Treatment/management/control

Antibiosis for 7–14 days (e.g. oxytetracycline, 'potentiated' penicillin). High-dose corticosteroid is given for severe laryngeal stertor to reduce the oedema and inflammation (e.g. starting dose of 0.5 mg/kg on day 1, reducing to 0.25 mg/kg on days 2 and 3, then 0.15 mg/kg on days 4 and 5). Tracheostomy may be necessary in cases that do not respond to steroid therapy. Occasionally, surgical drainage of abscesses may be necessary. Creating a laryngeal fistula, by splitting the cricoid cartilage length wise

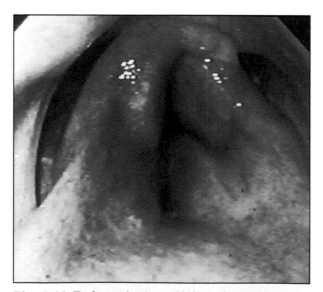

Fig. 6.11 Endoscopic view of bilateral necrotic laryngitis (calf). Note the thickened and ulcerated plaque on the arytenoid.

and suturing it to the skin opening, can also be used in refractory cases.

Aspiration pneumonia
Overview

Aspiration pneumonia affects individual animals, and has a guarded prognosis.

Aetiology

Common causes are regurgitation and inhalation of rumen fluid during sedation or anaesthesia, oral medication (e.g. propylene glycol) or milk or fluid therapy administered via a stomach tube. It can also arise in animals with compromised swallowing (e.g. listeriosis or rhododendron toxicity [see Chapter 16]).

Clinical presentation

Usually sudden onset of respiratory distress. Opportunistic pathogens such as *T. pyogenes* soon become established with the development of a severe pneumonia, leading to ventral consolidation of the lungs. Increased adventitious sounds, and decreased resonance on percussion of dependent parts of anterior lobes, are found. Pyrexia is common.

Diagnosis

History will support clinical suspicion. Radiography may be used to confirm the diagnosis.

Differential diagnosis

Acute infectious pneumonia is the main differential diagnosis. Traumatic causes, leading to haemothorax or diaphragmatic hernia, are ruled out through history and imaging techniques.

Treatment/management/control

Treatment consists of aggressive antibiosis (see Treatment principles), NSAIDs and general nursing care. Prevention relies on adequate starvation prior to GA and the use of cuffed endotracheal tubes, and proper technique when administering oral medication (see Chapter 1).

Pleural effusion
Overview

Pleural effusion is a potentially life-threatening condition, especially if severe and bilateral.

Aetiology

Haemothorax caused by trauma. A pyothorax is very occasionally seen secondary to traumatic reticulo-pericarditis or ruptured lung abscesses. Effusion may be due to inflammatory processes (e.g. broncho-pneumonia), hypoproteinaemia or severe uraemia.

Clinical presentation

Dyspnoea, detection of a fluid line on percussion and signs of impaired venous return. If pleuritis is present, signs of thoracic pain and friction sounds on auscultation. Additional signs depend on the cause, such as anaemia in cases of haemothorax or pain in the anterior abdomen with traumatic reticuloperitonitis.

Diagnosis

Confirmed with ultrasonography (**Fig. 6.12**), thoracocentesis and radiography.

Differential diagnosis

Any other respiratory condition for dyspnoea. A fluid line on percussion is practically pathognomonic.

Treatment/management/control

Treatment needs to address the primary problem, combined with drainage of the effusion. The latter can be difficult in ruminants because of their tendency to wall-off infection. Aggressive antibiosis (see Treatment principles) and NSAIDs.

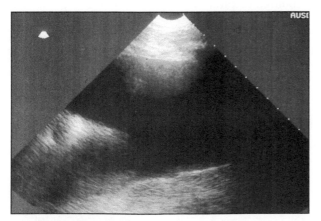

Fig. 6.12 Pleural effusion showing as dark (echolucent) fluid on ultrasonography. The lung lobe can typically be seen 'floating' back and forth in line with respiration on a real-time scan.

Pneumothorax

Overview

Pneumothorax is a serious but, if unilateral, rarely life-threatening condition.

Aetiology

May result from trauma, including to neonates during the birthing process, or from ruptured emphysematous bullae.

Clinical presentation

Because of the complete mediastinum, collapse tends to be unilateral. A disparity in lung sounds between left and right side is evident, with abnormal resonance on percussion (which may be high pitched). The goat displays inspiratory dyspnoea with marked abdominal effort, and possibly cyanosis. If traumatic in origin, rib fractures may be present, with pain on palpation evident. Subcutaneous emphysema is often present.

Diagnosis

Clinical signs are highly suggestive, with radiography used to confirm the diagnosis.

Differential diagnosis

A diaphragmatic hernia may present similarly and is ruled out using radiography.

Treatment/management/control

Wound closure and care as required, and prophylactic antibiosis if pneumothorax resulting from an external puncture is suspected. If possible, the air should be aspirated via thoracocentesis or via a thoracostomy tube. Otherwise, supportive therapy is provided until the air in the thoracic cavity has been absorbed.

Toxicities

Irritant gases or fumes

A variety of gases or fumes can cause an inflammatory response in the respiratory tract. Of particular interest is nitrogen dioxide (NO_2), generated in the first few days of silage fermentation. Crops of low dry matter or with high nitrate contents (e.g. rain close to harvest, late fertilisation) produce large amounts of the gas. It does not usually cause any problems in open, well-ventilated silage clamps, but cases of intoxication have occurred where animal housing is close to a clamp with poor ventilation. NO_2 is heavier than air and collects around clamp walls. Once inhaled, it dissolves in the moisture of the airways, forming a corrosive acid. It can be lethal to the animal, and is a work place hazard.

Snake bites

Snake bites commonly lead to pyrexia, tachypnoea and respiratory distress. Tracheotomy should be considered in severely affected animals. Supportive therapy includes corticosteroids and i/v fluids. Venom antiserum is given where the snake has been identified.

Neoplasia

In older goats metastatic tumour deposits may be identified in lung tissue, potentially compromising lung function. Other clinical signs will vary depending on the primary site and tissue affected. One of the most common sites for neoplasia to develop in older goats is the thymus gland. Some tumours are benign and usually well-differentiated/encapsulated (thymoma), others are more diffuse locally and may metastasise (thymic lymphosarcoma). Both can become very large and cause respiratory distress. This is described in more detail in Chapter 7.

INFECTIOUS DISEASES OF THE RESPIRATORY SYSTEM

Contagious caprine pleuropneumonia

Definition/overview

Contagious caprine pleuropneumonia (CCPP) is one of the most severe diseases of goats worldwide. It affects the respiratory tract and is extremely contagious and frequently fatal. In naive herds, the morbidity rate may reach 100% and the mortality rate can be as high as 80%. CCPP causes major economic losses in East Africa and the Middle East, where it is endemic. It is an OIE scheduled disease and is notifiable in many countries.

Aetiology

CCPP is caused by *Mycoplasma capricolum* subsp. *capripneumoniae*, a very fragile organism that is not able to exist for long in the external environment. On average it survives outside the host for up to 3 days in tropical areas and up to 2 weeks in temperate zones.

Pathophysiology

The incubation period under natural conditions is commonly 6–10 days, but may be prolonged (3–4 weeks). Some experimentally infected goats develop fever as soon as 3 days after inoculation and respiratory signs as early as 5 days, but others do not become ill until up to 41 days after exposure. CCPP is highly contagious: disease is transmitted during close contact by the inhalation of respiratory droplets. Chronic carriers may exist, but this remains unproven, although there are reports of outbreaks developing in endemic areas when apparently healthy goats were introduced into clean herds. Outbreaks of the disease often occur after heavy rains (e.g. after the monsoons in India), after cold spells or after transportation over long distances. This may be because recovered carrier animals shed the infectious agent after the stress of sudden climatic or environmental changes.

Clinical presentation

Affected goats may simply be found dead. In acute infection there is pyrexia (41–43°C), lethargy and anorexia, followed within 2–3 days by coughing and laboured respiration (**Fig. 6.13**). Coughing becomes

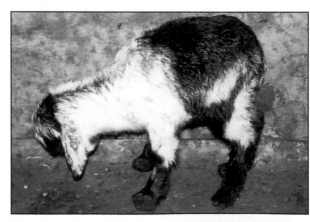

Fig. 6.13 Goat kid in the terminal stages of CCPP. (© Crown Copyright 2017. Used with kind permission of the Animal and Plant Health Agency.)

more frequent, violent and productive. In the final stages of disease, the goat may not be able to move and adopts a marked air-hunger position. Saliva can drip continuously from the mouth and the animal may grunt or bleat in pain. Frothy nasal discharge and stringy saliva may be seen terminally. Pregnant goats may abort.

Diagnosis

CCPP should be suspected in the field when a highly contagious disease occurs in a herd characterised by pyrexia of 41°C or greater, severe respiratory distress, high morbidity and mortality, and the characteristic gross pathology. At post-mortem examination (PME), there is invariably a large amount of straw coloured fluid within the chest cavity (**Fig. 6.14**), the result of a sero-fibrinous pleuritis (**Fig. 6.15**). There is marked consolidation/hepatisation of whole lung lobes, which is often unilateral. Pea-sized, yellow nodules may be found in the lungs, often surrounded by areas of congestion. Some long-term survivors have chronic pleuropneumonia or chronic pleuritis, with encapsulation of acute lesions and numerous adhesions to the chest wall.

A definitive diagnosis can be made by isolating *M. capripneumoniae* from lung tissue or pleural fluid at necropsy. Serology is considered to be of minimal value due to the acute nature of the disease and problems related to cross-reaction with other *Mycoplasma* spp.

Differential diagnosis

Diagnosis of CCPP can be complicated, particularly in those areas where it is endemic. The causative organism is readily contagious and fatal to goats of all ages and both sexes, but rarely affects sheep, and does not affect cattle where these are co-grazed. The primary differential diagnoses include:

- Peste des petits ruminants (PPR), to which sheep are also susceptible.
- Pasteurellosis, which can be tentatively differentiated at PME on the basis of the distribution of gross lung lesions.
- Contagious agalactia syndrome, in which the pneumonia is accompanied by prominent lesions in other organs, and is caused by another distinct mycoplasma organism.

Treatment/management/control

As CCPP is an OIE scheduled disease, most control, eradication, surveillance and reporting protocols are regulated on a country by country basis.

Pasteurellosis
Definition/overview

Pasteurellosis occurs in goats worldwide as either a primary or a secondary bronchopneumonia.

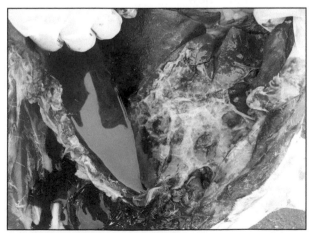

Fig. 6.14 Large quantity of clear fluid in the thoracic cavity in a case with CCPP. (© Crown Copyright 2017. Used with kind permission of the Animal and Plant Health Agency.)

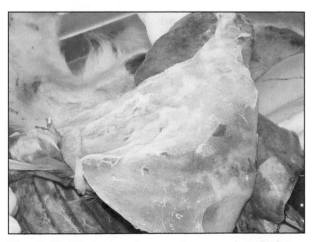

Fig. 6.15 Fibrinopurulent exudate covering the lung surface in a case with CCPP. (© Crown Copyright 2017. Used with kind permission of the Animal and Plant Health Agency.)

Aetiology

Caused predominantly by *Mannheimia haemolytica* or *Pasteurella multocida* singly or in combination.

Pathophysiology

Both organisms are commensal in the upper respiratory tract of many goats, with disease occurring following invasion of lung tissue. Although this invasion may be the result of concurrent infection with, for example, *Mycoplasma* spp., more commonly it occurs as a result of management induced stress factors. The disease occurs most commonly in young, intensively reared goats in which overcrowding, poor ventilation and a dusty environment are all contributing factors.

Clinical presentation

In peracute disease, affected goats can be found dead. More commonly, there is a rapid onset of clinical signs including pyrexia, lethargy, a mucopurulent nasal discharge, dyspnoea and coughing (**Fig. 6.16**).

Diagnosis

In the live goat, the clinical presentation is fairly characteristic. Ultrasonography may highlight the marked consolidation and pleurisy of the cranioventral lung lobes. Bacteriology of nasal swabs is of no real value as the causative organisms are commensal in this site. At PME, there is commonly a clearly demarcated bilateral cranioventral lung consolidation (**Fig. 6.17**), from which the causative organism can be cultured. Additional laboratory techniques may identify concurrent exacerbating infections such as mycoplasmosis (*M. ovipneumoniae* or *M. arginini*) or lungworm.

Differential diagnosis

The most important differential diagnosis is CCPP.

Treatment/management/control

In the face of an outbreak, attention should be paid to identifying the likely underlying stress factors and addressing any management shortcomings (e.g. reducing stocking rates, increasing ventilation without making buildings too cold or draughty, ensuring attention to dry bedding to reduce condensation). Treatment of clinical cases is based on anti-inflammatory therapy and parenteral antibiosis.

There are *Pasteurella/Mannheimia* vaccines available and these are used widely in the sheep sector, often marketed as a multivalent clostridial/pasteurellosis vaccine. In the UK, current advice is to vaccinate against clostridial infection and pasteurellosis in two separate programmes, rather than to use these combined vaccines (due to the perceived poorer immune response to vaccination in goats).

Parasitic pneumonia

Definition/overview

Parasitic pneumonia occurs in goats worldwide.

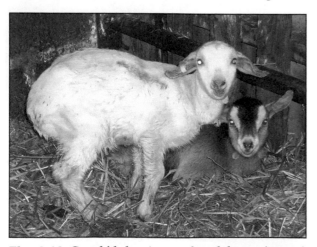

Fig. 6.16 Goat kid showing profound depression and respiratory distress.

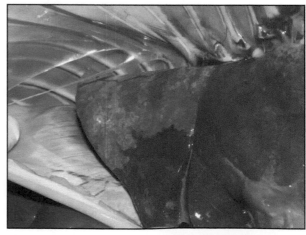

Fig. 6.17 Lungs showing severe cranioventral lung consolidation.

Aetiology

The two most common parasites are *Dictyocaulus filaria* and *Muellerius capillaris*. *D. filaria* has a direct life cycle: adults living in the airways produce 1st stage larvae (L1), which are coughed up, swallowed and appear in faeces on the pasture. Development continues to L3, and these can survive in a free-living form on pasture, completing the lifecycle if ingested. The life cycle of *M. capillaris* is an indirect one, involving a variety of slugs and snails acting as intermediate hosts for the infective larvae voided in faeces.

Pathophysiology

The physical presence of *D. filaria* in the airways causes irritation to the lining of the airways. Heavy infestation may lead to bronchitis/bronchiolitis and pulmonary emphysema. *M. capillaris* by comparison completes its life cycle in the deeper lung tissue at alveolar level, where in heavy infestations the developmental stages can be identified histologically.

Clinical presentation

Goats infected with *D. filaria* most commonly cough due to tracheal and bronchial irritation, which in heavy infestation leads to progressive dyspnoea and weight loss, often in association with secondary bacterial infection. In comparison, *M. capillaris* infestation in many goats may be asymptomatic and only identified as an incidental finding at PME. In heavy infestations, respiratory signs may be very subtle and easily overlooked, but cases have been described in which exercise intolerance was a feature, with infected goats lagging behind others when driven.

Diagnosis

In patent infections, larvae of both parasites can be readily identified in faeces by the Baermann technique. At PME, *D. filaria* parasites can be identified in the airways (**Fig. 6.18**), and other non-specific findings may include focal areas of consolidation near the caudal lung margins and emphysema. In heavy *M. capillaris* infestation, larvae can be readily identified histologically in lung sections (**Fig. 6.19**).

Differential diagnosis

Coughing due to *D. filaria* infestation needs to be differentiated from other causes, including pasteurellosis, aspiration pneumonia, allergic pneumonitis and congestive heart failure.

Treatment/management/control

The management, treatment and control of lungworm in goats should be a component part of the control strategy for parasitic gastroenteritis (see Chapter 5, pp. 154–157).

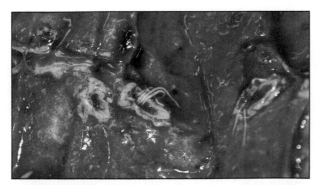

Fig. 6.18 *Dictyocaulus filaria* parasites visible in the airways on post-mortem examination. (Image courtesy RVC-AHVLA Surveillance Centre.)

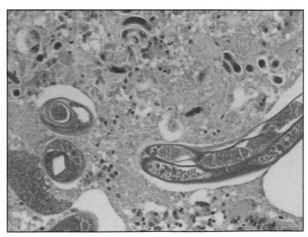

Fig. 6.19 *Muellerius capillaris* larvae evident histologically in lung tissue (in cross and longitudinal section).

MISCELLANEOUS CONDITIONS

Other *Mycoplasma* organisms

Respiratory infection can be a feature of contagious agalactia (see Chapter 12). *Mycoplasma ovipneumoniae* and *Mycoplasma arginini* can both cause relatively mild respiratory signs in isolation, but *M. ovipneumoniae* in particular is a common precursor to pneumonic pasteurellosis.

Peste des petits ruminants (syn. goat plague)

PPR presents with a sudden onset pyrexia, with severe depression, loss of appetite and initially a clear nasal discharge. The nasal discharge becomes thicker and yellow, often becoming so profuse that it forms a crust that blocks the nostrils, causing respiratory distress, and goats may sneeze persistently in an effort to clear the debris (see Chapter 5).

Caprine arthritis encephalitis

One of the many manifestations of caprine arthritis encephalitis is an interstitial pneumonitis (**Figs. 6.20, 6.21**). This may be mild and non-apparent clinically and only identified on PME. However, it can cause clinical signs, including an increasing dyspnoea, exercise intolerance and a mild cough, co-existing with other more typical signs (see Chapter 9).

Caseous lymphadenitis

Although caseous lymphadenitis typically presents as abscesses causing enlargement of the superficial lymph nodes, pulmonary abscesses and associated lymph node enlargement can occur in housed goats (**Fig. 6.22**) in which infection rates (and hence environmental contamination with the causative organism) can be high (see Chapter 7).

Tuberculosis

Although tuberculosis is generally considered to be less of a problem in goats worldwide than in cattle, goats can become infected, predominantly with *Mycobacterium bovis* or *Mycobacterium avium* (see Chapter 17). Typical caseous or more liquid pus-containing abscesses can develop in lung tissue (**Fig. 6.23**) and associated lymph nodes. Heavy infection can lead to respiratory distress and coughing, but infection can also be subclinical.

Fungal pneumonia/ allergic pneumonitis

Exposure to mouldy feed or bedding, particularly in poorly ventilated buildings, can lead to inhalation of fungal spores (e.g. *Aspergillus fumigatus*), resulting in a fungal pneumonia. This is most commonly confirmed at PME, when typical branching hyphae can be identified histologically colonising lung tissue. One other sequela, more commonly identified in older goats following repetitive

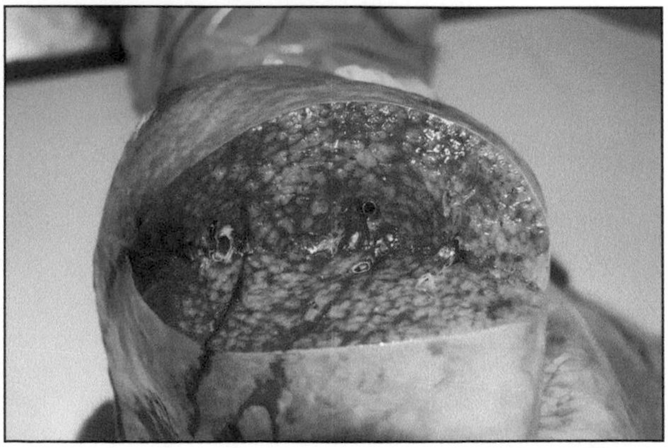

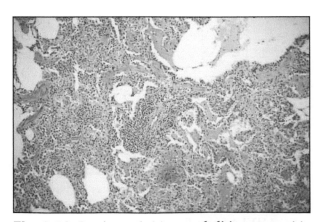

Fig. 6.20 Cut section of lung with caprine arthritis encephalitis pneumonitis. The lungs appear firm in consistency.

Fig. 6.21 Caprine arthritis encephalitis pneumonitis showing mononuclear cell infiltrates in the alveolar septae and the perivascular and peribronchial areas.

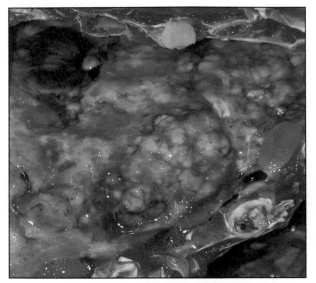

Fig. 6.22 Severe caseous lymphadenitis associated multifocal abscessation in lung tissue. *Corynebacterium pseudotuberculosis* was isolated.

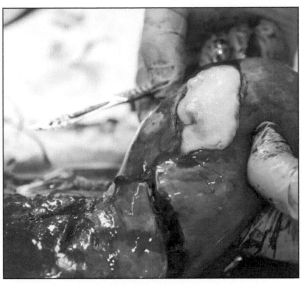

Fig. 6.23 Tuberculosis should be considered when presented with a caseous lung abscess.

exposure, is an allergic pneumonitis somewhat analogous to the condition referred to as farmer's lung in humans. This condition is worse during the winter housing period, but rapidly resolves when goats are turned out. It can vary from mild coughing to more severe respiratory distress in affected individuals.

Vena cava thrombosis

In this condition, emboli pass to the lungs, resulting in abscessation, chronic pneumonia and lesions in the pulmonary arterioles. Less acute cases may present with a painful cough, pallor of the mucous membranes, thoracic pain and increased lung sounds. (See Chapter 7 for a full description.)

CHAPTER 7

CARDIOVASCULAR DISEASE AND DISORDERS OF THE HAEMATOPOIETIC SYSTEM

NORMAL STRUCTURE AND FUNCTION

The goat's heart has a marked cone shape. It sits upright in the thorax, at almost 90 degrees to the sternum, with five sevenths lying to the left of the midline. It reaches from the 2nd to the 5th rib in width, with a height equivalent to approximately half the height of the thorax (the heart base is at the level of the midpoint of the first rib). Part of the left-hand side is not covered by lung lobes.

Of interest for post-mortem examination (PME) are a normal reference weight of roughly 0.5% of the animal's bodyweight and the typical patches of sub-endocardial fat tissue.

CLINICAL EXAMINATION OF THE CARDIOVASCULAR SYSTEM

Clinical assessment

Examination of any patient should include actively looking for signs of cardiovascular (CV) disease. General observations that may suggest a CV problem include dependent oedema (especially the brisket or mandible), dyspnoea, exercise intolerance or changes of parameters during exercise, weight loss or poor weight gain, poor or fluctuating milk yield, cold surface temperature or variable skin temperature between body areas, intermittent fever and postural abnormalities such as abducted elbows.

For adults, a normal heart rate of 60–80 bpm is commonly cited in the literature. However, several studies suggest a higher average resting heart rate of 95 bpm, with a range of 70–120. The heart rate may increase during pregnancy. Reported rates in kids are 200–220 bpm up to 1 month old, and 140 bpm up to 6 months old. The two heart sounds S1 and S2 are typically heard. Respiratory sinus arrhythmia is common in goats.

Auscultation also aims to establish adventitious sounds and, where present, their points of maximum intensity (PMI). For this it is useful to know the location of the heart valves. On the left, the pulmonary valve is in the 3rd intercostal space and the atrial and mitral valves in the 4th intercostal space, with the atrial valve dorsal to the mitral. The tricuspid valve is on the right in the 3rd intercostal space. In young tachypnoeic goats, palpation of the chest wall can be very useful to detect an abnormal cardiac thrill inaudible on auscultation. The heart beat may be palpable in the 4th intercostal space on the left, although this becomes difficult in goats in good body condition. A continuous rubbing sound could indicate pericarditis. Percussion may highlight an enlarged heart shadow. It helps cardiac assessment if the front leg is pulled forward.

The jugular veins are assessed for efficiency of filling, speed of deflation and evidence of permanent distension. A jugular pulse half way up the neck is often present in the normal goat standing with a lowered head. The femoral artery is useful for assessing pulse quality and possible deficits.

Normal mucous membrane colour is dark salmon pink and best assessed using the conjunctival membranes. Paleness suggests either anaemia or poor perfusion. Cyanosis is seen with severe respiratory disease or left-sided heart failure. Jaundice may be present with haemolytic anaemia. A capillary refill time of over 2 seconds suggests poor perfusion.

Typical signs of right-sided heart failure are caused by impaired venous return and venous stasis, and include filling abnormalities of jugular veins, brisket oedema, poor exercise tolerance and ascites. Ascites is rare without signs of ventral oedema. An abdominal fluid thrill can be readily elicited in affected goats. Left-sided failure typically causes pulmonary oedema, dyspnoea, further exercise intolerance and cyanosis.

Clinical signs may not be evident until an advanced stage of disease, which is an important consideration for prognosis.

Ancillary diagnostics
Ultrasonography
Ultrasonography is very useful for detecting valve anomalies, pericardial effusions, hypertrophy and ascites. A linear array probe will allow some assessment, but because of the narrow intercostal spaces, a sector probe is preferable. Colour flow imaging using Doppler is useful for defects such as ventricular septal defect, patent ductus arteriosus (PDA) or valve insufficiency.

Electrocardiography
Electrocardiography (ECG) can be used to establish rate, rhythm and some gross anomalies (**Fig. 7.1**). The considerable variation between goats (in particular in QRS pattern) means that further clinical application is limited. In addition, cardiac depolarisation is diffuse, therefore vectors are rarely used. Forestomach fill affects the heart axis.

A useful configuration is the base-apex lead system with RA over the heart base, LA over the apex and the N lead on the withers. The effect of position of the goat during ECG on readings is minor, and the pattern within an individual goat is quite constant from reading to reading.

Dysrhythmia may be associated with metabolic disease or septic foci, especially in the abdomen. Atrial fibrillation – with its characteristic F waves – is occasionally seen, and is almost always associated with metabolic problems including hypochloraemia, hypokalaemia and metabolic alkalosis.

Radiography
Some details of internal cardiac structures may be detected, but typically radiography is only useful for evaluating the overall size of the heart. A vena cava thrombus is sometimes detectable, as are radiopaque foreign bodies associated with traumatic reticulitis.

For positioning, it is important to pull the front legs as far forward as possible, to limit any shadowing.

Pericardiocentesis
Aspiration using a 5–10 cm long hypodermic needle through the skin and chest wall under local anaesthesia is a simple procedure. Ultrasound guidance is useful. Colour and odour of fluid may suggest infection, and the sample may be submitted for cytology, protein estimation and culture.

Blood sampling and basic in-house analysis
Blood is most commonly collected from the jugular vein, but the cephalic or saphenous veins are also suitable (following the same technique as in dogs). For a jugular sample from an adult, an assistant stands astride over the goat just in front of its shoulders, and with the goat's backend against a wall or corner. With one hand under the chin and the other on the poll, the assistant holds the head and neck in extension and as straight along the longitudinal axis as possible. The thumb of the non-dominant hand is pressed into the readily identifiable jugular groove, about halfway down the neck, to raise the vein. In heavily coated goats (where clipping is undesired), it can be useful to release and raise the vein a few times to identify its exact location. Surgical spirit is applied prior to needle insertion. A vacutainer or 5–20 ml syringe, with a 19–21 gauge, 2.5 cm (1 in) needle, is used.

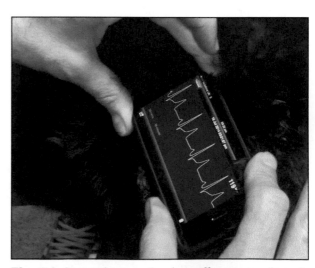

Fig. 7.1 Smartphone technology allows capturing of an ECG trace and posting to a specialist for analysis, if desired (e.g. AliveCor™).

With the exception of haematocrit and total protein, haematological and biochemical evaluation rarely gives useful information without a thorough clinical examination (see Appendix: Laboratory Reference Intervals). Blood culture may be attempted in cases of suspected endocarditis, but bacteraemia is often intermittent. *Table 7.1* shows how interpretation of haematocrit and total protein may be used to broadly differentiate disorders.

CARDIOVASCULAR DISEASE

There are few reports of primary heart disease in the goat worldwide, although cardiac failure and its sequelae may be a secondary feature in many systemic infections. The non-athletic nature of the species, and common group husbandry, may mask a higher incidence.

Specific CV conditions include:

- Congenital cardiac abnormalities.
- Nutritional muscular dystrophy (white muscle disease). Can affect cardiac muscle, resulting in sudden death (see Chapter 9).
- Foot and mouth disease. During an outbreak, kids may die suddenly as a result of a viral myocarditis (see Chapter 17).
- Cardiotoxic plants. These can result in heart failure and sudden death if ingested and include yew (*Taxus baccata*), foxglove (*Digitalis purpurea*) and oleander (*Nerium oleander*). Plant poisoning is discussed in more detail in Chapter 16.

- Heartwater (cowdriosis) is an infectious non-contagious tick-borne rickettsial disease of goats and other ruminants. Heartwater occurs in nearly all the sub-Saharan countries of Africa and in the surrounding islands. The disease is also reported in the Caribbean, potentially posing a threat to the American mainland.

Septal defects
Overview
Of the congenital defects affecting the heart, septal defects are the most common.

Aetiology
Ventricular defects are more common than atrial defects. Aetiology frequently remains unestablished. However, familial cases have been reported, suggesting a genetic component in some instances.

Clinical presentation
Ill-thrift, poor growth (**Fig. 7.2**), lethargy and exercise intolerance may be noted, but a number of affected animals show no marked CV compromise. An atrial defect typically causes more severe and acute clinical signs. A palpable thrill is often present over the thoracic wall, especially in kids.

A pansystolic murmur is heard on both sides of the chest, but especially on the right (direction of blood flow is from high pressure left ventricle to right). The PMI is on the right, and the murmur is 'diagonal' with greatest intensity towards the caudal aspect

Table 7.1 **Interpretation of haematocrit (Hct) in combination with total plasma protein (TP).**

HCT	TP	INTERPRETATION
Normal	Low	Protein-losing enteropathy or nephropathy; severe liver disease; vasculitis
	High	Increased globulin production (e.g. chronic inflammation); anaemia masked by dehydration
Increased	Low	Combination of splenic contraction and protein loss
	Normal	Splenic contraction; erythrocytosis; hypoproteinaemia masked by dehydration
	High	Dehydration
Decreased	Low	Substantial acute blood loss (recent or ongoing); overhydration
	Normal	Increased destruction or reduced formation of erythrocytes; chronic blood loss
	High	Inflammatory processes; multiple myeloma; lymphoproliferative diseases

Source: Adapted from Meyer DJ, Harvey JW (2004) *Veterinary Laboratory Medicine*. Saunders, Philadephia.

of the right side of the heart. Very occasionally there is also a diastolic murmur due to aortic valve insufficiency (because of lack of support for the valve by the defective septum). The degree of murmur varies depending on the size of the defect; in general, the smaller the defect the more turbulence and friction are caused and hence the louder the murmur.

Chronic changes include poor peripheral circulation and overload of the right ventricle (leading to hypertrophy) and pulmonary circulation. Fibrosis of pulmonary vessels can result, eventually leading to a right-to-left shunt. Endocarditis may result from turbulence.

Concurrent congenital defects may be present and should be checked for.

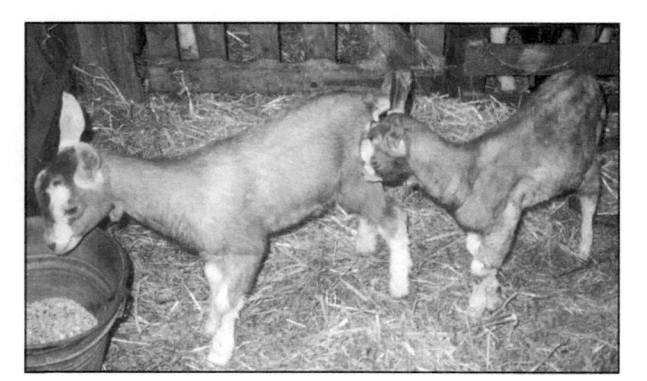

Fig. 7.2 Poor growth, as in the twin on the right, can indicate a congenital cardiac defect.

Diagnosis

The character of the murmur is suggestive, and ultrasonography is used to confirm the diagnosis (**Fig. 7.3**). Ventricular defects are often located very dorsally and can go unnoticed without thorough examination. Small defects may be overlooked during PME (**Fig. 7.4**).

Differential diagnosis

Other causes of cardiac murmurs such as PDA (continuous murmur of varying intensity ['machinery-like']), patent foramen ovale (closure may be delayed until 7–10 days old; loud murmur at level of heart base), endo- or pericarditis or more complex defects such as tetralogy of Fallot.

Treatment/management/control

Animals with a relatively small defect may reach adulthood and can carry pregnancies and lactate successfully for several years. However, the owner should be forewarned that sudden death is possible at any time.

Medical treatment is not effective and surgical intervention rarely undertaken. Euthanasia is the best option if severe compromise of cardiac function is present.

Endocarditis
Overview

Endocarditis is a common cardiac condition of adult animals, typically carrying a guarded prognosis.

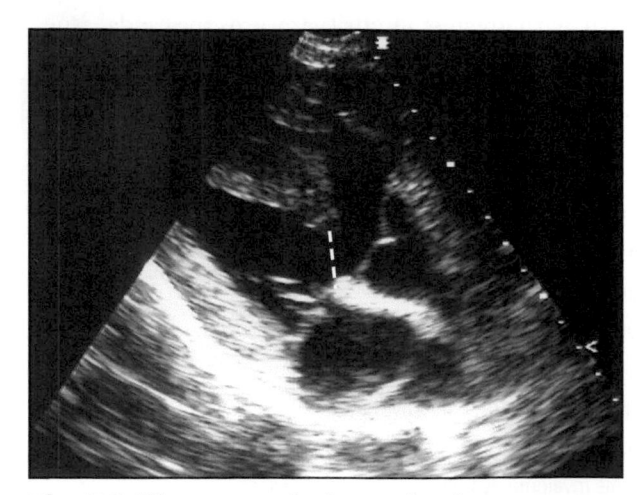

Fig. 7.3 Ultrasonography image showing a ventricular septal defect (dotted line).

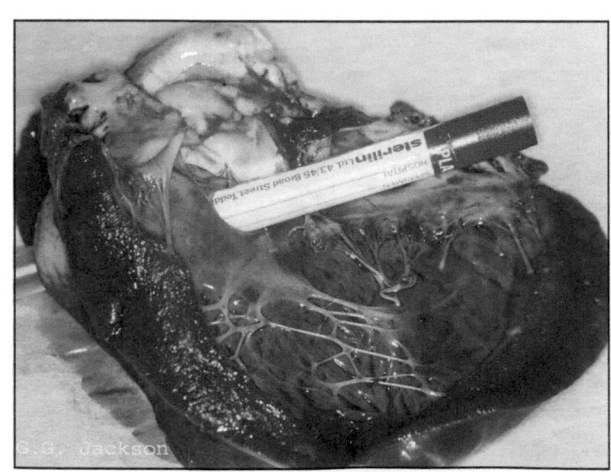

Fig. 7.4 Ventricular septal defect indicated by a sampling tube inserted into the defect. (Image courtesy Peter G.G. Jackson.)

Aetiology

Mostly bacterial, including *Trueperella pyogenes*, Group D streptococci, staphylococci and *Pasteurella* spp. The condition may arise from a septic focus elsewhere in the body (e.g. udder, uterus, subcutaneous abscess) or from poor intravenous injection technique. Circulating bacteria from such foci adhere to the endocardium, establishing infection. Valves, especially the tricuspid, are colonised with outgrowths developing and eventual compromise of valve function leading to cardiac failure. There is a risk of emboli breaking off from affected areas, leading to bacterial colonisation and emboli elsewhere.

Clinical presentation

Early signs are not necessarily cardiac in nature. Intermittent or persistent episodes of pyrexia with few other signs are common in the early stage, with an apparent response to antimicrobial therapy. Shifting leg lameness is occasionally seen. Later signs include poor exercise tolerance, positive wither's pinch test, heart murmur with the PMI over a particular valve and, occasionally, fluid sounds originating from pericardial sac effusion. Terminally, there are signs of right-sided heart failure (see earlier). Poor perfusion leads to compromised function of other organs (e.g. kidneys), with associated signs. Anaemia may be seen because of red blood cell destruction by blood turbulence around the affected valve.

Diagnosis

History, clinical signs and ultrasonography. Where pericardial effusion is present (**Fig. 7.5**), a centesis will yield clear fluid with a low cell count.

Differential diagnosis

Other causes of right-sided heart failure, especially pericarditis (cloudy fluid both on ultrasonography and centesis) and cardiomyopathies.

Treatment/management/control

May be too late by the time symptoms appear. Intense and prolonged antibiotic therapy can be tried in early cases. Blood culture prior to commencing antibiosis is ideal, but intermittent shedding can lead to lack of pathogen growth. Diuretic therapy may give short-term relief, but does not

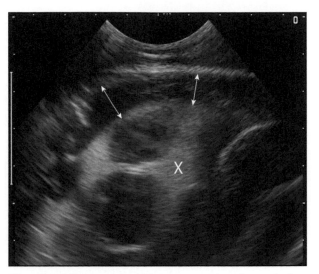

Fig. 7.5 Ultrasonographic cross-section through the heart (**X**), showing pericardial effusion (lines) in a case with mitral valve insufficiency.

delay terminal heart failure. An affected goat is unfit for slaughter for human consumption, because of recurrent bacteraemia.

Pericarditis

Overview

Pericarditis typically affects adult goats and carries a poor prognosis.

Aetiology

May arise sporadically from a focus of infection elsewhere in the body or as part of traumatic reticulopericarditis. With the latter, infection may also involve local lung tissue or cause a pyothorax. Pathogens involved include *T. pyogenes*, *Pasteurella* spp., *Histophilus somni*, staphylococci, streptococci and *Mycoplasma* spp. After accumulation of infected fluid and debris, fibrosis and adherence of the pericardium to the heart follow, leading to compression of the heart and compromised cardiac function (**Fig. 7.6**). Toxaemia may develop directly from the pericardial pathogens or as a result of organ failure caused by poor perfusion. Eventually, heart failure occurs.

Clinical presentation

In cases of traumatic reticulopericarditis, premonitory signs include a short episode of pyrexia of unknown origin, anorexia and rumen stasis (possibly

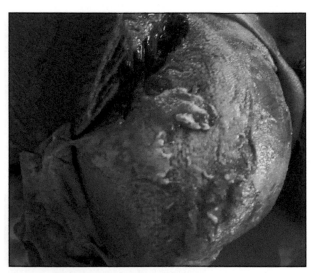

Fig. 7.6 Pericarditis causing fibrosis and adhesions. The pericardium has been peeled back from the heart.

associated with the initial foreign body penetration). The goat appears to respond to antibiosis, until the pericarditis becomes fully established.

In general, clinical signs often vary and progress with changing pathology. Early signs include the goat being uncomfortable and reluctant to move, with a fluctuating but marked pyrexia and reduced rumen activity. Thoracic pain is evident through an arched back, positive wither's pinch test, grunting associated with breathing (especially when recumbent) and pain over the thoracic wall. Auscultation often reveals a pericardial rub associated with heart movements, or tinkling sounds from fluid trapped in the pericardium. Heart sounds themselves are muffled. Later signs are associated with right-sided heart failure (see earlier). May see signs of toxaemia or septicaemia, and localised pleurisy and pneumonia.

Diagnosis
Clinical signs are often highly suggestive. Pericardiocentesis yields an often malodorous fluid with a high nucleated cell count; however, in advanced cases free fluid may be absent. Although neutrophilia with a left shift and elevated fibrinogen are common findings on haematology, these are not unique for this condition. Ultrasonography often shows echogenic pericardial contents and thickening of the pericardium.

Differential diagnosis
Pleural effusion may also result in muffled heart sounds and can be confirmed on ultrasonography.

Treatment/management/control
Prognosis is poor, in particular once signs of heart failure are present. High-dose antibiosis and drainage and flushing of the pericardium may give temporary relief. Diuresis can result in temporary relief and may be useful to support a dam to the end of gestation. Surgical stripping of the pericardium or fenestration carries a guarded prognosis. An affected goat is unfit for slaughter for human consumption.

Cardiomyopathies
Overview
Cardiomyopathies in young animals are associated with tocopherol (vitamin E) and selenium deficiency. There are other rarer causes in adults.

Aetiology
Cardiac hypertrophy and myocardial degeneration in young animals is associated with tocopherol (vitamin E) and selenium deficiency (see Chapter 15). A condition similar to dilated cardiomyopathy of adult cattle has been described in goats. Ionophore (e.g. monensin) poisoning may result in coagulative necrosis of cardiac muscle. Other reported toxins include avocado leaves (*Persea americana*) and members of the Rubiaceae family causing 'gousiekte' in southern Africa.

Clinical presentation
Exercise or excitement-induced sudden death with tocopherol (vitamin E)/selenium deficiency.

Cardiomyopathy in adults is typically characterised by signs of right-sided heart failure, often with extensive and severe dependent oedema and body cavity effusions (hydrothorax, ascites). Cardiomegaly with ventricular dilation (**Fig. 7.7**) and hypertrophy is common.

Diagnosis
See Chapter 15 for tocopherol (vitamin E)/selenium deficiency.

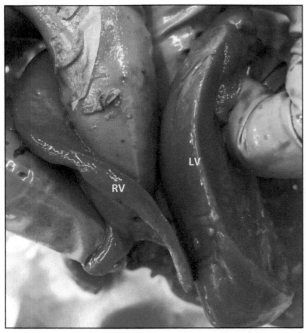

Fig. 7.7 Early stage right ventricular dilation in a yearling animal resulting in thinning of the wall (RV = right ventrical; LV = left ventrical).

Right-sided heart failure is evident on clinical examination; however, PME is required to establish the cause. On PME there is commonly extensive myocyte degeneration, atrophy, hypertrophy and muscle tissue fibrosis and necrosis. The blood vessels of heart, lung, kidney and lymph nodes may also show abnormalities.

Differential diagnosis
Neurological problems for weak or collapsed animals. Endocarditis or pericarditis for right-sided heart failure.

Treatment/management/control
No rewarding treatment is known. Whether dilated cardiomyopathy in the goat may be inherited, such as in cattle, is not known. Animals are usually affected as young adults, and therefore unlikely to successfully produce offspring.

Other conditions
Cor pulmonale has been reported secondary to respiratory disease. Cardiac neoplasia appears to be very rare.

DISORDERS OF BLOOD VESSELS

Venous thrombosis
Overview
Venous thrombosis may affect any of the major superficial veins and is often iatrogenic and therefore preventable.

Aetiology
Local inflammation or infection, commonly after intravenous injection or catheterisation leading to trauma of vessel wall, irritation from injected substances (e.g. calcium) or introduction of infection. May also result from external trauma of veins (e.g. compression caused by poor restraint or entrapment).

Clinical presentation
Obvious swelling over affected vessels. Initially painful and warm, later becoming hard and fibrous.

Complications may include tissue necrosis and sloughing, leaving the vein exposed. Proliferative growth of a thrombus may arise if a jugular catheter is left *in situ* for too long, leading to sudden death because of occlusion of the right atrium.

Embolus formation (and pulmonary embolism) appears to be rare.

Diagnosis
Clinical signs or, in the case of sudden death, thrombus detected on PME.

Differential diagnosis
Localised haematoma, foreign body reaction or insect sting. History and ultrasonography is useful to distinguish.

Treatment/management/control
Warm water bathing may help speed up the healing process. Also consider local (e.g. topical corticosteroid in non-pregnant animals, dimethyl sulfoxide) or systemic anti-inflammatories, possibly antibiotics.

After accidentally injecting an irritant substance perivascularly, dilute by injecting saline into the perivascular tissue.

If the vein has become exposed after tissue sloughing, healing mostly follows with routine wound care, and circulation is typically not compromised.

Prevention includes good i/v injection technique, in particular where irritant solutions are involved: adequate restraint of patient, discarding needle after drawing up the solution and inserting a new clean needle into the vein, and intermittently drawing back to check that the needle is still in the vessel.

For i/v catheter placement, attention is paid to aseptic preparation and adhering to the maximum dwell time for the type of catheter chosen (e.g. not more than 72 hours for short-stay catheters).

Caudal vena cava thrombosis
Overview
Caudal vena cava thrombosis is an occasional sequela to ruminitis and liver abscessation.

Aetiology
The following sequence of events has been suggested: rumenitis (e.g. caused by rumen acidosis; **Fig. 7.8**) leads to seeding of bacteria into the liver and/or caudal vena cava (either direct diffusion through rumen wall or via portal circulation). Where initially just liver abscesses form, a resulting localised phlebitis in the hepatic portion of the caudal vena cava creates abscessation in the vessel (**Fig. 7.9**). From this, emboli pass to the lungs, producing abscessation, chronic pneumonia and lesions in the pulmonary arterioles. Arteritis and thromboembolism occur and aneurysms may develop in the pulmonary artery. These rupture, causing severe haemorrhage into the alveoli and bronchial tubes. Organisms involved include *Fusobacterium necrophorum* and *T. pyogenes*.

Clinical presentation
Sudden death in peracute cases, with blood appearing at the mouth and nostrils. In less acute cases, possible signs include a painful cough, haemoptysis, pale mucous membranes, thoracic pain, increased lung sounds and a haemic murmur. Some animals may show signs of cardiac failure with liver enlargement and ascites.

Diagnosis
The sporadic and often peracute nature of the disease prevents easy diagnosis, although haemoptysis and anaemia are suggestive. The vena cava abscess may be seen on radiographs (close to the diaphragm) or with ultrasonography.

Differential diagnosis
Anthrax for sudden death with bleeding. Other causes of anaemia, thoracic pain or cardiac failure.

Treatment/management/control
Antibiosis is typically unrewarding, with prognosis very poor especially where haemoptysis is evident. Others in the group on a similar diet are likely to have suffered rumenitis and liver abscessation as well, and

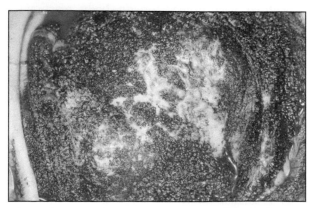

Fig. 7.8 Signs of rumenitis: loss of papillae and scarring (post-mortem specimen).

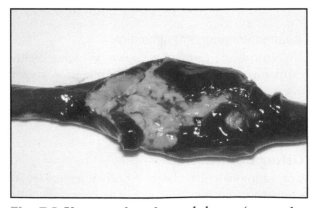

Fig. 7.9 Vena cava thrombus and abscess (removed from vessel).

disposal in the near future should be considered. If taken to slaughter, the owner should be prepared for carcase condemnation.

Control involves prevention of rumenitis, in particular rumen acidosis (see Chapter 5).

Other vascular abnormalities

Arterial thrombosis, or vasculitis resulting in occlusion of peripheral capillaries, may be seen with severe bacteraemia or septicaemia (e.g. salmonellosis) and some toxins (e.g. ergot). This may lead to necrosis of peripheral tissue, such as the ear tips, or the coronary band, resulting in loss of the horn capsule. A thrombus in the middle uterine artery is an occasional incidental finding and typically regresses slowly.

Trauma to superficial vessels may occur from fighting amongst animals, predator or dog attack, or sharp objects in the animal's environment. The mammary vein in the lactating doe is particularly vulnerable. Any severe haemorrhage is treated accordingly, including blood transfusion where necessary. Resulting haematomata are best left alone.

Portosystemic shunts have been reported in a variety of breeds, in kids from 1 month to 1 year of age. Typical signs include poor growth and a hepatic encephalopathy resulting in neurological signs.

Calcification of blood vessels can be caused by toxicosis with calciferol (vitamin D) or golden oat grass (*Trisetum flavescens*).

DISORDERS OF THE HAEMATOPOIETIC SYSTEM

Normal structure and function
Blood forming organs
Primary haematopoiesis (i.e. formation of the three lineages of blood cells, namely erythroid cells, lymphocytes and myelocytes) takes place in the long bones in young animals and mainly in the pelvis, sternum and vertebrae in adults. Involved in secondary, or extramedullary, formation are the spleen, thymus and lymph nodes (maturation of cells, and activation and some proliferation of lymphoid cells). In the fetus, the liver is important for haematopoiesis.

Thymus
The thoracic part of the thymus lies in the dorsal mediastinum in front of the heart. Most of the cervical part lies in the lower one-third of the neck, with bilateral limbs reaching all the way to the larynx. Whether the thymus continues to grow in the kid up to puberty, as in the lamb, is unknown. Although the thymus does involute as the animal matures, a considerable thoracic remnant can still be found in 5-year-old goats.

Lymph nodes
Table 7.2 shows details of the main external lymph nodes, plus a selection of internal lymph nodes that may be of interest during PME.

Anaemia
Overview
Anaemia is a common and potentially life-threatening condition, with a multitude of aetiologies.

Aetiology
Common causes include endoparasites (blood sucking or blood losing such as *Haemonchus contortus*, liver fluke [and other trematodes], coccidiosis), ectoparasites (lice, ticks), blood parasites (babesiosis, anaplasmosis), chronic inflammatory disease (including heavy endoparasite burden), haemolysis and haemorrhage. *Table 7.3* gives an overview of the more common causes.

Clinical presentation
Pale to completely white mucous membranes are the main clinical indicator (**Fig. 7.10**).

Diagnosis
Haematology will confirm anaemia. In cases of haemolytic anaemia, an animal-side urine sample can be indicative (urine discolouration and abnormal urine dipstick reactions). Where blood parasites are suspected, it is important to prepare an air-dried smear immediately after collecting the blood sample.

Endoparasite burden should always be investigated, bearing in mind that a faecal egg count (FEC) may give a false-negative result (e.g. larvae sucking blood in haemonchosis, severe pathology in the

Table 7.2 **The main external and selected internal lymph nodes of the goat.**

NAME	LOCATION	SIZE (MM)	PALPABLE?
Parotid	Caudoventral to mandibular joint, covered by the parotid gland	10–50	If enlarged
Mandibular	Caudoventral mandibular ramus	15–35	Yes
Retropharyngeal (lateral)	Below wing of atlas, 2–3 nodes each side	7–28, disc-shaped	If enlarged
Prescapular	At the cranial edge of the supraspinatus muscle, two-thirds down the shoulder blade	35–60	Yes
Popliteal	2.5 cm deep between the semitendinosus and glutaeobiceps muscles	10–25	If enlarged
Subiliac	Cranial to quadriceps muscle, about halfway between the tuber coxae and patella	50	Yes
Supramammary (superficial inguinal)	In female: two nodes at base of udder (near pudendal vessels)	Bean-sized	If enlarged
Caudal mediastinal	Unpaired in midline between thoracic aorta and oesophagus	Small node: 10–30; large node: 100–130	Internal
Jejunal	In mesenterium, between jejunum and ascending colon; typically about 12 nodes (2–25)	Average 35 (range 3–300)	Internal
Intestinal – other	Associated with the various sections of small and large intestine	Average 15–20	Internal

Source: Compiled based on data from: Vollmerhaus B (2005) Lymphatisches System. In: *Nickel, Schummer, Seiferle - Lehrbuch der Anatomie der Haustiere, Band III*, 4th edn. (eds K-H Habermehl, B Vollmerhaus, H Wilkens *et al.*) [Lymphatic system. In: *Textbook of Anatomy of Domestic Animals, Vol. III*, 4th edn.] Parey Verlag, Stuttgart.

Table 7.3 **Known or potential causes of anaemia in goats.**

CAUSE	COMMENTS
Inflammatory process	In particular chronic processes. Blood protein levels often changed
Parasitism	In particular *Haemonchus contortus* and liver fluke, but potentially any severe worm burden. Severe lice or tick burden
Haemorrhage	External (e.g. dog bite, accident) or internal (e.g. accident, obstetrical). (**Note:** Thick fleece may hide external injuries.) Also extensive abomasal/duodenal ulceration
Iron deficiency	Rare in grazing adults. Possibly microcytosis and hypochromia, especially in chronic cases
Blood parasites	If suspected, prepare an air-dried smear immediately after taking blood sample. Examine with Giemsa stain
Haemolysis	Nitrate/nitrite ingestion. Red maple leaves (presents with intravascular haemolysis and Heinz bodies). Onions or brassica species. Haemolytic crisis in chronic copper toxicity
Copper deficiency	
Bone marrow	Neoplasia or functional abnormalities (e.g. myelodysplastic syndrome)
Coagulopathies	*Mycoplasma mycoides subsp. mycoides*, inherited afibrinogenaemia (factor I deficiency in Saanen goats), secondary to severe liver disease. Also possibly snake venom, warfarin, mycotoxins or sweet vernal grass (*Anthoxanthum odoratum*) toxicosis

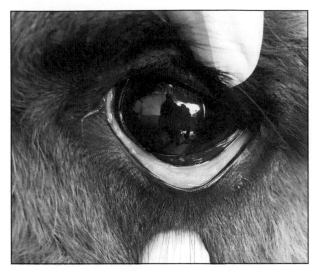

Fig. 7.10 Pale mucous membranes (here conjunctiva) indicate either anaemia or poor perfusion.

pre-patent period with coccidiosis and liver fluke, less correlation between FEC and worm burden in adult goats). Hypoproteinaemia may be present, especially with coccidiosis.

If anaemia is the result of inflammatory disease, finding the primary cause can be a challenge. A thorough clinical examination, blood biochemistry and further diagnostic aids, such as ultrasonography, are of immense value and may have to be repeated if a diagnosis cannot be established first time round.

For prognosis and treatment, establishing whether the anaemia is regenerative or non-regenerative is of interest. Signs of regeneration include anisocytosis, polychromasia, reticulocytosis and increased numbers of metarubricytes. However, these are not consistently present and sometimes may be present in clinically normal animals. In cases with a chronic, non-regenerative anaemia a bone-marrow biopsy is of value. Under local infiltration anaesthesia, a suitable biopsy needle is inserted into the thick part of the sternum. Bone marrow is harvested by 2–4 strong pulls on a 10-ml syringe. A smear is prepared immediately. Additional sample material can be stored in EDTA.

Differential diagnosis

The main one to consider is CV compromise, often presenting with the following clinical findings: delayed capillary refill time, weak pulse (as opposed to thready character with anaemia), pulse deficit, cold extremities and heart murmur (although anaemia-induced murmurs can occur).

Treatment/management/control

The primary cause is treated as appropriate, with supportive nursing care including high-quality nutrition.

A blood transfusion should be considered in cases with either severe anaemia (PCV <0.12 l/l) or rapid blood loss. It may also be of benefit outside the emergency situation, in particular where there are no signs of regeneration. Goats have at least five major blood group systems with a substantial degree of polymorphism, making exact matching of donor and recipient difficult. However, in the field cross-reactions appear rare, especially during the first transfusion. Suitable donor animals include non-breeding males or non-pregnant females, at least 2 years of age, clinically healthy and ideally from the same breed and herd. A human blood collection set and its needle are suitable (see **Fig. 4.11,** p. 92). A 60 kg goat can easily donate 500 ml (from the jugular vein; sedated if necessary). As a rule-of-thumb, one litre of blood will increase the haematocrit of the recipient by 5%.

Milk goitre/thymic enlargement
Overview

Milk goitre/thymic enlargement is a self-curing marked swelling of the cervical parts of the thymus. Anglo-Nubian and Boer goats appear more susceptible.

Aetiology

Unknown. Blood and dietary iodine levels are normal. Investigated cases have been negative for a variety of pathogens.

Clinical presentation

Large bilateral swelling just caudal to the mandibular ramus and sometimes underneath the lower jaw as well. Swelling develops from about 1 week of age, and typically starts regressing from 4–6 months of age. If severe, discomfort and change in vocalisation may be seen. The swelling must be differentiated from thyroid enlargement.

Diagnosis

Clinical signs and PME. The cervical part of the thymus may reach around 200 g in weight. Histology is normal.

Differential diagnosis

Caseous lymphadenitis (CLA) is ruled out by culture. General abscessation is confirmed with ultrasonography and aspirate. Severe upper respiratory tract infection leading to reactive lymph node enlargement will show associated clinical signs.

Treatment/management/control

None. The apparent success of iodine supplementation is highly ambiguous. In addition, forced reduction of the thymus may negatively influence immunocompetence.

Neoplasia of lymph nodes or thymus

Overview

Multicentric, sporadic or thymic lymphoma or lymphosarcoma (**Fig. 7.11**), and thymoma are recognised.

Aetiology

Sporadic forms of lymphoma/lymphosarcoma appear to be more common than multicentric ones in goats. Aside from lymph nodes, almost all other tissues may be affected, including synovial membranes and meninges. Sometimes associated with bovine leukaemia virus, and occasionally there is neoplastic involvement of the bone marrow.

The thoracic part of the thymus is retained well into adulthood, and thymoma is a common neoplasia in mature goats.

Clinical presentation

Typically, a progressive debilitating presentation in goats over 2 years old. Weight loss and increasing weakness are common. Some goats are alert, others depressed and inappetent. Depending on the lymph nodes involved, other signs may include ataxia, dysphagia, abdominal pain, dyspnoea, reduced milk yield, diarrhoea, exophthalmos, pyrexia and enlargement of superficial lymph nodes.

For mediastinal lesions, tachypnoea and dyspnoea, tachycardia with uni- or bilaterally muffled heart sounds, and pleural effusion are common findings, as is a pronounced jugular pulse. However, a considerable number of goats with thoracic thymomas show no obvious associated signs.

Diagnosis

Imaging for internal lesions. Palpation and fine needle aspirate or biopsy for lesions of external lymph nodes. Lymphocytosis may be evident on haematology. Gross evidence of thymic enlargement is evident at PME (**Fig. 7.12**).

Differential diagnosis

The main specific conditions to consider are: Johne's disease, CLA, dental disease and endoparasitism for progressive weight loss; CLA and pneumonia for dyspnoea. In cases with ataxia, a full neurological examination to locate the lesion is indicated, and caprine arthritis-encephalitis should be considered.

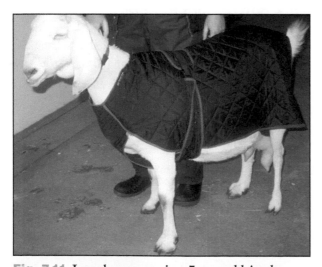

Fig. 7.11 Lymphosarcoma in a 7-year-old Anglo-Nubian doe. Retropharyngeal and submandibular lymph nodes were visibly enlarged (note swelling near throat). Internally, lesions were present in lung, liver and kidneys (and their associated lymph nodes).

Treatment/management/control

Symptomatic treatment may be tried, but is often without noticeable effect. Chemotherapy (cyclophosphamide) has been described in sheep.

Swelling disease

Overview

Swelling disease is recognised in multiple countries, including the UK, mainly affecting young animals and fibre breeds.

Aetiology

Remains unestablished, with hypotheses including proteinaemia/hypoalbuminaemia, tocopherol (vitamin E) or selenium deficiency, stress (like shearing) and vasoactive substances.

Clinical presentation

Oedema affecting the caudoventral abdomen (**Fig. 7.13a**), limbs (**Fig. 7.13b**) and udder, with up

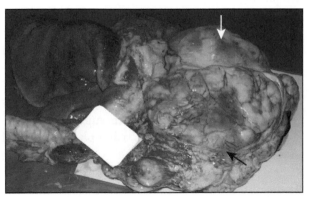

Fig. 7.12 A thymic lymphosarcoma at post-mortem examination (white arrow = heart; black arrow = thymoma).

to 5 kg of fluid accumulation reported. Affected animals may be lame and show signs of anaemia. Appetite often remains good and rectal temperature typically within normal range. Goats usually recover within 3–4 days, but recurrent episodes are possible.

Diagnosis

Clinical signs. Changes on haematology may include relative neutrophilia, basophilia and low total protein or albumin or albumin:globulin ratio. Biochemistry parameters tend to be within normal limits.

Differential diagnosis

For dependent oedema, consider chronic liver disease, cardiac problems, endoparasitism, Johne's disease and plant poisoning.

For anaemia, see above.

Treatment/management/control

Supportive only.

Caseous lymphadenitis

Definition/overview

CLA is a chronic bacterial infection affecting both goats and sheep. It causes superficial and visceral lymphadenopathy and has a worldwide distribution. It is a potential zoonotic pathogen.

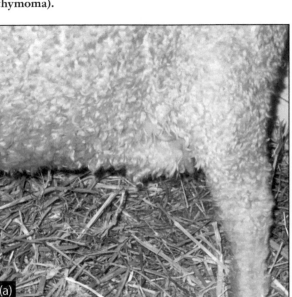

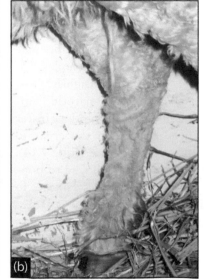

Fig. 7.13 Two Angora goats with swelling disease showing varying degrees of oedema.
(a) Along the ventral abdomen up to the udder;
(b) in the limbs.

Aetiology

The causative agent in both species is *Corynebacterium pseudotuberculosis*, a facultative anaerobic organism.

Pathophysiology

The organisms gain access mainly through wounds or small breaks in the skin and mucous membrane, but occasionally in heavy infections by inhalation into the lung tissue and associated lymph nodes. They are carried to regional lymph nodes, in which they can remain, resisting normal host immune mechanisms. The incubation period from infection to superficial lymph node enlargement becoming apparent due to abscess formation may be as long as 6 months, although 2–3 months is more typical. Abscesses may rupture and drain spontaneously or, if prominent, may rupture due to mechanical insult. This is usually followed by apparent resolution. In heavily infected herds, internal abscesses may develop in a number of sites, particularly the bronchial and mediastinal lymph nodes following inhalation, but have been reported in many other sites including renal and hepatic nodes. It is important to emphasise that once infected, a goat will probably never be free of infection, even if a lymph node has become enlarged, has ruptured and apparently healed. Disease can theoretically flare up at any stage.

Clinical presentation

In many affected goats, there is little or no impact on their general health and productivity, because typically it is only the superficial lymph nodes that are affected, although these are unsightly. The most common superficial nodes are parotid, submandibular and prescapular, reflecting the greater likelihood of superficial trauma in the areas to which these nodes provide drainage (**Fig. 7.14**). Infected lesions in the hind legs will lead to popliteal lymph node enlargement, and damage to the skin of the udder and teats may cause enlargement of the supramammary node. However, if infection levels in the herd increase, abscess formation becomes more widespread, internal

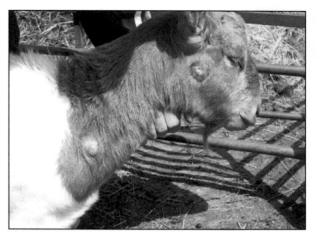

Fig. 7.14 A young Boer kid showing caseous lymphadenitis lesions in the parotid and prescapular lymph nodes.

organs and lymph nodes are affected, and clinical signs will vary depending on the site of bacterial multiplication.

Diagnosis

The presence of one or more superficial swellings anatomically linked to a lymph node should raise a strong suspicion of CLA. Culturing *C. pseudotuberculosis* will confirm the diagnosis. If an abscess is burst, a swab inserted into the abscess and rubbed over the abscess capsule is ideal, although there is a greater chance of contaminating bacterial overgrowth. If no burst abscesses are available, then after shaving and sterilising the skin surface, a wide bore needle is inserted into the abscess and pus aspirated, although this may be very thick. It is important while waiting for results that any goats with discharging abscesses, including any that were subjected to needle aspiration, are isolated to minimise spread. Serological tests are available and are being used to manage outbreaks, although false-negative results in early infection can be problematic.

Differential diagnosis

The condition is fairly characteristic, but should be differentiated from Morel's disease, lymphosarcoma or bacterial abscesses due to other pathogens such as *Staphylococcus aureus* or *T. pyogenes*.

Treatment/management/control

Treatment of individual goats of economic or sentimental value can be attempted, but is of questionable value as a tool for control in infected herds. There are two approaches: either surgical or by the use of antibiotic (or a combination of the two).

Surgical treatment involves either draining or excising infected lymph nodes. Mature abscesses can be incised at a dependant point, and the contents flushed out with a weak disinfectant solution. The content is infectious and should be collected and disposed of away from other livestock. The goat is then kept in isolation until the abscess has healed. Excision is a safer option for disease control, but care must be taken to avoid major blood vessels located near the parotid gland in particular. The main problem with the surgical approach is that only visibly enlarged nodes are dealt with. Allowing the abscesses to mature and burst naturally is to be discouraged, as the leaking pus can contaminate the building fixtures and fittings (such as feed troughs) on which the organism can survive for up to 10 weeks (and up to 6 months in contaminated soil). Because of the potential zoonotic risk, protective gloves should always be worn.

Antibiotic treatment of infected goats has been attempted, but can give disappointing results, mainly because antibiotics cannot penetrate into the centre of abscesses where the organism resides.

Control in infected herds is based on identification of infected goats (by clinical evidence of abscess formation, or positive serology) and a strict culling policy. This approach has been reportedly successful. Attention should be paid to possible environmental trauma predisposing to new infections, such as projecting nails, barbed wire or gate hinges. Ectoparasitic infestations should be controlled – they will predispose to rubbing, potentially compromising skin integrity, which may allow the causative bacteria to enter. Because the organism is so resistant in the environment, control by segregating known infected goats from 'clean' goats is difficult. Infection can be readily transferred from one group to another on weigh crates, hurdles, feed troughs and in the milking parlour. Thorough cleaning and disinfection with an approved disinfectant should be undertaken regularly, including shearing equipment in fibre herds.

There are commercial vaccines available in some countries, and some success has also been reported following the use of autogenous vaccines. Keeping new infection out of clean herds is of paramount importance, but is problematic due to the long incubation period when goats are outwardly healthy. All incoming goats should be examined for evidence of enlarged lymph nodes while in quarantine, but an effective quarantine period for this disease should be 2–3 months. Serological screening of incoming goats is a further tool, although false-negative results are a problem in the early stages of disease. Where possible purchases are made only from herds where no clinical disease has been recorded.

Babesiosis
Overview
Babesiosis is caused by intraerythrocytic protozoan parasites of the genus *Babesia*. Transmitted by ticks, babesiosis affects a wide range of domestic and wild animals worldwide. It is a particular problem in cattle, but the disease has been described in goats.

Aetiology
Goats can be infected by several species of *Babesia*. The two most important ones are *B. ovis* and *B. motasi*, transmitted by the ticks *Rhipicephalus bursa* and *Haemaphysalis* spp., respectively. Infection is of importance in the Middle East, southern Europe and some African and Asian countries.

Clinical presentation
Infection leads to erythrocyte destruction, often preceded by a non-specific pyrexia. This erythrocyte damage leads to inappetence, anaemia, jaundice, weight loss and increased respiratory rate together with haemoglobinuria in the terminal stages.

Diagnosis
Diagnosis is based on the clinical signs, often with ticks still evident on the skin surface. Examination of Giemsa-stained, air-dried smears prepared immediately after sampling from peripheral blood (e.g. ear) will demonstrate the dark staining intraerythrocytic inclusions. Serological and PCR tests are being adapted for

detection of disease in cattle, and these may be available and validated for use in goats in affected countries. At PME, splenomegaly is often a feature accompanied by evidence of jaundice and anaemia.

Differential diagnosis
Other causes of haemoglobinuria (see *Table 10.1*).

Treatment/management/control
Treatment commonly utilises the diamidine derivatives, with a single i/m dose of diminazine (3 mg/kg) or imidocarb (1–2 mg/kg). Control is aimed at tick control. Vaccination using live, attenuated strains of the parasites has been used successfully in a number of countries.

CHAPTER 8

NERVOUS SYSTEM DISORDERS

CLINICAL EXAMINATION OF THE NERVOUS SYSTEM

A good understanding of the nervous system and a methodical approach to examination is essential to pinpoint the lesion to a particular part of the system, thereby narrowing down the multitude of differential diagnoses. Exact location may remain elusive in some patients because of overlap of neurological function between areas or concurrent disorders.

Consciousness, alertness and behaviour

For clinical cases, the following simplistic approach is usually sufficient. The fore- and midbrain and part of the brainstem are responsible for mental state, behaviour and sensory functions. The hindbrain (cerebellum) governs coordination. *Table 8.1* details

Table 8.1 **Central nervous system regions and their associated functions.**

REGION	FUNCTION
Frontal cortex	Mentation, behaviour, fine motor function
Parietal cortex	Pain, proprioception
Occipital cortex	Vision
Temporal cortex	Behaviour, hearing
Hypothalamus and pituitary gland	Autonomic and endocrine function
Limbic system	Inherent behaviour
Cerebellum	Coordination of voluntary movements, subconscious proprioception
Brainstem (reticular activating system)	Consciousness, alertness

the important areas and functions of the central nervous system (CNS). Severe impairment of vision or hearing can lead to fear-induced behavioural abnormalities.

Reflexes, upper motor neurons and lower motor neurons

A simple reflex pathway triggers a motor response without CNS contribution. It is important that all components of the pathway are intact: sensory receptor (e.g. a stretch receptor in the patella tendon), corresponding sensory neuron in the dorsal ganglion, internuncial neuron (which effects muscle contraction via an efferent motor neuron), nerve endings, neuromuscular junction and muscle. A malfunction in any of these parts could be the reason for a reflex being absent. For example, an absent menace reflex in an animal with listeriosis is not necessarily because it cannot see, but because it cannot blink due to facial nerve paralysis.

The motor neuron part in these reflexes is largely alpha neurons, also called lower motor neurons (LMNs), located in the ventral grey matter of the spinal cord and brainstem. Signs of a LMN lesion include loss of reflexes, severe weakness and in particular extensor muscle weakness, muscle atrophy, and flaccid paralysis (i.e. loss of voluntary movement). The extensor weakness commonly results in a short stride length, with a bouncing or 'bunny-hopping' gait.

The upper motor neuron (UMN) system has the following roles:

1 It receives feedback from the sensory input of the reflex arc on pain, touch and proprioception. It is important to observe the animal for generic signs of pain, such as

vocalisation, twitching, body movements or head jerk, particularly when conducting deep pain tests, where a defect in the peripheral nerve or executing muscle may lead to absence of the expected localised response.

2 It controls voluntary movements, particularly initiation of movement and flexor muscle strength. Therefore, UMN lesions typically manifest as slow onset of the swing phase, a long stride and decreased joint flexion (leading to 'marching soldier' gait in extreme cases).

3 Lastly, it has a calming effect on reflexes. Therefore, a lesion cranial to a reflex arc will result in an exaggerated response, potentially to the point of spastic paresis. Ataxia, and hypoalgesia in affected areas, may also be seen. A small lesion often has a marked effect, and depending on its location (e.g. off-centre, unilateral, bilateral) signs are restricted to one side of the animal or not (e.g. hemiparesis versus tetraparesis). In large animals, even marked lesions in the motor centres of the cerebral cortex do not appear to exert any severe or long-term effect other than fine motor function.

Normal head/cranial nerve reflexes include:

- The response to noise is to look towards source. A high-pitched sound is best to elicit a response.
- Menace reflex is present, but is a learned response and therefore may not be seen in neonates. Care must be taken not to create airflow towards the eye when testing the menace reflex.
- Palpebral and corneal reflexes are always present.
- Facial sensation can be tested by tickling the hairs on the muzzle or introducing a pen or similar into the nostril.
- Gag reflex can be elicited by palpating the larynx, then observing the swallowing response.
- Suck reflex is present in healthy kids.
- Eyes follow nose when the head is moved.
- Indirect and direct pupillary light reflexes are present; however, the pupil rarely constricts fully.
- *Table 8.2* shows the connection between the type of blindness and location of lesion.

Normal limb reflexes include:

- The patellar reflex, with the animal in lateral recumbency, is reasonably reliable. Gastrocnemius, cranial tibial, biceps, or triceps reflexes show variable responses.
- The stoic nature of goats means that the withdrawal reflex is very unreliable. Stimulation consists of pinching the interdigital space or coronary band. When present, an initial delay is common.

Table 8.2 **Guidelines on type of blindness and likely location of lesion.**

REFLEX	LOCATION OF LESION
PLR present	'Higher' lesion (i.e. CNS) Cases of cerebrocortical necrosis (CCN) or poisoning with sodium, sulphur or lead
PLR lost	Retinal, optic nerve or optic chiasm
Pupils dilated	Optic nerve trauma, retinol (vitamin A) deficiency
Strabismus present	Cranial nerves III, IV, VI (**Fig. 8.1**)

PLR = pupillary light reflex.

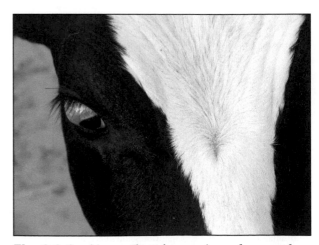

Fig. 8.1 Strabismus (here in a cow) may be caused by lesions affecting cranial nerves III, IV or VI, or a space-occupying lesion in the orbit.

Body region reflexes include:

- The panniculus reflex is usually present, but may be difficult to appreciate in thick coated goats.
- The goat should dip its back in response to stimulation of the withers region.
- Anal/perineal reflex is variable. Stimulation of the ventral vulva or base of penis may also be tried.

Proprioception may be assessed by:

- Asking the animal to move up and down a kerb, or over obstacles.
- Making the moving animal stop suddenly.
- Pulling a foot away from the body with the aid of a piece of paper, cardboard or towel placed underneath (paper slide test). However, it is not uncommon to see considerable sideways movement of the leg before the goat corrects the position
- Knuckling reflex. Care must be taken not to support the goat's weight, otherwise a poor response is likely.
- 3-legged walking and hemi-walking should result in hopping movements. Variable results are more a function of logistics, with adults often resentful to handling and neonates collapsing in response.

Vestibular syndrome

This is caused by lesions affecting the inner ear, cranial nerve VIII, the medulla oblongata or parts of the cerebellum. Common causes are head trauma and otitis interna or media. Clinical signs include head tilt (versus head aversion with forebrain lesions), strabismus, changes to the normal nystagmus, leaning, falling, drifting sideways, wide-based stance and deliberate movements. There is a mild, regular irregular ataxia, but no hypermetria. Blindfolding exacerbates signs. Bilateral lesions may present more like cerebellar signs. Because the facial nerve travels in part parallel to cranial nerve VIII, facial paralysis may also be present (**Fig. 8.2**). Neck pain (e.g. after injection site reaction to an i/m injection) must be ruled out as cause of apparent head aversion or reluctance to bend the neck.

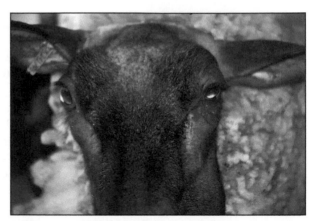

Fig. 8.2 Vestibular signs in a ewe with otitis media. Mild head tilt and facial nerve compromise shown by a drooped left ear, lowered upper left eyelid and food impaction in the left cheek.

REGION	CLINICAL SIGNS
C1 to C5	All four legs affected, but spastic paresis often more pronounced in the hind legs compared with the front legs
C2 to T2	All four legs affected, but front legs worse than hind legs. Front legs show reduced muscle tone and reflexes (versus normal to increased in hind legs). If both grey and white matter are affected, a 'two engine' gait results: LMN component in front legs resulting in short and/or bouncing stride; UMN component in hind legs resulting in slow onset, long stride
T3 to S2	Trunk and hind legs affected. May see specific peripheral nerves or muscles affected (e.g. lesion at L4 resulting in femoral nerve deficits)
S1 to S5	Abnormal signs associated with rectum, anus, perineum and bladder function

Table 8.3 **Spinal cord lesions and their associated clinical signs.**

C = cervical vertebra; T = thoracic vertebra; S = sacral vertebra.

Spinal lesions

Table 8.3 is a basic guide to pinpointing which part of the spinal cord is affected, depending on the signs seen.

Peripheral nerves

Hyperflexion or hyperextension of particular joints typically allows identification of the compromised

Table 8.4 **Lesion location and associated gait and postural abnormalities.**

ABNORMALITY	CHARACTERISTIC FOR LESION OF	USUALLY PRESENT WITH LESION OF	USUALLY ABSENT WITH LESION OF
Postural deficit	Cerebrum, vestibular	Brainstem, cerebellum, UMN, LMN, spinal cord, peripheral nerve	
Paresis	LMN, peripheral nerve	Brainstem, UMN, spinal cord, musculoskeletal	Cerebrum, vestibular, cerebellum
Ataxia	Cerebellum	Brainstem, vestibular, UMN, spinal cord	Cerebrum, musculoskeletal
Hypometria		Brainstem, vestibular, UMN, spinal cord, some LMN	Cerebrum
Hypermetria	Cerebellum, some LMN	Brainstem, UMN, spinal cord	Cerebrum, vestibular, musculoskeletal

LMN = lower motor neuron; UMN = upper motor neuron.
Source: Adapted from Mayhew J (2009) *Large Animal Neurology*, 2nd edn. Wiley-Blackwell, Ames.

peripheral nerve (see *Table 8.5*). To differentiate nerve malfunction from muscle malfunction, skin sensation is tested (being absent if nerve is involved, **Fig. 8.13**). Close observation for muscle atrophy is also useful to detect peripheral nerve disorders.

Specific assessment considerations
Gait and posture
Abnormalities in gait and posture may help to establish what part of the nervous system is affected (*Table 8.4*)

Differentiating ataxia and weakness
With ataxia, there is a lack of order or an inconsistent order (i.e. proprioceptive dysfunction). This results in irregular and unpredictable movements. The ataxia is exaggerated by circling or moving backwards or on an incline.

Weakness, or paresis, presents with consistently changed movements. Lifting one leg will often make the weakness worse, inducing muscle tremors on the contralateral leg. The swing phase is shortened or delayed, and the animal cannot resist a tail pull.

Using challenging movements
Forcing the animal to make unusual movements can highlight ataxia or any unilateral character of a deficit, and is useful to differentiate lameness from a neurological disorder. Circling and weaving during the swing phase forces a change to the normal flight-path of the leg. If the goat is ataxic, it may result in stepping on the other foot, crossing over or circumduction etc.

Moving the animal backwards, or up and down an incline, highlights ataxia and may exacerbate UMN signs (such as 'marching soldier' gait). A similar result can be achieved by holding the goat's head high. This helps to detect UMN input, as several parameters are changed like the visual horizon.

Pulling on the lead rope or tail is a good test to detect extensor or flexor muscle weakness. If the goat can resist the pull while standing, but not while circling, a UMN lesion is likely (e.g. a cervical lesion in a wobbler case). In contrast, inability to resist a pull while standing indicates an extensor muscle weakness (i.e. likely a LMN lesion [e.g. resistance to a tail pull is poor in a lesion at lumbar vertebrae 3–5]). The pull should be applied in a constant manner, not a sharp jerk, and with force appropriate for the goat's size.

Blindfolding
This is a useful technique to accentuate abnormalities arising from the brain or inner ear lesions (in particular vestibular syndrome). It is also useful to establish unilateral blindness. It should be performed on soft ground or with an assistant ready to prevent falling. The left and right eye are blindfolded in turn, followed by complete blindfolding.

The recumbent patient

Neurological assessment of the recumbent goat is often difficult. Unless a fracture is suspected, every effort should be made to lift up the animal, or encourage it to stand, to facilitate examination. Flaccid attempts to take its own weight after lifting suggest a LMN lesion or severe depression. Spastic attempts suggest UMN involvement.

If the goat can get into a dog-sitting position and is using its front legs well, including extending the legs, in an attempt to stand, it likely has a lesion caudal to T2. Otherwise, the lesion is cranial to T2. If the goat is lifting its head, but not the neck, the location is in the cranial cervical cord.

Spinal reflexes can be tested quite well in the recumbent patient. However, it must be remembered that muscle tone and reflexes are often poor in the limb the goat has been resting on. Flaccid muscle tone suggests an LMN lesion.

For progress monitoring of a patient undergoing treatment, the tail, anal and perineal reflexes should be checked regularly. Contusion and oedema of the lower spinal cord often result from prolonged recumbency, dog-sitting posture or suspension in a sling.

The neonatal goat

Mentation and sensory function adjust within 24 hours post partum in the neonate, and behaviour within 2–7 days. A mild wide-based stance (see **Fig. 4.9**, p. 91) and somewhat jerky movements or mild hypermetria are normal in neonates. They usually have a dominant extensor tendon strength, and this may result in hyperreflexia. As mentioned earlier, the menace reflex is a learned response and is typically absent in kids less than 1 week old. A neurological neonate may demonstrate sham-chewing, lip curling, star gazing, yawning and 'rag-doll' limpness (**Fig. 8.3**).

Common non-neurological disorders may present with a similar clinical picture to nervous system disorders. In particular, tendon hyperextension or contraction, septicaemia, hypothermia, hypoglycaemia and parturition-induced anoxia. These common conditions should always be ruled out. Particular attention should be paid to ensuring passive transfer in a neurological neonate.

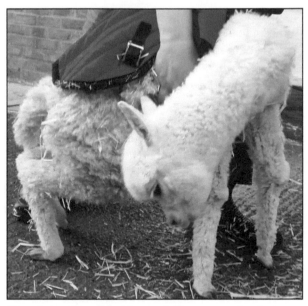

Fig. 8.3 Limp, flaccid 'rag-doll' presentation in a neonatal alpaca with a brain lesion.

Cerebrospinal fluid collection and analysis

Indication

Cerebrospinal fluid (CSF) collection and analysis is useful in most cases with neurological signs or suspected spinal trauma. Collection from the lumbosacral space (as described here) can be safely carried out in the field. Collection from the cisterna magna requires general anaesthesia and carries a higher risk of adverse reaction.

Preparation and equipment

The lumbosacral area is clipped and surgically prepared. A hypodermic or spinal needle, 19 or 20 gauge, 2.5 cm (1 in) for kids, 3.75–5 cm (1.5–2 in) for adults, plain and EDTA sampling pots, a 5–10 ml syringe and surgical gloves are required.

Restraint

Conscious, possibly lightly sedated goat in sternal recumbency. An assistant kneels facing backwards over the withers of the goat, with the goat's head and neck between their legs (taking care not to exert too much pressure onto the withers). The assistant grasps a hind leg in each hand, pulling them forwards so that they come to lie along either side of the goat's abdomen. This results in downward tilting of the spine and opens the lumbosacral space (**Fig. 8.4**).

Local anaesthetic (1 ml in a kid or 2–3 ml in an adult of 2% lidocaine HCl or 5% procaine HCl) is injected subcutaneously and into the muscle.

Technical description

The lumbosacral space can be felt just caudal (1–2 finger-widths) to an imaginary line connecting the tuber coxae (**Fig. 8.5**). When placing the index finger onto the dorsal spinous processes just cranial to this line, and then drawing it caudally with some pressure, the finger will 'fall' into the space.

Kneeling behind the animal, the surgeon introduces the needle precisely midline into the space at an angle of 75 degrees to the skin (i.e. slightly off perpendicular with the hub angled caudally). With the wrist resting on the animal, the needle is steadily advanced while appreciating the layers it penetrates, namely: skin, subcutaneous tissue and muscle, interarcuate ligament and ligamentum flavum (slight 'pop') followed by entering the epidural space, then dura mater (another slight 'pop') to enter the subarachnoid space. Placing a drop of local anaesthetic into the needle hub once the skin has been penetrated is useful to establish that the epidural space has been entered. After entering the subarachnoid space just a little deeper to this, CSF will typically well up after about 10 seconds and can be collected free-flow or with a syringe (break seal of syringe plunger before connecting). It is important to not advance the needle too deeply, as penetration of the conus medullaris will elicit a pain response (**Fig. 8.6**). If two attempts (using a fresh needle) fail, the procedure should be abandoned.

One to 2 ml is placed into an EDTA and a sterile sample pot. A rough assessment can be undertaken on farm: orange discolouration suggests haemorrhage into the spinal canal. Vigorous shaking of the sample may lead to precipitation if the protein contents is increased. (**Note**: Precipitation renders the sample unsuitable for running through an analyser.)

Normal values for common CSF parameters in ruminants are: protein, <0.4 g/l; nucleated cells, 0–8/µl; red blood cells, none; bacteria, none.

Aftercare

The penetration site should be protected from contamination.

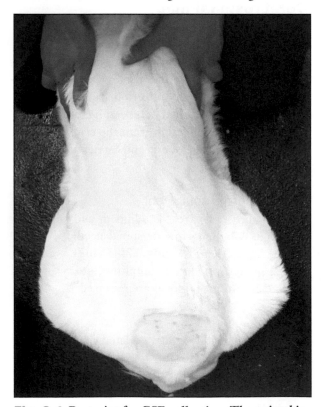

Fig. 8.4 Restraint for CSF collection. The animal is held in sternal recumbency, with an assistant pulling both hind legs forward alongside the body.

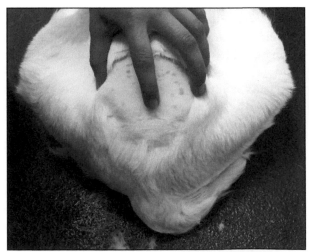

Fig. 8.5 The person's index finger rests on the lumbosacral space, which is 1–2 finger-widths caudal to a line between the tuber coxae (indicated by person's thumb and middle finger).

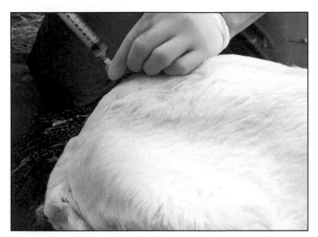

Fig. 8.6 The needle has been advanced at 75 degrees to the skin and, after entering the subarachnoid space, a syringe attached to collect the CSF.

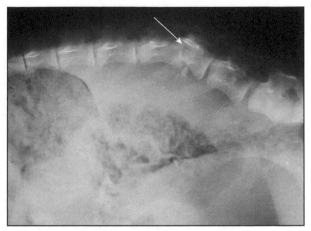

Fig. 8.7 Vertebral fracture in the lumbar region, obvious on a plain radiograph (arrow).

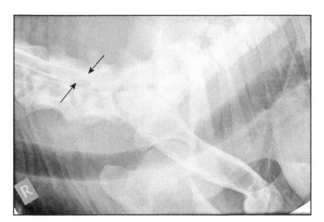

Fig. 8.8 Myelogram highlighting a space-occupying cervical spine lesion. The contrast material does not progress caudally (arrows indicate its end point).

Potential complications

Haemodilution of sample if needle is placed laterally. Pain response if needle is placed too deep. Mild to moderate haemorrhage at site if goat moves during procedure. Spinal abscess or meningitis if asepsis is not observed.

Imaging and further diagnostics

Radiography is useful to detect fractures, osteomyelitis and bone malformations in the spinal column (**Fig. 8.7**). It may also highlight parasite-induced pathology (e.g. coenurosis or calcification in muscles caused by sarcocystosis). Interpretation must take into account normal variations and incidental findings.

Myelography (**Fig. 8.8**) has largely been superseded by CT and MRI. MRI is the most useful imaging modality for nervous tissue abnormalities, otitis and brain lesions. Electromyography (EMG) is useful to further investigate peripheral nerve deficits. The brainstem auditory evoked response (BAER) test aids diagnosis of deafness and cranial nerve VIII deficits.

NON-INFECTIOUS DISEASES

Central nervous system

Disbudding injury

Because of the thin skull in kids, prolonged (over 3–4 seconds at a time) application of a disbudding iron may lead to thermal insult of the meninges (**Fig. 8.9**). Clinical signs typical of encephalitis develop within 2–3 days of disbudding, usually followed by death. Treatment with anti-inflammatory or intracranial pressure reducing drugs may be tried but is unrewarding.

Acquired storage disease
Overview

Acquired mannosidosis is reported from several regions around the world, but in particular South America.

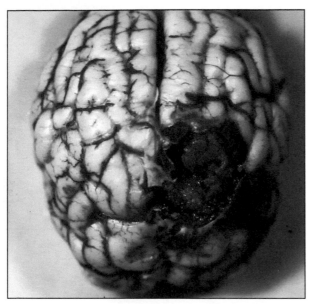

Fig. 8.9 Circular thermal trauma to the brain following disbudding. The affected kid died within 15 minutes of the procedure.

Aetiology

Plants containing swainsonine (so called locoweeds), such as *Ipomoea* spp., *Astragalus* spp., *Oxytropis* spp., *Delphinium* spp. and also *Solanum* spp,. have been associated with these poison-induced neurological disorders. Ingestion of both fresh and dried plant material appears poisonous. Feeding 0.8 mg/kg swainsonine (equivalent to 4 g/kg of dried *I. verbascoidea* leaves) for 40–55 days leads to irreparable damage.

Pathology consists of vacuolation of Purkinje cells in the CNS, but also cells in the pancreas, liver, kidney, thyroid gland and lymphoid organs.

Clinical presentation

The first clinical signs appear after about 3 weeks of ingestion. General signs include weight loss and inappetence. Neurological signs include ataxia, dysmetria, intention tremors, head tremors and postural abnormalities including a wide-based stance. Handling, moving or other stimuli may trigger pronounced signs and lead to the goat falling over.

Diagnosis

Anaemia is often present, and depending on the organs involved, other biochemistry parameters may be elevated (e.g. AST). Histopathology shows vacuolation and atrophy of Purkinje cells, with lectin binding typical of alpha-mannosidosis or other glycoproteins.

Differential diagnosis

Other cerebellar or brainstem disorders.

Treatment/management/control

There is no specific treatment other than removing goats from affected pastures. Goats may recover if ingestion was over a relatively short period (3–4 weeks), but about one quarter of those retain some abnormalities such as head tremors and a staggering gait. Euthanasia is often required.

Goats have been observed to develop compulsive eating of *Ipomoea* plants. Long-term control relies on eradication of the plant.

Inherited central nervous system disorders

Few reports on neurogenetic disorders exist in the goat. However, beta-mannosidosis (see Chapter 4) and cerebellar abiotrophy have been identified.

Abiotrophy leads to ataxia, wide-based stance and hypermetria in affected kids. Head tremors and nystagmus are common. Thinning of the cerebellar vermis may be detected on MRI. Other cerebellar disorders need to be considered as differential diagnoses. There are no treatment options.

Swayback (syn. enzootic ataxia)

See Copper deficiency (Chapter 15).

Polioencephalomalacia (syn. cerebrocortical necrosis)

Definition/overview

Polioencephalomalacia (PEM), also referred to as cerebrocortical necrosis (CCN), is a sporadic condition affecting growing ruminants worldwide including goats. It is most often encountered on units in which young goats are being intensively reared.

Aetiology

PEM is a descriptive term for the pathology encountered, which is essentially softening or necrosis of the grey matter of the cerebral cortex. Although there are a number of causes for this condition, the term is most closely linked and most commonly associated with disturbances to thiamine (vitamin B1) metabolism. In healthy goats, thiamine is produced in the rumen by microbial activity, providing the daily requirements without the need for ration supplementation. Dietary factors resulting in rumen acidosis will result in a change in the rumen microflora. Under this type of change, PEM is thought to result from a reduction in thiamine producing bacteria, coupled with an overgrowth of other bacteria that produce a thiaminase enzyme, further degrading available thiamine and resulting in deficiency. Other reported causes of the condition include sulphur toxicity and water deprivation or salt poisoning, although these mechanisms and biochemical pathways remain poorly understood. The condition can often be encountered sporadically alongside an outbreak of enterotoxaemia, both conditions essentially precipitated by dietary imbalance.

Pathophysiology

Thiamine is an important co-enzyme (as thiamine pyrophosphate) in a number of important biochemical pathways related to brain function. The degenerative change in brain tissue results most likely from accumulation of sodium in the cerebrocortical cells, leading to water ingress, cell swelling and cell death.

Clinical presentation

The clinical condition is seen most frequently in growing goats and young adults. The presentation most often seen is one of acute onset, although clinical signs may be more protracted over 24–48 hours following an initial period of depression and inappetence. Affected goats become excitable, staring upwards ('star-gazing'), and they begin to wander aimlessly, often in circles (**Fig. 8.10**). Teeth grinding and blindness may also be features before collapse into lateral recumbency with profound opisthotonus. In these later stages, affected goats become hyperaesthetic, develop extensor muscle rigidity of the limbs and can convulse violently. If untreated, affected goats will die in 24–48 hours.

Diagnosis

The clinical signs, age of the goat and past history of a dietary change are all highly suggestive of PEM. In the early stages, a response to i/v thiamine therapy may give further support to the diagnosis. The acute nature of the disease means that laboratory tests are of limited value overall, although measurement of blood erythrocyte transketolase (an indirect measure of thiamine activity) may be offered by some laboratories. At post-mortem examination (PME), lesions are confined to the brain, which shows flattening of the cerebral gyri, with areas of yellowish discolouration. Examination of the sagittally sectioned brain in a darkened room under UV light can show very clearly delineated areas of tissue necrosis (**Fig. 8.11**). Histological examination confirms laminar necrosis.

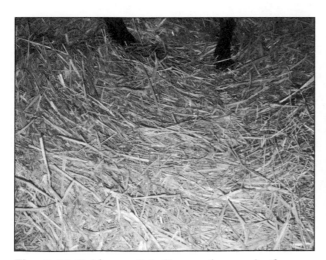

Fig. 8.10 **Evidence of circling can be seen in the straw bedding in this goat's pen.**

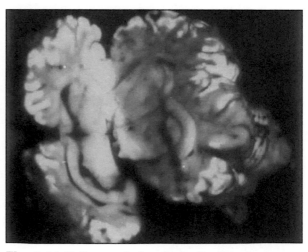

Fig. 8.11 **Polioencephalomalacia showing autofluorescence under UV light in a dark room.**

Differential diagnosis

Includes listeriosis, enterotoxaemia and bacterial meningitis in the early stages. As the condition progresses, the limb rigidity often exhibited can be confused for tetanus. The convulsive stages need to be differentiated from rabies, Aujeszky's disease (pseudorabies) and chemical poisoning.

Treatment/management/control

Rapid and decisive treatment with intravenous thiamine (10–15 mg/kg thiamine hydrochloride every 4–6 hours) can be very effective in the early stages, and should be repeated twice daily for the next 48 hours. Multivitamin preparations can be used, but with the dosage calculated based on the thiamine content of the product. Nursing is vital to prevent injuries while convulsing and in prolonged lateral recumbency. Any other concurrent problem (such as rumen acidosis, enterotoxaemia) should also be treated.

Prevention is problematic due to the sporadic nature of the condition, but is best aimed at ensuring that any dietary changes are made gradually, particularly at weaning. It is important to ensure that all goats can feed on concentrate or grain simultaneously (to avoid individual goats engorging), and ensuring that feed stores are goat proof. Although its role is poorly understood, the overall sulphur content of the ration may need to be explored if an outbreak continues.

Floppy kid syndrome

See Chapter 4.

Peripheral nervous system

Peripheral nerve paralysis

Overview

Paralysis of various peripheral nerves is occasionally observed.

Aetiology

Trauma anywhere along the nerve's path is the most common cause. For example, obturator or peroneal nerve paralysis may be a sequela to dystocia caused by feto-maternal disproportion. In dystocia cases, excessive traction may also result in nerve damage in the neonate. Brachial plexus compromise may result from a goat becoming trapped over a gate or bar with its front leg. Unstable leg fractures can cause secondary nerve damage, as can casting a leg or pressure during prolonged anaesthesia. Other causes include localised abscess formation, injection site reaction, neoplasia or haematoma. Space-occupying lesions in the spinal cord at the level of the nerve roots may also occur. In the case of spinal canal abscessation, a secondary pathological fracture can lead to further nerve insult (**Fig. 8.12**).

Clinical presentation

The immediate effect is an abnormal leg angulation. *Table 8.5* shows the normal action of the main peripheral nerves. Where nerve compromise is present, the opposite would be observed (e.g. flexion or knuckling of the fetlock with peroneal paralysis). Skin sensation over the nerve's sensory supply areas is absent (**Fig. 8.13**). Longer term, atrophy of the muscles that receive motor supply from the affected nerve is seen.

Diagnosis

Clinical signs are highly suggestive. CSF analysis and imaging where a spinal disorder is suspected as the cause. EMG to confirm.

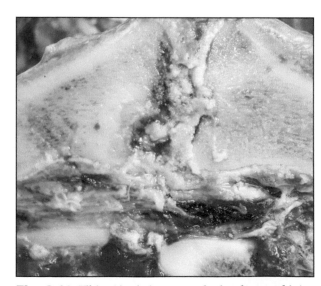

Fig. 8.12 This spinal abscess at the lumbosacral joint in a cow led to bilateral tibial nerve paralysis.

Table 8.5 **Major peripheral nerves of the front and hind legs, and their main action.**

	MAIN MUSCLES RECEIVING MOTOR SUPPLY	JOINT ACTION	MAIN ABNORMALITY SEEN WHEN COMPROMISED
Front leg nerves			
Suprascapular	Supraspinatus, infraspinatus	Shoulder extension and lateral stabilisation	Shortened stride, abduction of leg
Axillary	Deltoideus, teres major and minor	Shoulder flexion	
Musculocutaneous	Biceps, proximal end of brachial	Elbow flexion	
Median and ulnar	Carpal and digital flexors	Carpus and digit flexion	'Goose-stepping', hyperextension of carpus and fetlock
Radial	Triceps, distal end of brachial, digital extensors	Elbow, carpus and digit extension	Dropped elbow, inability to extend lower limb, dragging of leg
Hind leg nerves			
Obturator	Adductors	Limb adduction	Recumbent, 'frog-leg position'
Femoral	Quadriceps	Hip flexion, stifle extension	Dropped stifle resulting in vertical line of upper limb, often unable to support weight (**Fig. 8.14**)
Tibial	Gastrocnemius, digital flexors	Hock extension, digit flexion	Dropped hock, hock has more acute angle than normal (**Fig. 8.14**)
Peroneal	Cranial tibial, digital extensors	Hock flexion, digit extension	'Knuckling' of fetlock

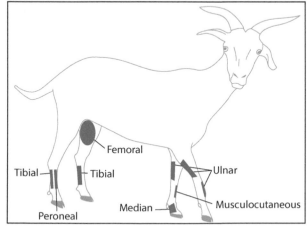

Fig. 8.13 Autonomous zones of skin innervation. (Adapted from: Mayhew J (2009) *Large Animal Neurology*, 2nd edn. Wiley-Blackwell, Ames.)

Differential diagnosis

Abnormal angulation caused by muscular, tendon or ligament disorders, dislocations or fractures. Skin sensation will be intact and often there is localised swelling (although this may also be present with nerve damage). Crepitus is present in fractures and dislocations.

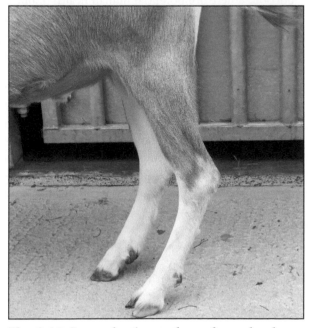

Fig. 8.14 Stance showing moderate femoral and tibial nerve compromise in a goat with a suspected thoracolumbar lesion. The upper limb is straighter and the hock more flexed than usual, resulting in the hind feet being placed deeper underneath the body.

Treatment/management/control

Anti-inflammatory therapy is often successful if instigated early. Corticosteroids (e.g. starting dose of methylprednisolone at 30 mg/kg or dexamethasone at 2 mg/kg) may be more effective in nerve damage cases than NSAIDs (providing they are not contra-indicated [e.g. a pregnant doe]). Spinal lesions carry a poor prognosis.

Control relies on using caesarean section for feto-maternal disproportion, providing a safe environment for goats, good i/m injection technique (appropriate needle length, correct insertion angle and site) and casting technique, adequate positioning and padding during anaesthesia, and good nursing care of recumbent animals.

INFECTIOUS DISEASES

Listerial encephalitis

Definition/overview

Listeriosis is an important neurological disease of goats worldwide, and can also be associated with other clinical syndromes including septicaemia and abortion. There are potential human health implications associated with the production and sale of dairy products, particularly soft cheeses. Septicaemic goats may excrete the organism in milk, and infected vaginal discharge following abortion may contaminate the udder, teats and hands of the milker, and hence the milk. Milk excretion is less likely to occur in the encephalitic form of the disease, but has been reported in latent carriers, that can be found particularly in endemically infected herds. Even a small inoculum in unpasteurised milk may rapidly proliferate when the milk and resulting dairy products are stored at fridge temperatures.

Aetiology

Listeria monocytogenes is a small, gram-positive, aerobic and facultative anaerobic rod-like organism. It grows at a wide range of temperatures from 3°C to 45°C, with active proliferation at fridge temperatures (a useful technique when isolating the organism in a laboratory). It can be subclassified into a number of serotypes (and subtypes), with serotypes 1/2a, 1/2b, 4b and 5 (*Listeria ivanovii*) most commonly associated with disease in goats. The organism is ubiquitous in the environment and can be found in the faeces of wild animals and birds (potentially contaminating feeds), soil and other organic matter, thereby being a potential risk factor in the process of silage making.

Pathophysiology

Clinical disease in goats can often be initiated by stressful insults such as sudden changes in weather conditions or by overcrowding coupled with keeping them in a dirty contaminated environment. The introduction of a feedstuff (particularly silage) contaminated with *Listeria* organisms is a significant risk factor, particularly in intensively managed herds. Goats kept on overgrazed pasture may inadvertently ingest contaminated soil. Sporadic incidents will occur, however, even in the absence of any of these risk factors. As an example, one author encountered encephalitic listeriosis in two of three goats that had been eating brambles growing over a stacked heap of horse manure and bedding.

In the encephalitic form of the disease, the organism gains entry to nerve endings in the mouth via breaks in the oral mucosa (e.g. abrasions caused by coarse feed [brambles, thistles or browsings]), dental or gum abnormalities, or teeth loss or change. Infection ascends along the cranial nerves to the brain, resulting in focal microabscess formation. The incubation period may be as long as 3–4 weeks. The onset of septicaemic listeriosis is more rapid, with an incubation period as short as 1–2 days, probably resulting from organisms gaining access to the blood stream via a damaged gut mucosa. If pregnant, septicaemic goats may abort. Ocular listeriosis may result from contaminated feed (principally silage) falling into the eyes as goats feed from raised containers.

Clinical presentation

Outbreaks of clinical disease tend to feature only one manifestation of the infection, although there are reports of encephalitis, septicaemia and abortions all occurring in the same incident.

The encephalitic form tends to develop slowly, with initial signs confined to depression, anorexia and reduced milk yield. Incoordination then develops, with stumbling and an increasing tendency to lean, move or fall in the same direction.

Other characteristic signs include a drooped ear, ptosis, nystagmus, protruding tongue, flaccid buccal muscles and an increasing inability to prehend food and to swallow (**Fig. 8.15**). Weakness, progressive dehydration and recumbency (**Fig. 8.16**) follow, and if untreated the mortality rate can be high.

The initial presentation in the septicaemic form is similar, but progression is rapid and neurological signs are usually not a feature. Diarrhoea, often haemorrhagic, is a common finding and affected goats deteriorate rapidly over a few days. If pregnant, septicaemic goats may abort, but not all goats that abort show other clinical signs. In the ocular form, both keratoconjunctivitis and anterior uveitis (silage eye) have been reported (see Chapter 13).

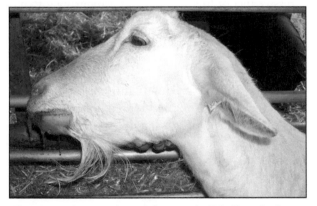

Fig. 8.15 Saanen doe with encephalitic listeriosis showing drooping of the ear and eyelids and hypersalivation. Marked nystagmus was also evident.

Diagnosis

The clinical signs in encephalitis cases are fairly typical. Bacteriological and cytological examination of CSF may be of benefit, but haematology is of limited value due to the localisation of the infection. Available serological tests are of limited value in clinical cases due to cross reaction with other gram-positive organisms, but may be of benefit for herd screening exercises.

At PME there are few gross lesions evident. Confirmation of infection is based on the laboratory isolation of the organism from brain tissue of encephalitic cases and from multiple sites in septicaemic carcases. Histological examination of brain tissue will demonstrate focal microabscessation and perivascular lymphoid cuffing as the primary features (**Fig. 8.17**).

Differential diagnosis

Differential diagnoses for the encephalitic signs include bacterial meningitis, brain abscesses, PEM, coenurosis and early rabies. For septicaemic cases presenting with haemorrhagic diarrhoea consider enterotoxaemia, salmonellosis and yersiniosis.

Treatment/management/control

To be successful, treatment must be instigated rapidly and decisively. High doses of antibiotic administered i/v for the first 24 hours should be followed

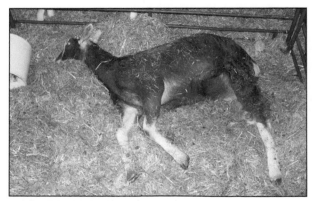

Fig. 8.16 Lateral recumbency in a case of advanced encephalitic listeriosis.

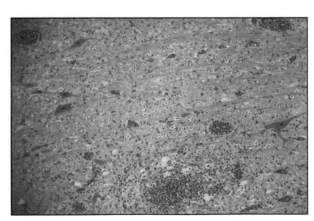

Fig. 8.17 Encephalitic listeriosis showing perivascular cuffing with mononuclear cells and focal microabscessation histologically.

by i/m antibiosis for 3–7 days. Suitable antibiotics include penicillin, tetracycline and potentiated sulphonamide. Supportive therapy includes NSAIDs and fluid therapy (orally or i/v) to combat both dehydration and rumen acidosis resulting from the inability to swallow saliva and the loss of its rumen buffering capacity. Nursing, particularly of recumbent goats, is essential.

In an outbreak, attention is directed at identifying the source of infection and likely risk factors identified for future herd control measures. If contaminated silage or other feed is suspected, this should be removed and replaced. For prevention, uneaten silage should routinely be discarded after 24 hours. If silage is the source, the production process is reviewed: excessive soil contamination must be avoided during the ensiling process (mole hills are commonly incriminated, and cutting blades are often set too low). Ensure the silage clamp or bags/wraps are airtight. Silage pH should be around 3.8–4.3. Silage with a pH of 5 or greater will be of high risk. Avoid feeding wet bales of either hay or pea straw, and avoid the use of wet bales for bedding. Vaccines are available in some countries.

Bacterial meningitis/encephalitis
Definition/overview
This condition is seen most commonly in young kids as part of a spectrum also including septicaemia and joint ill resulting from umbilical infection and/or concurrent hypogammaglobulinaemia (see Chapters 4, 5 and 9). In mature goats, there are occasional reports of brain abscesses and specifically abscesses of the pituitary gland.

Aetiology
Escherichia coli is the most common isolate, although other possible (essentially environmental) pathogens include *Streptococcus dysgalactiae, S. zooepidemicus, Pseudomonas aeruginosa, Trueperella pyogenes* and *Corynebacterium pseudotuberculosis.*

Pathophysiology
In young kids infection will most often develop following a bacterial septicaemia and localisation of infection within the meninges, predominantly overlying the brain and, more rarely, the spinal cord.

The development of a brain or pituitary abscess is most likely the result of haematogenous spread from a cutaneous, visceral or foot septic focus or following middle ear infection.

Clinical presentation
Affected kids may exhibit depression, incoordination, ataxia, teeth grinding, hyperaesthesia and blindness, leading to recumbency often with opisthotonus and extensor rigidity, although the front legs are usually flexed. Signs related to umbilical infection may be evident including umbilical inflammation and joint effusion and pain. Clinical signs related to brain abscess formation will vary depending on the size and location of the abscess, but may include progressive incoordination, aimless wandering (often in one particular direction), head pressing, blindness, abnormal pupillary responses and dysphagia.

Diagnosis
Diagnosis is based predominantly on the spectrum of clinical signs in young kids, combined with CSF analysis. Brain abscess diagnosis is almost always presumptive and confirmed at PME or with diagnostic imaging such as MRI or CT.

Differential diagnosis
One of the main differentials is thermal damage and resulting infection following disbudding injury (**Figs. 8.9, 8.18**). Brain abscesses need to be differentiated from other space-occupying lesions such as those caused by trauma or parasitic cysts, and from CCN, listeriosis, neurological signs of *C. perfringens* enterotoxaemia or lead poisoning. Tetanus may cause a similar picture of recumbency with extensor rigidity affecting all four legs.

Treatment/management/control
Treatment of affected kids is most successful in early cases, with more advanced cases carrying a poor prognosis. The use of broad-spectrum antibiotics, or those with activity against gram-negative organisms, capable of crossing the blood–brain barrier, such as potentiated sulphonamide, ampicillin or cephalosporin at high dose rates i/v, has been advocated. Supportive therapy with NSAIDs and/or agents reducing intracranial pressure should be

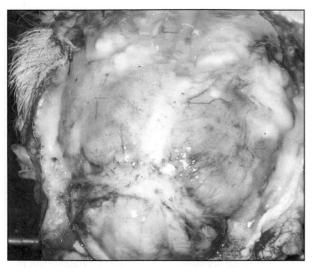

Fig. 8.18 Trauma, necrosis and suppuration (penetrating into brain tissue) as a result of a disbudding injury.

given, and affected kids kept in a well-bedded dimly lit hospital pen, and turned frequently if recumbent to avoid pressure sores and hypostatic lung congestion Force feeding may be required. Treatment of brain or pituitary abscesses is rarely successful. Neonatal problems in general can be prevented by reviewing overall management (see Chapter 4).

Tetanus

Definition/overview
Tetanus is a well-documented condition affecting many animal species and humans worldwide, causing tetanic muscular spasms, convulsions and death. It is easily preventable by strategic vaccination.

Aetiology
Caused by *Clostridium tetani*, a highly resistant gram-positive, anaerobic, spore-forming organism found widely in animal faeces and soil.

Pathophysiology
As the organism proliferates at the site of entry, it produces and releases a potent neurotoxin. This can occur, for example, when spores are introduced from the environment into a deep penetrating wound or necrotic lesion encouraged by the localised anaerobic environment within the lesion itself. Neurotoxin tracks up the local peripheral nerve trunks to the spinal cord, leading to sustained discharge of motor neurons, resulting in the clinical signs of tetany. In addition to accidental wounds or injuries, infection can also be acquired as a result of a variety of managemental procedures such as disbudding, dehorning, castration (both surgical and via an elastrator ring), ear tagging and obstetrical procedures. It occasionally results from i/m injection of certain drugs (e.g. prostaglandin-F$_2$-alpha).

Clinical presentation
Clinical signs are highly variable, depending on the location of the primary focus of proliferation and the size of the goat (both influencing the distance toxin must travel along peripheral nerves). Onset of signs may vary from days to several weeks. An early sign may be mild unexplained rumen tympany. Affected goats become reluctant to move, developing both front and hind leg rigidity, and major muscle groups may feel firm. The ears are held high and may not move in response to a noise. The third eyelid becomes more prominent and hyperaesthesia develops, with an exaggerated reaction to sounds. Constipation may be present. The disease progresses to convulsions, recumbency and death usually from respiratory failure.

Diagnosis
There are no laboratory tests in the live goat and no specific post-mortem signs. Bacteriology is of limited value as the organism remains at the site of entry, but the typical 'drumstick' morphology of the organism may be evident in Gram-stained smears taken from the primary lesion.

Differential diagnosis
The disease is fairly characteristic in the later stages. In the early stages, stiffness could mimic either laminitis or muscular dystrophy, and other causes of rumen tympany must be ruled out. Hypomagnesaemia causes hyperaesthesia, but does not result in continuous muscle spasm.

Treatment/management/control
Treatment of clinical cases is usually disappointing unless detected early. Crystalline penicillin given i/v has a rapid mode of action, and may be followed

by procaine penicillin (30,000–40,000 IU/kg i/m q12h for 2–3 days). Tetanus antitoxin, where available, is given i/v or intrathecally. Persistent rumen bloat is addressed by placing a trocar or surgically creating a rumen fistula (see Chapter 5). The latter also facilitates instilling feed and water into the rumen if swallowing is impaired. Sedatives when convulsing are useful, as is analgesia to counteract the marked pain caused by muscle spasm (preferably opioids, with NSAIDs or acepromazine having some effect). Euthanasia on welfare grounds should be considered if cases do not improve. Prevention is based on a sound tetanus vaccination regime (e.g. a multivalent clostridial vaccine providing cover for both tetanus and enterotoxaemia), good techniques for routine procedures and prompt attention to wounds.

Enterotoxaemia

C. perfringens toxins can lead to CNS signs as a result of focal symmetrical encephalomalacia changes in the brainstem and cerebral oedema (**Fig. 8.19**). These changes can result in profound neurological signs including ataxia, blindness, opisthotonus, convulsions and death, in addition to the more typical signs described in Chapter 5.

Scrapie and bovine spongiform encephalopathy

Definition/overview

Scrapie is one of the transmissible spongiform encephalopathies or prion diseases that can affect sheep and goats. Although scrapie has been reported in sheep for over 200 years, the first case of natural scrapie in a goat was only confirmed in 1975. The emergence of bovine spongiform encephalopathy (BSE) in the UK in 1986, and in particular the subsequent links to human health, resulted in a worldwide interest in this group of diseases. Extensive monitoring of cattle, sheep and goat brain material followed across Europe, focussing on healthy animals entering the food chain and on stock that died on farm. Initially, BSE was confined to cattle brain and scrapie to sheep and goat brain, but in 2002, BSE was confirmed in the brain tissue of a goat in France, and a second case was subsequently identified in a goat from Scotland. At the time of

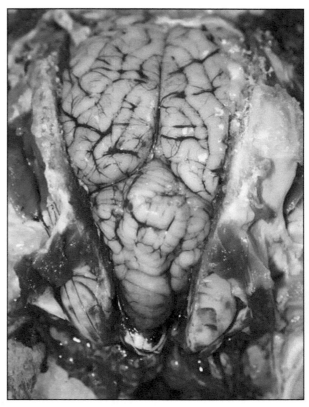

Fig. 8.19 Cerebral oedema. Note the cerebellar herniation through the occipital condyles.

writing, no further natural cases of BSE have been identified in goats, and the BSE epidemic itself is undoubtedly on the decline.

Scrapie is still endemic in goats (and sheep) in the UK and other countries in Europe, in Iceland, and in the USA and Canada, although many of these countries are developing successful control and monitoring programmes. Cases have also been reported in many other countries, but most often with links to sheep imports from the UK. Australia and New Zealand have subsequently both eradicated the disease.

Aetiology

It is generally accepted that scrapie and BSE are caused by the expression of an abnormal form of the naturally occurring cellular protein referred to as prion protein (PrP), found throughout the body but being of clinical relevance in the nervous system. Disease appears to be associated with replication of this abnormal protein, although this is only one factor in what is a highly complex and still incompletely understood process. Most cases of natural scrapie in goats occur as a result of lateral spread between sheep and goats, although the rate of goat to goat transmission has been reported to be high in intensively housed animals in the UK.

Pathophysiology

The infective PrP agent present in the placenta and uterine fluids of either goats or sheep (and a risk if co-located) appears to be the primary source of new infection for newborn kids, although other minor transmission routes may also exist. As goats are fastidious about clearing up and consuming the placenta after kidding, this behavioural trait may in part explain the rapid spread among housed goats once infection is present in the cohort.

The agent is notoriously resistant in the environment, and thorough cleaning and disinfection of buildings in which infected goats have been housed is important, particularly after kidding or lambing has taken place. Following oral ingestion, it is thought that the infectious agent enters via Peyer's patches, then colonises the lymphoreticular system and other body tissues including the brain, where further replication occurs. The incubation period is variable, but usually 12 months or more.

Clinical presentation

Clinical signs will not usually develop until infected goats are at least 18 months old, and even then progress very slowly over a period of several weeks. Early signs are easily overlooked, but may include subtle changes in behaviour towards other goats or their owners such as lack of interest/recognition or increased irritability. This is followed by progressive ataxia, difficulties in leg placement and stumbling when moved forward, particularly when made to deviate their course. Although pruritus is a common presentation in sheep, it is more rarely reported in goats. The ears and tail are often held aloft. Reaction to sound and other stimuli is often exaggerated. A gradual decline in body condition is followed by eventual recumbency, by which time most goats will have been destroyed on humane grounds.

Diagnosis

A presumptive diagnosis in the live goat is based on the clinical signs described. There is no detectable immune response. A number of experimental tests are now being used diagnostically in live sheep and goats, such as the rectoanal mucosa-associated lymphoid tissue (RAMALT) test, in which a biopsy specimen is taken from the rectum and subjected to immunohistochemical testing. There are no gross lesions on PME. Definitive diagnosis is based on histological examination of brain obex tissue (in which vacuolar/spongiform change is evident; **Fig. 8.20**) or by brain immunohistochemistry or immunoblotting. These latter techniques will also distinguish between scrapie and BSE.

Differential diagnosis

The slow rate of development of clinical signs is highly typical of scrapie. Other causes of progressive ataxia include space-occupying lesions in the brain or spinal cord.

Treatment/management/control

There is no treatment. Scrapie and BSE are both on the OIE list of notifiable diseases, and any suspicion should be reported to the relevant national authority, which in turn will initiate a full epidemiological investigation and instigate their own national control and advisory plan. In the sheep sector, the use of genetic selection of scrapie resistant breeding stock has become a well-established disease control option in scrapie-affected flocks and has been

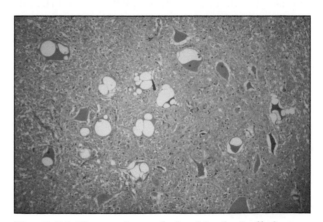

Fig. 8.20 Neuronal vacuolation histologically in a confirmed scrapie case.

highly successful. The genetics of scrapie resistance in sheep, however, are significantly different to that of goats. Collaborative work within the EU is ongoing to establish genetic resistance in goats, although this has been hampered somewhat by the wide genetic variation within goat breeds.

Rabies

Definition/overview
Rabies is a viral disease that can infect all warm blooded mammals, including on very rare occasions goats. In those countries in which rabies is present, it should be considered as a differential diagnosis in neurological cases. It also has important zoonotic implications.

Aetiology
Rabies is caused by a neurotropic rhabdovirus, which is excreted in saliva and transmitted by the bite of a rabid animal such as a dog. Goats are effectively end hosts and rarely transmit the disease when infected, although there is always the possibility of infected saliva gaining access to cuts and abrasions on the hands and arms of human handlers – hence its potential importance as a zoonotic infection, although there appear to be no reports of human infection acquired from goats.

Pathophysiology
After a bite, the virus replicates at the site of the lesion, before tracking along peripheral nerves to the CNS. The distance of the bite from the CNS dictates the incubation period, with bites on the face resulting in clinical disease developing more rapidly than one on the distal limb. The virus continues to replicate within the CNS, resulting in the expression of clinical disease.

Clinical presentation
Clinical disease is rare, but signs have included an increase in aggressive behaviour, excessive vocalisation, salivation, ataxia and recumbency.

Diagnosis
Diagnosis is problematic due to the often vague initial presenting signs, with a presumptive diagnosis in known rabies areas resulting from elimination of other potential causes.

Differential diagnosis
Includes listeriosis, tetanus, brain abscess, scrapie, Aujeszky's disease (pseudorabies), lead poisoning and some plant poisonings.

Treatment/management/control
There is no treatment for rabies. It is on the OIE list of notifiable diseases, and any suspicion should be reported to the relevant national authority, which in turn will initiate a full epidemiological investigation and instigate their own national control and advisory plan.

Aujeszky's disease (syn. pseudorabies)

Definition/overview
Aujeszky's disease is primarily a condition of pigs that can pass to goats kept in close contact. Individual cases are invariably sporadic, but morbidity and subsequent mortality within outbreaks may be high.

Aetiology
Caused by a herpesvirus that is excreted in saliva and nasal droplets and can remain active in a damp warm environment for several months. Indirect transfer has been reported via transport vehicles previously used for pigs.

Pathophysiology
Goats that become infected are almost always housed with or close to pigs in which infection is established. Virus is picked up either via aerosol inhalation or contamination of skin abrasions. The incubation period is very short (less than 5 days), after which the virus has a predilection for CNS tissue.

Clinical presentation
Severe pruritus is a very common finding, with intense rubbing, scratching and licking leading to self-inflicted trauma. In acute infection goats may simply be found dead or show marked pyrexia and profound depression, leading to recumbency, rumen tympany and death with or without pruritus.

Diagnosis

The clinical presentation of acute disease, pruritus and contact with pigs all lead to a presumptive diagnosis. Serology is of limited value as goats rarely live long enough to mount an immune response. There are no gross lesions at PME, and confirmation is based on the typical histological picture of a severe focal non-suppurative encephalitis and myelitis and subsequent immunohistochemistry.

Differential diagnosis

Cases in which pruritus is a feature need to be differentiated from skin disease (see Chapter 11), and scrapie and rabies, which can both cause neurogenic pruritus. Acute cases need to be differentiated from CCN, acute listeriosis and poisoning.

Treatment/management/control

There is no treatment. Control is based on avoiding keeping goats near potentially infected pigs. Many countries have control and eradication measures in place for the disease in pigs, which has a direct effect on reducing the risks to goats.

Caprine arthritis encephalitis

See Chapter 9.

Louping ill

Louping ill is caused by a tick-borne flavivirus, most commonly seen in sheep in the UK, but capable of causing clinical disease in goats. It is characterised by an initial febrile viraemic stage, which may be accompanied by depression and anorexia, followed in susceptible animals by neurological signs. In goats with encephalitis, the clinical signs may include muscle tremors and/or rigidity, incoordination, ataxia, hypersensitivity, salivation and nervous nibbling, progressing in some cases to head pressing, posterior paralysis, recumbency, convulsions and/or coma. It is a differential diagnosis for other neurological conditions such as scrapie.

Coenurosis (syn. gid)

Definition/overview

Coenurosis is a space-occupying lesion in the brain (and occasionally in the spinal cord) of ruminants caused by a metacestode parasitic cyst.

Aetiology

The metacestode stage found in the CNS of an infected goat is *Coenurus cerebralis*, the intermediate stage of the carnivore tapeworm *Taenia multiceps*.

Pathophysiology

The tapeworm segments are passed in the faeces of the dog or fox. If these are ingested by a grazing goat, the *Taenia* eggs are released and penetrate the gut wall, entering the blood stream. Those metacestode stages that reach the brain begin to develop and increase in size, although it is usually only one that outgrows the remainder over a period of several weeks, developing into a thin-walled, fluid-filled cystic structure in which the developmental scolices may be seen within the cyst wall (**Fig. 8.21**). If the goat dies or is slaughtered, and its head is eaten by carnivores thus consuming the cystic structure, a new wave of *T. multiceps* will develop to complete the life cycle.

Clinical presentation

The clinical presentation depends on the size of the cyst and its location. In the early stages, signs may be very vague, including dullness, apathy, inappetence and an unsteady gait. As the cyst grows, the intracranial pressure will increase, with signs determined by its location. A cyst found in the cerebellum tends to produce the most dramatic signs, including opisthotonus and a severe loss of balance. Cysts in the cerebral cortex can be quite large, even destroying

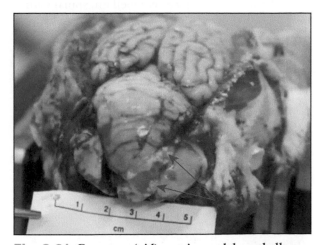

Fig. 8.21 Coenurus (gid) cyst in caudal cerebellar tissue. Note the scolices (arrows) evident on the cyst wall between the occipital condyles.

(by pressure necrosis) 50% or more of the total cortex, with only minimal signs. If the cyst is present on one side of the cortex, the goat will tend to move or circle to that side, with blindness in the opposite eye. In established cases, softening of the skull overlying the cyst may be apparent, and gentle downward pressure may exacerbate the clinical signs. Cysts developing in the spinal cord will result in gradual leg weakness (depending on location) and progressive paresis.

Diagnosis

Diagnosis is based on the clinical signs, and the knowledge that the pathogen is present in the locality. There are no reliable laboratory tests, but MRI or CT scans are useful in valuable animals (**Fig. 8.22**). At PME, thin-walled cystic structures can be clearly identified within the CNS tissue.

Differential diagnosis

Once established, the condition needs to be differentiated from other space-occupying lesions such as brain abscesses, the pituitary abscess syndrome and trauma.

Treatment/management/control

There is no medical treatment for the condition. A thorough neurological assessment enables identification of the location of the cyst. If located in the cerebral cortex, it can be removed quite successfully. Cysts present in the cerebellum, spinal cord or elsewhere carry a poor prognosis. Surgery is most successful when there is obvious thinning of the skull overlying the cyst. The goat is sedated or anaesthetised, and an incision is made down to the bone over the cyst location. Using a bone trephine, a circular hole is created. If the cyst has been correctly located, it should be seen beneath the dura mater and will begin to protrude when the dura is cut. Using blunt forceps, the cyst wall is grasped (**Fig. 8.23**), with its removal facilitated by holding the goat's head upside down. The skin is closed over the incision.

Prevention is based on ensuring that dead sheep and goats are not left in the open for carnivores to consume, and that goat and sheep offal (particularly the head) is not fed. If gid is a known problem, then regular worming of all dogs in the locality against tapeworms should be encouraged.

Cerebrospinal nematodiasis (syn. meningeal worm)

Cerebrospinal nematodiasis is reported in goats in Switzerland, occurring mainly in winter. Goats present with progressive ataxia in the hind legs and proprioceptive deficits, circling, vestibular syndrome and eventually recumbency, but with normal appetite. CSF may contain eosinophils. *Elaphostrongylus cervi* and *Parelaphostrongylus tenuis* are nematodes suspected to be involved. *P. tenuis* has occurred in llamas in the UK. Treatment with albendazole may be tried. Monthly ivermectin treatment is used for prevention in camelids in the US.

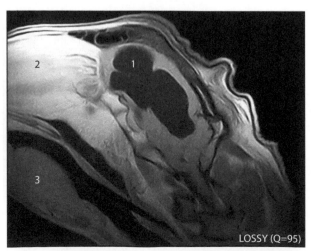

Fig. 8.22 MRI showing a cerebral coenurus (gid) cyst in a ram (1 = cyst; 2 = nasal septum; 3 = tongue).

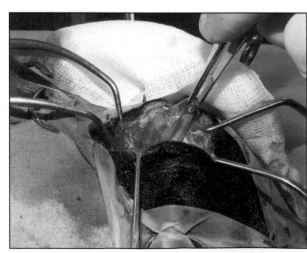

Fig. 8.23 Surgical treatment of gid. The cyst wall is grasped and the cyst removed.

CLINICAL EXAMINATION OF THE MUSCULOSKELETAL SYSTEM

Clinical assessment

History and environment

Speed of onset can give an indication as to the likely cause; for example, slow onset in degenerative joint conditions as opposed to sudden onset in fracture cases. Establishing current environment (**Fig. 9.1**) as well as recent management procedures, and observation of animal behaviour is important for prevention of further cases (handling, transport, oestrus etc.; **Fig. 9.2**). Diet analysis is important where metabolic bone or cartilage disease is suspected. For infectious causes, potential breaches in biosecurity and disease prevention should be investigated.

Gait and posture

The goat is assessed while walking. A weight-bearing lameness presents with a shortened stride of the normal leg, and lesions tend to affect the lower limb or involve fractures or joint infection. At the point of weight-bearing, the head is lifted up if a front leg is involved or dipped down if a hind leg is involved. A swinging leg lameness presents with a shortened stride of the affected leg, and usually indicates an upper limb problem. The degree of lameness (on a scale of 1 to 5 or 1 to 10) gives an indication of likely pathology, and should be recorded in case notes to allow monitoring of progression.

Resting of one particular leg may be obvious when the goat stands still (**Fig. 9.3**). Limb angulation and position are judged for normal appearance. Noting any asymmetry between the left and right

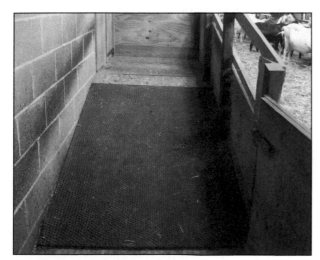

Fig. 9.1 A rubber mat on the ramp into the milking parlour provides good grip, thereby reducing the risk of slipping.

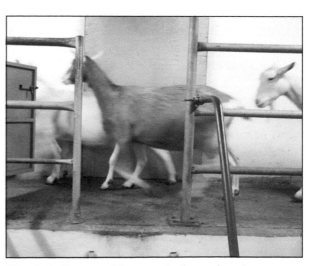

Fig. 9.2 Goats rushing to exit the parlour increases the risk of musculoskeletal trauma. The green gate swung into the goats' path poses an additional injury risk.

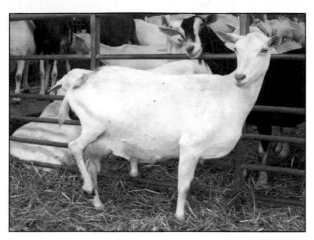

Fig. 9.3 Non-weight-bearing lameness caused by a foot abscess in the right hind leg.

body sections is very useful and indicates muscle atrophy or tissue swelling.

Palpation

Ideally, the goat should be in lateral recumbency for further assessment (using sedation if necessary). Attention is paid to any hair loss, skin abrasions, soiled areas or discharge. Palpation establishes excessive or reduced range of movement, heat or coldness, pain, crepitus and any swelling. Joints are assessed for effusion. If pain is detected, care must be taken to manipulate the leg very gently and to move one joint at a time, so that the affected region can be accurately determined. Auscultation while moving the leg can be useful in heavily muscled animals to detect any crepitus in the shoulder or hip region.

General assessment

Some infectious causes affect additional body systems or vital signs. Where a traumatic aetiology is suspected, the patient is examined for systemic problems, such as ABC (airway, breathing, circulation), hypo- or hyperthermia, shock or hypovolaemia, and haemorrhage.

Ancillary diagnostics

Flexion tests

Applying maximum flexion to a joint can exacerbate lameness. Starting with the most distal joint, flexion is held for 2 minutes, followed by the animal moving off at a trot. For goats that are not halter trained,

placing a companion animal at a distance may encourage the patient to trot away from the observer.

Imaging

Radiography is useful to establish bone integrity and position and the presence of joint effusion or degenerative changes, as well as soft tissue swelling and integrity (e.g. gas shadows in open fractures). A view of the contralateral leg is invaluable if one is unsure about normal radiographic anatomy or appearance (e.g. open growth plates in young goats; **Fig. 9.4**).

Ultrasonography is useful for tendon injuries and investigation of swellings (e.g. differentiating an abscess from a haematoma). It can also be used successfully to demonstrate an interruption in bone outline (e.g. in a pelvic fracture).

Other imaging modalities include MRI, CT, arthroscopy, thermography and scintigraphy.

Arthrocentesis

This is easiest performed with the goat in lateral recumbency. The site is clipped and thoroughly surgically prepared. Asepsis must be strictly maintained throughout. A 20 or 21 gauge needle (3.75 cm [1.5 in] long for stifle, 1.8–2.5 cm [3/4 to 1 in] long for other joints) is inserted into the joint cavity. Having broken the seal, a 2 or 5 ml syringe is attached and joint fluid aspirated. The synovial fluid is transferred into EDTA and plain sample containers and assessed for nucleated cells and protein, plus bacterial culture where required. When interpreting results, communications between joint compartments must be taken into account.

Average values for normal synovial fluid of the goat are 20 g/l protein and a nucleated cell count of 50/µl, of which most are lymphocytes or monocytes.

Nerve and joint blocks

To allow accurate interpretation, lameness must be shown consistently. The blocks are carried out in a distal to proximal sequence along the leg. Thorough surgical preparation of the injection site and aseptic technique throughout are absolutely essential. Using a 23–25 gauge, 1.8 cm (3/4 in) long needle, 1–2 ml of lidocaine or mepivicaine is injected either over the nerve or into the joint. To maintain asepsis, a new bottle of local is used for each joint block. Loss of skin sensation confirms the onset of a successful

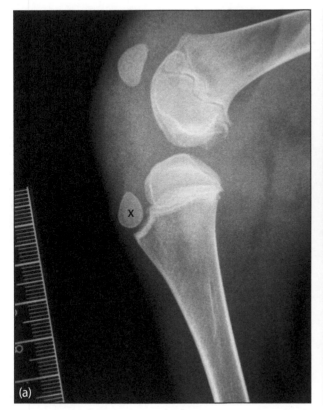
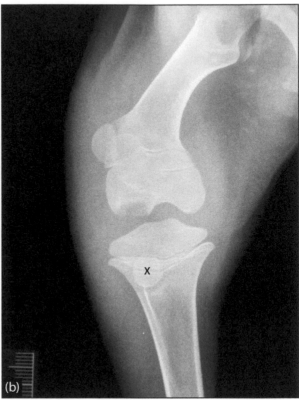

Fig. 9.4 Lateral (a) and dorsoplantar (b) radiographs of the stifle of a 1-month-old lamb showing open growth plates and the secondary centre of ossification of the tibia (X). Osteomyelitis is present in the lateral condyle of the femur.

nerve block. Deep pain, mechanical lameness or learned behaviour may lead to unsuccessful isolation of the affected region or joint. If blocks are conducted in multiple legs, care must be taken not to reach the toxic dose for local anaesthetic (see Chapter 18), and the animal may be ataxic for a few hours.

NON-INFECTIOUS DISEASES

Nutritional muscular dystrophy/ white muscle disease

Selenium/tocopherol (vitamin E) deficiency (see Chapter 15).

Rickets

Definition/overview

Rickets is a disease of young growing goats (mainly those kept indoors) associated with a failure of bone mineralisation in the epiphyses of the long bones.

Aetiology

The condition is classically linked to calciferol (vitamin D) deficiency, but has also been linked to long-term deficiencies of calcium or phosphorus when calciferol levels have been considered adequate.

Pathophysiology

Inadequate mineralisation results in a structural weakness of bone tissue, which is most apparent in the long bones, resulting in visible distortion and 'bowing' of legs and prominent end plates.

Clinical presentation

Affected goats initially develop a stiff gait and are reluctant to move. When viewed from the front, there is visible 'bowing' of the front legs (angular limb deformity [ALD]; **Fig. 9.5**) and swelling of the carpi. Palpation of the epiphysis often elicits pain, and palpable enlargement of the costochondral junctions may also be apparent. Within an affected

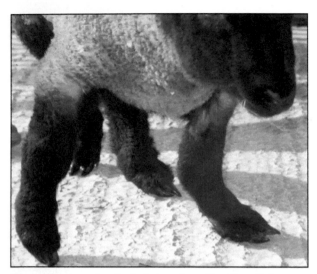

Fig. 9.5 Angular limb deformity affecting all four legs in a lamb. This may be congenital, but rickets should be ruled out.

cohort, there may be goats showing severe abnormalities alongside others with subclinical disease.

Diagnosis
Diagnosis is based on clinical signs and a review of feeding and management practices. Elevated serum alkaline phosphatase (SAP) is a consistent finding. There may also be a reduction in serum calcium and phosphorus and other minerals such as copper and zinc. Radiographic examination may confirm poor bone density in long bones, with widening of the growth plates.

Differential diagnosis
The clinical presentation is quite characteristic. Congenital ALD or a poorly aligned healed fracture should be considered.

Treatment/management/control
Severely affected goats may need to be culled on humane grounds. Those less severely affected may respond to management changes aiming to correct the mineral imbalance and allowing access to daylight if this has been deprived. This approach will also prevent further cases developing. Calciferol (vitamin D) administration at 1,000–2,000 IU/kg given twice (1 month apart as injection or 2 weeks apart as oral paste) is beneficial in some cases.

Osteodystrophy of mature bone
Overview
Metabolic bone diseases occur with reasonable frequency in young adult or mature goats.

Aetiology
A deficiency or imbalance of the minerals calcium, phosphorus and copper, and the calciferols (vitamin D). Calcification, and bone tissue and cartilage formation, are impaired. In the mature bone, this may lead to poor mineralisation of the trabecular structure at the ends of weight-bearing bone (osteomalacia) or bone cortices (osteoporosis). Enzootic calcinosis is also recognised in goats, typically caused by plant poisoning or by excessive calcium intake or cholecalciferol (vitamin D3) supplementation. Little information is available on renal failure-induced mineral imbalance causing osteodystrophy in the goat.

Clinical presentation
Stiffness, increased periods of recumbency, reluctance to move or rise and increased incidence of long bone fractures are common signs. Milk yield and body condition are often reduced. Where vertebrae are affected, lordosis and kyphosis are seen. Swelling of joints (especially hock) and epiphyses (especially with copper deficiency) is reported.

Diagnosis
Most useful for a definitive diagnosis are post-mortem findings including histopathology and bone ash concentration. Serum calcium may be low and SAP is often elevated because of bone pathology. Thinning of cortices may be seen on radiographs. Ration analysis is important to establish the cause. Typically, several animals are affected over a period of time.

Differential diagnosis
Other causes of fractures such as trauma, discospondylitis for spinal presentation, septic arthritis for joint swelling (with associated increased cellular content of joint fluid), other infectious causes of musculoskeletal problems.

Treatment/management/control
Euthanasia in severely affected animals, otherwise there is usually a good response to a balanced diet,

with recovery over 2–3 weeks. Control relies on adequate mineral and vitamin supplementation, in particular on farms using home grown cereal based diets (cereals have a high phosphorus:calcium ratio).

Fractures

Overview

Fractures comprise one of the more common musculoskeletal disorders associated with marked pain.

Aetiology

Trauma is the most common cause of fractures in livestock. However, spontaneous fractures may occur, especially as a sequela to osteodystrophy. A cluster of long-bone fractures in a group of animals should prompt assessment of the diet for mineral imbalances (e.g. hypophosphataemia). Pathological fractures may occur in bone weakened by infection or necrosis.

Clinical presentation

Typically, acute onset non-weight-bearing lameness. Muscle tone in the affected leg is lost and the leg may hang limply, possibly showing abnormal angulation. Unusual and abnormal movement of adjacent parts of the leg may be present. There may be severe soft tissue swelling in upper leg fractures, caused by haematoma formation. Crepitus is evident when the leg is moved (this should be performed very gently). Pain on manipulation is not always present. Superficial soft tissue damage may be present, and in open fractures a bone fragment may protrude from the wound.

Diagnosis

Even though the diagnosis is usually obvious based on clinical findings, radiographs should be taken whenever possible. Assessment of alignment, fracture direction (straight, spiral etc.), and joint involvement is important for choice of treatment and prognosis. Gas shadows in the tissues surrounding the site suggest an open or infected fracture. Follow-up radiographs will demonstrate callus formation, union or complications such as osteomyelitis (**Fig. 9.6**). In young animals with open growth plates, comparative views of the unaffected contralateral leg are often helpful for interpretation.

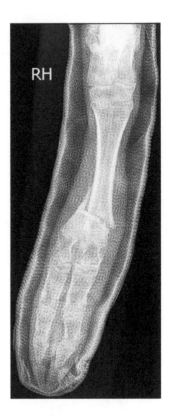

Fig. 9.6 Follow-up radiography (taken through the cast) showing poor callus formation at a metatarsal fracture in a lamb. Insufficient stabilisation, poor blood supply or infection of the fracture are the main considerations.

Differential diagnosis

Decreased weight bearing and gait abnormalities may be caused by septic arthritis, joint dislocation, tendon or ligament rupture and neurological deficits. Tendon, ligament or neurological problems should also be considered for abnormal angulation (see **Fig. 8.14**) or excessive movement in the limb.

Treatment/management/control

First aid is important to prevent further displacement and soft tissue trauma. The patient's movements are restricted (e.g. tying up, hurdles). If transport is necessary, a Robert-Jones bandage or splinting is imperative (*Table 9.1*), and the patient is placed with two sound legs forward in the vehicle (which is padded out to limit movement). Failure of passive transfer needs to be considered in neonatal fracture patients.

Treatment is governed by the type of fracture, expertise and available equipment, as well as costs and future purpose of the patient. Techniques used in companion animal orthopaedics can generally be applied in the goat. In brief, options include:

• Box rest. For fractures involving the humerus or femur. Box rest may only be considered if there

Table 9.1 **Splint positioning in relation to fracture site.**

FRACTURE REGION	SPLINT DETAILS
Front leg	
Foot up to and including carpus	One splint each on the lateral and palmar aspect of the leg, reaching from the foot to the elbow
Proximal carpus up to and including the elbow	Single splint on the lateral aspect of the leg, reaching from the foot to the top of the shoulder blade (with the holding bandage extending as high into the axilla as possible)
Above the elbow	No splint. A Velpeau sling may be appropriate in some cases
Hind leg	
Foot to proximal metatarsus	One splint each on the lateral and plantar aspects of the leg, reaching from the foot to mid-tibia
Between and including the hock and stifle	Single splint on the lateral aspect of the leg, reaching from the foot to the hip joint (with the holding bandage extending as high into the groin as possible)
Above stifle	No splint. An Ehmer sling may be appropriate in some cases

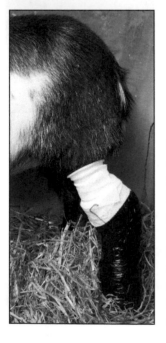

Fig. 9.7 **A cast used to stabilise a metatarsal fracture. Elastic bandage has been applied at the proximal end to stop bedding getting between cast and leg. Note that deep straw bedding can make it difficult for a goat with a cast to move freely.**

is no displacement, no joint involvement and the animal is ambulatory. Because a good degree of muscle mass is required to stabilise the fracture, it is rarely suitable for goats. Appropriate analgesia must be provided.

- Amputation may be considered in open or severely comminuted fractures. Goats are nimble and lightweight and cope well with an amputated leg. The technique is the same as for companion animals.
- External coaptation involves the application of a cast, splint or Robert-Jones bandage. The support must include the joints either side

of the fracture, and therefore is only suitable for lower limb fractures up to the level of the carpus or proximal metatarsus (**Fig. 9.7**). Deep sedation and analgesia must be provided to allow pain-free manipulation of the limb in order to achieve good alignment and prevent movement during cast setting. In growing animals, the foot is not included in a cast and the support replaced after 10–14 days.

- Hanging pin casts (also called transfixation pin casts) are an intermediary between coaptation and external skeletal fixation. It is a useful technique for comminuted fractures with many or small fragments, or where the distal fragment is very small or close to a joint.
- External skeletal fixation (ESF) is useful for comminuted and open fractures (**Fig. 9.8**). General anaesthesia is required to allow proper placement of the pins. While a technique readily achievable in private practice, it requires familiarity with the art and science behind it. ESF does have the disadvantage of creating some motion at the bone–pin interface, creating pain. Compared with internal fixation, less reduction and anatomical alignment of the fracture is achieved.
- Intramedullary pins are suitable for some types of fractures, such as simple mid-shaft upper limb ones. They do not provide much stability against rotational forces and the pin is a potential tract for infection. They sometimes can be used successfully in combination with cerclage wires for comminuted fractures.

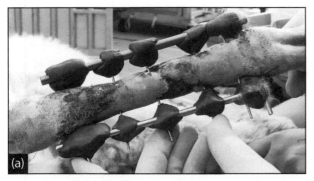
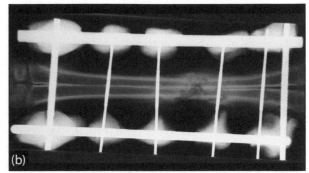

Fig. 9.8 (a) External skeletal fixation for an open metacarpal fracture in an alpaca cria, allowing ongoing wound care. (b) The corresponding radiograph showing pin placement in relation to the fracture site and adjacent joints.

- Internal fixation in the form of ASIF plates and screws requires special equipment and expertise. Neonates can pose a special problem, with their thin bone cortices offering little holding power to screws.

Good nursing care is essential. Especially, young animals require help in standing up for the first few days. Malodour, increased heat in the limb, pyrexia or a period of weight-bearing followed by protecting the leg indicates a problem, and should prompt re-assessment. Disuse atrophy after extended immobilisation is commonly seen, and it is important to provide support of decreasing strength after cast/fixation removal, such as a Robert-Jones bandage or splint, or removing ESF pins gradually.

Complications include nerve damage, nonunion, osteomyelitis, abnormal bone growth and nursing complications. Blood supply to the portion distal to the fracture may also be compromised. Prognosis is generally better in young animals (less body weight, better bone healing, better mobility), distal limb versus proximal limb, closed versus open and simple versus comminuted fractures. Quite often there is a delay in presenting goat patients, reducing prognosis.

Bone sequestrum
Overview
A bone sequestrum results from the loss of periosteal or cortical blood supply to a small section of long bone, with concurrent infection. Surgical treatment is indicated to achieve long-term resolution.

Aetiology
The typical cause is trauma to the leg and is the reason why the metacarpus and metatarsus are most often affected (with little 'soft tissue padding' over these particular bones). However, haematogenous spread of infection is also recognised as a cause, potentially leading to several sequestra (**Fig. 9.9**). Where a haematogenous aetiology is

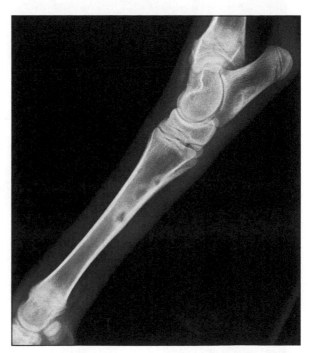

Fig. 9.9 Multiple areas of osteomyelitis in the right metatarsus of a lamb. Similar lesions were also present in the left metatarsus and tibia and both metacarpi, suggesting a haematogenous aetiology.

suspected, other potential abscessation sites, such as liver or heart valves, need to be examined. The pathogens involved tend to reflect those in the animal's environment.

Clinical presentation

A bone sequestrum should be suspected in non-healing wounds of the lower limb (**Fig. 9.10a**), recurrence of discharge through a fistula or recurrent lameness with pain on palpation over a small area of one of the long bones. The degree of lameness can vary from mild to severe.

Diagnosis

Confirmative diagnosis is via radiography. No radiographic changes will be seen for the first few weeks after the insult. Then, the cortices appear disrupted over the area in question, with lysis around the dead piece of bone and diffuse new bone formation in the area. To aid later surgical approach, it is of great help to position 2–3 three radiodense markers (e.g. skin staples or drawing pins secured with clear adhesive tape) onto landmarks such as a discharging tract or particular anatomical feature (**Fig. 9.10b**).

Differential diagnosis

For a discharging fistula, foreign body embedment or soft tissue abscess. For pain on palpation, fracture (acute or non-union) or ostitis/periostitis.

Treatment/management/control

Surgical removal of the sequestrum gives the best long-term prognosis. A temporary resolution of any discharge may be achieved with antibiosis,

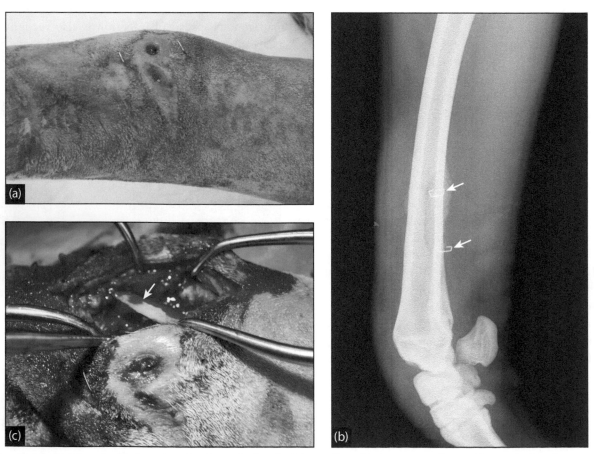

Fig. 9.10 (a) Chronic discharging fistula at the level of the radius. (b) Corresponding radiograph showing a bone sequestrum. Two skin staples (arrows) were placed either side of the fistula to aid orientation. (c) The sequestrum (arrow) in the process of being removed. Note the circumcision of the fistulous opening.

but invariably the foreign body nature of the sequestrum will lead to a flare up. In addition, the loss of blood supply leads to poor drug penetration of the area. Prognosis for surgical resolution is about 80% in cattle (no figure known for goats).

Surgery may be carried out under general anaesthesia or sedation and i/v regional anaesthesia (although the latter was found to carry a lower prognosis in cattle). A longitudinal skin incision is made over the sequestrum. Where this coincides with any discharging tract, the fistulous opening is circumcised. Exploration follows to locate a loose edge of the sequestrum. Occasionally, a bone chisel is required to loosen the piece of dead bone (**Fig. 9.10c**). After removal, any remaining abnormal soft bone in the area is removed with a curette. The skin incision is closed in a routine fashion. Leg support is necessary for 2–4 weeks; a Robert-Jones bandage, cast or splint are all suitable.

Joint dislocation
Overview
Dislocation typically affects the upper limb joints: hip, stifle, shoulder or elbow. Patellar luxation has also been described in the goat.

Aetiology
Joint dislocation usually occurs as a result of excessive rotational force caused, for example, by the leg becoming trapped, inaccurate handling or dismounting in the male. The female appears to be at particular risk of hip dislocation in the periparturient period and during oestrus. Patellar luxation, in particular bilateral medial, may be congenital.

Clinical presentation
Severe, acute-onset, swinging leg lameness with markedly reduced anterior phase. With hip dislocation in a craniodorsal direction, the animal usually remains ambulatory, whereas dislocation in a caudoventral direction results in recumbency. Pain on palpation, increased joint movement, swelling in the joint area and crepitus are commonly present.

Diagnosis
Comparison of angulation, position and joint space with the contralateral, unaffected leg shows dissymmetry; comparison with anatomical landmarks

shows abnormal distances. Radiography with flexed, extended and skyline views is used to confirm.

Differential diagnosis
Fracture of the affected joint or nearest long bone (e.g. femoral fracture in hip dislocation), confirmed by radiography.

Treatment/management/control
Best prognosis is achieved when the patient is attended to within 12 hours. Closed or open reduction is suitable for hip, shoulder and elbow dislocations. A Velpeau (front leg) or Ehmer (hind leg) sling is applied prior to recovery from sedation or general anaesthesia for several days to provide stability following reduction. The goat should receive suitable analgesia and box rest for several weeks.

For patellar luxation and ruptured cruciate ligament, surgical techniques used in the dog are suitable.

Tendon injuries
Overview
Flexor tendon injuries appear to be most common.

Aetiology
A traumatic insult is common in farmed livestock. Spontaneous rupture may result from excessive rotational or weight-bearing force. Occasionally, prior infection leads to weakening of a tendon. The role of hypophosphataemia or compartment syndrome is not known in the goat. Multiple tendons may be involved.

Clinical presentation
A physical, external insult (e.g. from farm machinery) typically results in a wound. Rupture as a result of excessive force (e.g. involving the gastrocnemius tendon) may be 'closed', with the overlying skin intact. The angulation of the leg is changed, with overextension of the immediately affected joint, resulting in overflexion of other joints. Swelling may be present over the rupture site.

Diagnosis
Clinical signs such as visible trauma to the tendon or abnormal limb angulation are usually diagnostic.

Differential diagnosis

Changed joint angulation caused by peripheral nerve deficiency will show loss of skin sensation over the area innervated by the relevant nerve (see **Fig. 8.13**).

Treatment/management/control

First aid consists of stabilising the leg in a flexed position (using a splint or Robert-Jones bandage). Where a wound is present, this is treated in the standard way using lavage, debridement and bandaging, combined with antibiosis (systemic, i/v regional or intraosseus) and anti-inflammatory therapy. Depending on the site of the wound, joint involvement must be ruled out.

Options for stabilising the tendon include splinting, casting (once tissue infection is under control, or using a fenestrated cast), tenorrhaphy or a combination of these. Prognosis for traumatic ruptures in the lower limb is good, but convalescence may be several months. Chronic lameness and digit hyperextension are the most common complications. Upper limb tendon ruptures carry a guarded prognosis.

Cartilage disorders

Overview

Hip dysplasia, osteochondrosis (OC) and degenerative joint disease (DJD) fall into this category.

Aetiology

In goats, factors such as age (young adult for OC and DJD), gender (males) or breed disposition, as recognised in other species, are not established. Fast growth and excessive body weight are likely to play a role. OC is a complex arthropathy. Its aetiology is still poorly understood, but a heritable component is present in other species and it may be a precursor for DJD.

Clinical presentation

Animals with hip dysplasia present with a shortened stride and pain on palpation and extension of the hip joint. While usually a bilateral condition, one leg is often affected worse. When looking from behind, the stifle and fetlock are rotated outwards and the hock inwards. The dorsal acetabulum and femoral head are affected in hip dysplasia (**Fig. 9.11**).

OC commonly affects the atlanto-occipital and femoropatellar joints, but also the hip joint, and tends

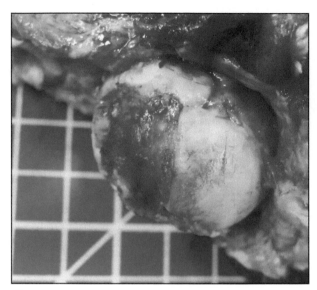

Fig. 9.11 Severe erosion of the femoral head cartilage, presumed secondary to hip dysplasia (alpaca specimen).

to be bilateral. Lameness may not be obvious until osteochondrosis dissecans is present.

DJD is a severe, progressive arthropathy, typically affecting the fetlock and carpal joints.

Diagnosis

Radiography is a useful first-line imaging modality, followed by ultrasonography, MRI or CT if required. DJD lesions may appear aggressive and septic on radiography, but tend to be focal, and there is usually little joint effusion. Joint fluid analysis is either within normal limits or shows mild inflammation and mildly increased protein levels.

Differential diagnosis

Septic arthritis results in joint effusion and joint fluid with marked cellularity and high protein. Osteoarthritis is a differential to DJD, but typically affects older animals.

Treatment/management/control

For hip dysplasia, the conservative and surgical options used in the dog may be considered. Conservative treatment of OC includes box rest for 3–6 months, combined with NSAIDs and possibly intra-articular hyaluronic acid or polysulfated glycosaminglycan. Surgical options include debridement and forage or microfracture. Prognosis is poor if radiographic signs of DJD are present at the commencement of treatment. For DJD, arthroscopic debridement, lavage and NSAID therapy may be tried, but is likely to result in temporary relief only. In general, because high motion joints are involved, arthrodesis is not feasible for these cartilage disorders.

Affected goats should be removed from the breeding pool, in particular males.

INFECTIOUS DISEASES

Caprine arthritis encephalitis

Definition/overview

Caprine arthritis encephalitis (CAE) is a viral disease caused by CAE virus (CAEV). It is an important disease of goats worldwide, causing a spectrum of clinical presentations and was only identified in the early 1970s. Many countries have instigated voluntary or compulsory control and eradication programmes.

Aetiology

A lentivirus in the family Retroviridae, a genus causing a group of slowly developing insidious conditions such as CAE and maedi visna (MV) of sheep, the two diseases often referred to collectively as SRLV (small ruminant lentivirus). Although the two viruses cause different clinical presentations in their respective host species, cross-species infection can occur and is an important factor in CAE control programmes.

Pathophysiology

CAE is transmitted predominantly via the ingestion of infected colostrum or milk from infected does. There are, however, many other important routes of infection such as via nose to nose contact and aerosol transfer, via 'infected milk impacts' at the teat end in the milking parlour, or through shared use of equipment such as drenching guns or tattooing equipment. Transplacental infection can occur but is thought to be at low levels, and although both embryo transfer and artificial insemination may pose only a minimal risk of transferring infection, both practices need to be risk managed if eradication is being attempted. Increased infection rates will occur in housed and intensively managed goats

because of close contact. Feeding pooled colostrum and milk (**Fig. 9.12**) in dairy herds can also lead to increased infection rates as one infected doe can infect the pool, and hence potentially a large number of kids.

The development of any clinical disease after infection will be slow and protracted, and as such is associated with a high prevalence of latent inapparent infection, in which goats remain fit, healthy and productive. The incubation period between infection and the development of clinical signs can be very variable. Infection induces a strong humoral response, but the antibody produced is not protective, and an infected goat is essentially both virus and antibody positive. The colostrum from infected dams will contain both virus and antibody, the latter affording no maternal protection.

After infection is acquired by whatever route, the virus quickly enters the reticuloendothelial system, carrying virus to target tissues such as the synovial membrane, lung, choroid plexus and udder where virus replication and lymphoproliferation continues.

Clinical presentation

After initial infection, goats may be asymptomatic for many months or even years before clinical disease is seen. There are a number of different clinical presentations that may be encountered either singly or in combination.

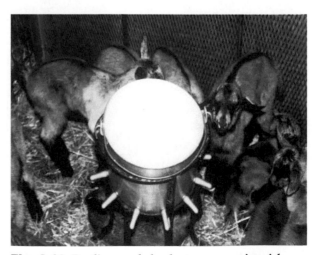

Fig. 9.12 Feeding pooled colostrum, a major risk factor for CAE transfer in infected herds.

Arthritis

Seen most commonly in mature goats aged 12 months and older. The onset may be acute or more slowly developing. All leg joints are susceptible, as is the atlanto-occipital joint. The carpal joint appears to be the most common site (**Fig. 9.13**), followed by the tarsal, stifle and fetlock joints. Single or multiple joints may be affected. Most affected joints are enlarged, often visibly, but not always painful. Signs will include obvious lameness, unwillingness to move, increased recumbency with inappetence and reduced milk production in lactating goats.

Leucoencephalomyelitis

A slowly developing presentation confined to young kids mainly from 1–6 months of age. Early signs include incoordination and poor leg placement progressing to paresis, with the hind legs most commonly affected. They may manage to drag themselves around, and remain relatively bright and alert in the early stages. Other CNS signs described include blindness, nystagmus and abnormal head carriage.

Interstitial pneumonitis

A slowly developing condition that may initially only cause exercise intolerance progressing to dyspnoea and weight loss, although often with other

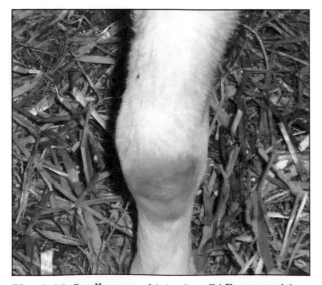

Fig. 9.13 Swollen carpal joint in a CAE-seropositive goat from a herd with a high prevalence of infection.

manifestations of CAE in the individual or herd. Secondary bacterial infection may be a sequela.

Mastitis

Referred to colloquially as 'hard udder', CAE infection has been linked to the development of an indurative mastitis in which the udder tissue becomes firm and shrunken and milk production from the affected half progressively ceases. The condition is usually insidious in onset. Mastitis is also discussed in Chapter 12.

Progressive weight loss

May occur in goats in which other manifestations of the disease are apparent, but CAE-seropositive illthriving goats in which no other more typical signs are present can also be identified in herd investigations into CAE.

Diagnosis

Diagnosis is based on the clinical signs, a previous indication of CAE in the herd and positive CAE serology. The possibility of new infection should be considered when investigating any group of goats with an increased incidence of ill thrift, particularly if there is evidence of increased lameness due to swollen joints, reduced milk yields and udder induration. For serological diagnosis of CAE it is recommend targeting up to 10 older goats exhibiting clinical signs, as infection is usually well established when clinical signs become evident. At post-mortem examination (PME), findings may include lesions within the joints such as visible thickening of the joint capsule, and in more chronic cases calcification of the tendon sheaths, joint capsules and bursae can occur. There may also be evidence of an indurative mastitis and enlarged supramammary lymph nodes. Less commonly, there may be lung pathology and the lungs may be heavy and swollen. A diagnosis at PME can be made by histopathological examination of tissues in combination with serological testing.

Differential diagnosis

Depends on the clinical presentation: arthritis in mature goats needs to be differentiated from degenerative arthritis or from trauma in more acute conditions. Nervous signs need to be differentiated from swayback and spinal trauma. The signs of indurative mastitis are fairly typical and distinct from other causes of mastitis.

Treatment/management/control

There is no treatment for CAE and no commercial vaccines are available at the time of writing. Control is therefore based predominantly on developing a test and cull policy. Determination of the disease prevalence is the first step. Ideally, all mature goats in the herd over 12 months of age should be tested using a validated CAE serological test. If this is not financially viable, a proportion of the herd could be tested ensuring that goats of all age groups (over 12 months) are included. Once the level of infection is established, an eradication or control programme can be instigated. If the infection is ignored and no control methods are put in place, it is likely with time that the infection will lead to significant production losses.

Culling of seropositive animals with or without their progeny has been used successfully to reduce herd prevalence. This approach involves blood testing all goats over 12 months at regular intervals (every 3–6 months) and removing all seropositive animals at each test. After two tests six months apart, where no antibody positive animals are identified, the herd can be classed as free of CAE, providing sensible biosecurity procedures have been followed and no goats of unknown health status have been purchased.

If the prevalence of disease is high in a herd (or the affected goats are not being kept commercially) and culling of the seropositive animals is not possible, the herd can be separated into two groups (one 'dirty' containing seropositive animals and one 'semi-clean' containing seronegative animals). Seronegative animals cannot be guaranteed to be uninfected as some could be in the early stages of infection. The 'semi-clean' group should therefore be tested on a 6–12 monthly basis and any seroconverted animals moved to the 'dirty' group. Any animals showing clinical signs of CAE should be culled as they are likely to be excreting high levels of CAEV.

For this approach to work successfully the two groups have to be managed completely separately and strict biosecurity measures put in place. Equipment should not be shared, which can be more difficult in the dairy situation. In a dairy herd the semi-clean group should be milked first and the dirty group second. Ideally, the equipment is disinfected between milkings. At parturition, the clean group should be kidded separately. Kids from the 'dirty' group could be snatched at birth before they have been licked or suckled, but as intrauterine transmission can occur in a small proportion of infected dams, further screening of these kids as they get older would be required.

Heat treating or pasteurising has reportedly been a useful supportive measure: milk or colostrum is held at 56°C for 60 minutes. Commercial pasteurisers are available.

There is evidence of natural cross infection between goats and sheep with CAE and MV, respectively. The most likely risk factors are ingestion of virus-contaminated ovine colostrum and milk by goats and vice versa, as well as close contact between the species in overstocked housing. It is unclear at what rate these viruses spread within the 'heterologous' host population, but there is consensus that SRLV infection across the species barrier must be taken into account in any control programme. Any control programme in goats that ignores sheep kept in close contact may not be successful.

Bacterial arthritis (syn. joint ill)
Definition/overview

A condition most commonly encountered in young kids, referred to as 'joint ill', and encountered worldwide, particularly where goats are reared intensively. It most commonly results from rearing in unsanitary conditions, allowing bacterial colonisation of the umbilicus and resulting septicaemia, especially if combined with failure of passive transfer.

Aetiology

A wide variety of organisms have been incriminated, most commonly *Escherichia coli*, *Streptococcus dysgalactiae*, *Trueperella pyogenes*, *Erysipelothrix rhusiopathiae*, *Pasteurella* spp. and *Klebsiella* spp.

Pathophysiology

Most infections arise following intensification, with few cases seen in kids born outdoors. A combination of overcrowding, environmental pathogen build-up, lack of umbilical hygiene at birth and hypogamma-globulinaemia are all contributing factors. Infection gains entry most commonly via the umbilicus, causing septicaemia with organisms settling in a number of predilection sites such as joints.

Clinical presentation

Swollen painful joints in young kids, often with a thickened necrotic umbilicus. The carpus and stifle are most commonly affected, followed by the hock and fetlock.

Diagnosis

Clinical signs and presenting history are typical. Joint aspirates taken aseptically (or at PME) may appear turbid and will show elevated protein and nucleated cell counts. Bacterial culture of joint fluid is useful, but false-negative results are common.

Differential diagnosis

Joint ill should be differentiated from mycoplasma infection and tick pyaemia and from joint trauma.

Treatment/management/control

Treatment can be disappointing unless instigated at an early stage by use of broad-spectrum parenteral antibiosis at a high dose rate. Joint lavage is beneficial in valuable or pet goats, but should be considered early on in the disease process for best prognosis.

Control centres on good neonatal kid care (see Chapter 4).

Mycoplasma arthritis

Definition/overview

Mycoplasma spp. organisms are responsible for a variety of conditions in goats. Contagious caprine pleuropneumonia is described in Chapter 6 and contagious agalactia in Chapter 12. Mycoplasma arthritis can occur in isolation as a result of localisation in joints of a septicaemic infection, but it can also be one of the clinical presentations in a multisystemic infection such as contagious agalactia.

Aetiology

Our understanding of *Mycoplasma* spp. is dynamic; new species are being identified and known species reclassified and often renamed. They are quite distinct from bacteria, do not possess a cell wall and are difficult to grow in the laboratory. Isolation rates have been improved by new molecular techniques such as denaturing gradient gel electrophoresis (DGGE). The primary species involved in polyarthritis are *M. capricolum* subsp *capricolum*, *M. mycoides* subsp *capri*, *M. agalactia*, *M. arginini* and *M. mycoides* subsp *mycoides*, and the distribution of each of these organisms varies from country to country.

Pathophysiology

Mycoplasma arthritis most commonly occurs in multiple joints because of localisation of infection from an initial septicaemia.

Clinical presentation

Although arthritis can occur at any age (particularly with the more virulent *Mycoplasma* spp. organisms), it is encountered more commonly in kids and young immature goats. Joint involvement is most often seen in association with other clinical signs within the spectrum of mycoplasma-associated disease in the herd, including pneumonia, ocular infections, mastitis, abortion and agalactia. Carpal, tarsal and stifle joints are most commonly affected and become swollen, painful and often warm to the touch, causing marked lameness and reluctance to move.

Diagnosis

Clinical signs are fairly characteristic. Joint aspirates can be subjected to laboratory testing for mycoplasma by culture or DGGE. Affected and recovered goats may demonstrate seroconversion. At PME, joint fluid is initially clear before becoming turbid and blood tinged (**Fig. 9.14**), and there is evidence of a necrotising synovitis histologically.

Differential diagnosis

Joint ill and tick pyaemia are the main differentials. *Mycoplasma* spp. infection should always be suspected if polyarthritis and joint enlargement are seen in association with pyrexia and other clinical signs within a group of goats.

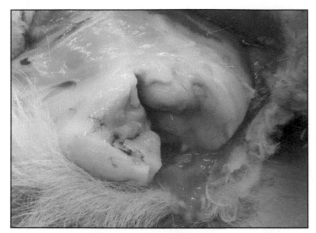

Fig. 9.14 Turbid and blood-tinged joint fluid in infectious arthritis.

Treatment/management/control

Treatment can be disappointing, particularly if joint lesions are advanced or there are other accompanying systemic signs. Prolonged courses (5 days minimum) of, for example, tetracyclines (15 mg/kg) or tylosin (20–40 mg/kg) have been recommended.

Control should be aimed initially at keeping the important *Mycoplasma* spp. infections out, by applying strict biosecurity with quarantine and laboratory testing of incoming goats. Contagious agalactia, if confirmed, will be controlled by the imposition of statutory control measures as a reportable OIE disease. Vaccines are available in some countries, and should be used alongside management procedures to minimise spread of infection if confirmed. If infection is widespread, a strict culling policy of infected groups of goats may be beneficial, as infection is seldom restricted to individual goats within a cohort.

Clostridial myositis

Blackleg and malignant oedema caused by the proliferation of *Clostridium chauvoei*, *Clostridium septicum*, *Clostridium novyi* and *Clostridium sordellii* in muscle tissue singly or in combination is relatively common in cattle and sheep worldwide, but relatively uncommon in goats. Its absence as a cause of disease in the UK, for example, is the reason '4 in 1' clostridial vaccine is generally advised (as opposed to more multivalent vaccines). In those countries in which it is occasionally recorded, goats affected with blackleg may simply be found dead. Those with malignant oedema usually present with a localised tissue swelling, often at the site of a wound or injury. In both conditions, gas accumulates under the skin in the affected areas, causing crepitus. Disease is confirmed most often at PME in which typical gas-gangrenous change to muscle tissue and associated oedema are features. If seen alive, very high doses of i/v penicillin (20,000 iu/kg q12h) should be administered, with multiple incisions into affected tissue to allow aeration and drainage. Prevention is by the implementation of a multivalent clostridial vaccine regime.

Arbovirus infection (Akabane, Schmallenberg)

These viruses can cause leg and joint abnormalities in newborn and neonatal kids (see Chapter 2).

FOOT DISORDERS

Laminitis
Definition/overview

Laminitis is an aseptic inflammation of the sensitive laminae beneath the foot horn. It can present as an acute attack causing severe lameness or can be chronic causing long-term damage to the foot architecture.

Aetiology

The causes of laminitis have been investigated in many livestock species, including goats, and opinions still vary as to the exact aetiological basis. Cases tend to occur predominantly in intensively managed herds or in goats kept as pets with excessive or unsuitable supplementary feeding (e.g. biscuits). Any sudden change in the ration, particularly excessive feeding of cereal grain (or inadvertent access to stored grain), can lead to lactic acidosis and to laminitis change. It can also occur following an episode of acute toxaemia resulting from, for example, metritis, retained placenta or mastitis.

Pathophysiology

The principle lesion appears to be an engorgement of the vessels in the sensitive corium, resulting in intense pain in the foot in acute cases and insidious changes to the foot architecture in mild (and possibly asymptomatic) cases leading to more long-term chronic change. These changes include rotation of the third phalanx and progressive distortion of new horn growth.

Clinical presentation

In acute cases, affected goats will either stand motionless unwilling to move or be recumbent and unwilling to stand, and there may be other signs of illness related to the primary insult. The condition is almost always bilateral, and front feet tend to be affected more than hind feet, but all four feet may be affected at the same time. The digits feel warm, particularly around the coronary band, and any pressure applied to this area is resented. Lameness may only be obvious if one individual foot is painful, otherwise a change in gait and stance is more apparent. Frequent weight-shifting may be seen, and goats may walk on their knees (**Fig. 9.15**) or shuffle along lifting affected front feet in an exaggerated manner. When hind feet are affected, these are placed forward of their natural position. Chronic cases tend to follow a series of earlier laminitic episodes, which may or may not have been apparent. The claws in chronic laminitis progressively become 'box shaped', and the horn becomes abnormally hard and may

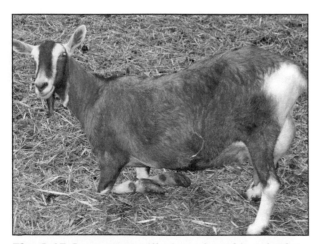

Fig. 9.15 Lame goats will often adopt this attitude, and may even move around on their knees, although some goats may naturally feed like this and develop superficial abrasive lesions as a result.

show horizontal grooves. If the third phalanx has rotated, horn overgrowth may result in 'slipper foot' formation. Chronic laminitis can be a particular problem in geriatric goats.

Diagnosis

Diagnosis is based on the clinical signs described and the history suggesting sudden diet change or toxaemia.

Differential diagnosis

Other causes of lameness need to be eliminated, but laminitis should always be suspected if more than one foot is affected.

Treatment/management/control

In acute laminitis, any potential underlying factors should be identified and managed. Treatment is aimed predominantly at controlling the pain and discomfort by the use of analgesics and NSAIDs. If a dietary cause has been identified, rapidly fermentable carbohydrates should be removed from the diet (or reduced as much as possible in lactating does) and replaced by good quality hay or other forage. In chronic cases, attention should be directed to identifying and removing any underlying causes, and to regular foot trimming to address overgrowth and re-establish the correct foot shape. Analgesics and NSAIDs are used if required, with culling on humane grounds in elderly goats in which there is no improvement. Prevention is focused on avoiding any sudden dietary changes.

Scald and footrot

Definition/overview

Footrot is a potentially severe and highly contagious foot disorder affecting both goats and sheep worldwide, with cross infection and spread between species. The condition is more prevalent in temperate climates, particularly if goats are kept outdoors with warm wet conditions underfoot. Severe outbreaks have also been described in goats kept indoors on deep litter, when rapid transfer from goat to goat can occur. Scald or interdigital dermatitis is generally classified as a milder form of the condition (**Fig. 9.16**).

Aetiology

The primary pathogen of both these conditions is *Dichelobacter nodosus*, with *Fusobacterium necrophorum* as a co-existing secondary pathogen in footrot cases. *D. nodosus* is an obligate anaerobe, easily adapted to foot tissue, and was originally thought not to survive in the environment for long. Recent work in the sheep sector, however, has indicated that *D. nodosus* can survive for up to 14 days at 5°C in soil, and at least 24 days when hoof material is present, depending on ambient weather conditions. This factor is important when developing any footrot and scald control programme.

Pathophysiology

Weaker strains of *D. nodosus* are now thought to be involved in the development of the interdigital lesions typical of scald and more virulent strains with footrot, although these pathogens are often found in association with *F. necrophorum*, an environmental organism that is able to colonise damaged foot epithelial tissue. *D. nodosus* strains possess varying degrees of keratolytic enzyme activity which, in the development of footrot lesions, effectively erodes the thin keratin layers, beginning at the horn–skin junction in the interdigital space and heels and extending to involve large areas of the hoof matrix. Because the sensitive lamina and its network of capillaries are destroyed by the infection, the hoof wall's corium loses its blood supply and anchorage to the underlying tissue, progressively compacting with soil and faecal debris and becomes detached, causing underrunning of the wall. This often results in the affected claw being shed, a process referred to as 'thimbling' (**Fig. 9.17**).

Clinical presentation

This will vary depending on the severity of the condition and the number of feet affected. In scald, when damage may be mild, there may be little or no lameness. In established footrot cases, lameness becomes more apparent with affected goats reluctant to move. If both front legs are affected, goats may move around and feed on their knees or remain recumbent. Other sequelae include loss of condition and reduced milk yield.

Diagnosis

Initial diagnosis is based on localisation of any lameness to the foot, followed by differentiation from other causes of foot lameness. The changes described above are fairly typical in both conditions.

Differential diagnosis

When a number of goats suddenly become lame, foot and mouth disease, bluetongue and laminitis should be considered.

Treatment/management/control

As the condition is contagious, the primary aim is to keep infection out by examining the feet of any

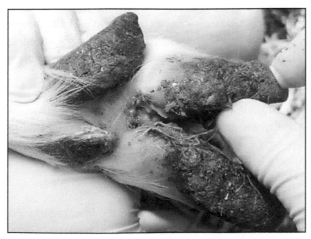

Fig. 9.16 Scald, evident in the interdigital cleft of the foot of this sheep.

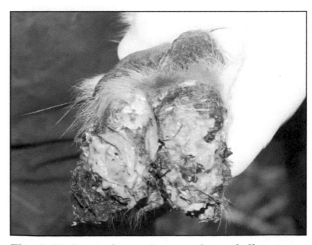

Fig. 9.17 Severe footrot in a goat housed all year on deep litter.

purchased goat on arrival and taking swift action if footrot is suspected. Once identified in a group, the first step is to isolate any affected goats immediately to prevent further spread of infection, while monitoring the remainder of the group for developing infection. Treatments for footrot in sheep are constantly under review and undoubtedly influence the current approaches used in goats. Treatment of individual cases with systemic antibiosis has proved successful in sheep, but is unproven in goats, with the added problems of milk withhold for dairy goats. Although paring away the infected and underrun tissue has been a traditional approach to treatment, this is now being challenged in the sheep sector as being counterproductive. Proprietary antibiotic sprays are used widely, but have only a short duration of action and are probably ineffective in deep-rooted infection. Footbathing is an extremely useful approach for both affected and in-contact goats, and footbaths can be easily installed in race exits from milking parlours or buildings.

Footbathing is only effective if carried out correctly:

1   Feet must be clean before entering the footbath (ideally sprayed with water).
2   Zinc sulphate 10% is the treatment of choice, although there are a number of other commercial products available worldwide.
3   Goats must stand in the solution and not run straight through.
4   Traditionally, formalin has been used in footbaths, but this product is painful on open foot lesions, it poses safety risks to the operator and disposal is difficult.
5   Antibiotic footbaths should only be used where there is a specific clinical indication such as contagious ovine digital dermatitis (CODD). An appropriate milk withdrawal period must be observed.
6   Footbath content should be replaced regularly.
7   Goats must stand on a dry, hard surface (ideally concrete) after footbathing until the feet are dry.
8   Animals should be moved to clean pasture, or cleaned and disinfected pens, after treatment.
9   A sponge mat soaked in footbath solution on the base of the bath can be an effective way of ensuring that all the feet are immersed.

Footrot vaccines are available, but should be part of an overall foot health programme; they cannot replace it. Culling of any goat that does not respond to treatment, or whose welfare is severely compromised, is recommended.

Treponeme-associated foot disease
Definition/overview
CODD is a highly contagious foot disorder first identified in sheep and reported in the UK (by one of the authors [DH]) in 1997. Although the characteristic clinical signs identified in sheep have not been encountered in goats, a virulent and apparently contagious presentation with a similar mixed aetiology has been reported in dairy goats by veterinary researchers in the UK at both the University of Liverpool and the University of Bristol.

Aetiology
Consistent isolates have been species of *Treponema* organisms, which have also been incriminated in CODD and in digital dermatitis of cattle. Outbreaks have been associated with three cultivatable digital dermatitis treponeme phylogroups: *Treponema medium*, *Treponema phagedenis* and *Treponema pedis*. It is still not known whether the treponeme bacteria are the only cause of the disease in goats, or whether there are other factors as yet unidentified.

Pathophysiology
Treponema organisms can survive in faeces and contaminated bedding, thus facilitating spread between goats. Histopathological examination of early lesions confirms a morphological diagnosis of chronic lymphoplasmacytic, suppurative and ulcerated pododermatitis.

Clinical presentation
To date there is no single consistent description of the disease presentation; however, a common finding appears to be severe, non-healing toe, wall or sole ulcers (**Figs. 9.18, 9.19**).

Diagnosis
Diagnosis is currently based on the clinical signs identified, the sudden emergence within a group of goats and its rapid spread within that group. There are currently no commercially available diagnostic tests.

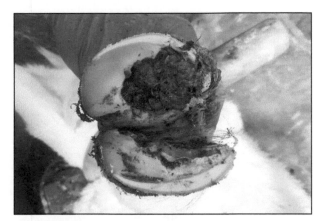

Fig. 9.18 Treponeme-associated solar ulcer. (Image courtesy Hayley E. Crosby-Durrani.)

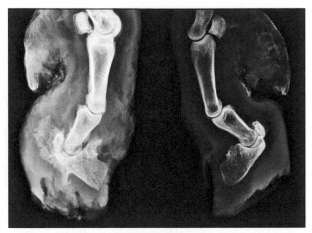

Fig. 9.19 Radiograph of a chronic lesion suspected to be associated with *Treponema* spp. (leg on left). Note the severe bone reaction around, and partial destruction of, P3. Of note in the control foot (leg on right) is the normal club-shape and almost plantigrade position of P3. (Image courtesy Hayley E. Crosby-Durrani.)

Differential diagnosis

The condition needs to be differentiated from other causes of foot lameness, specifically sporadic toe ulcers.

Treatment/management/control

Treatment and control is currently extrapolated from measures developed to control both CODD in sheep and digital dermatitis in cattle. These include:

- The rapid identification and isolation of affected goats.
- Topical and/or parenteral antibiotic or antibiotic foot bathing.
- Improved underfoot hygiene (keeping deep litter yards clean and dry).
- A review of foot trimming practices – ensuring extra care is taken with routine hoof trimming, never over trimming feet and never causing bleeding and hoof damage.
- Cleaning and disinfecting hoof clippers between goats (**Fig. 9.20**) and handling area after a trimming session to avoid spread between goats and premises.

Overgrown claws

Overgrown claws can be a particular problem in intensively managed goats kept on deep litter (**Fig. 9.21**). Wall growth rates can be as high as 6 mm per month. If left untreated, they can lead to abnormal stresses on joints and other soft tissue structures, leading to pain and an unwillingness to

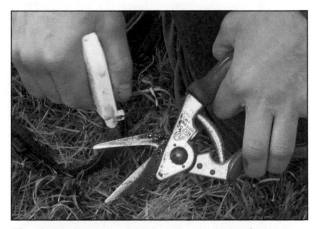

Fig. 9.20 Foot trimming equipment must be disinfected between animals and herds, particularly where infectious conditions are present.

move around. Under normal circumstances, feet are worn down by contact abrasion with the walking surface. The problem can be controlled by regular monitoring of claw length and shape, with foot trimming undertaken where necessary.

Routine foot trimming

This is a skilful procedure and should only be undertaken by trained personnel – in untrained hands overtrimming can have disastrous results. Foot examinations should be carried out regularly on at least

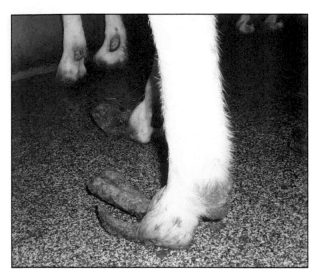

Fig. 9.21 Foot overgrowth. Note the excessively elongated claws. (Image courtesy Kathy Anzuino.)

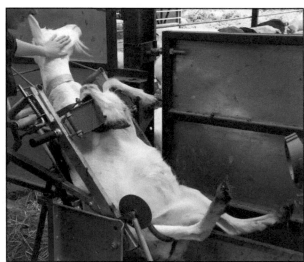

Fig. 9.22 Goat restrained for foot trimming. Such a device is useful on large units. (Image courtesy Kathy Anzuino.)

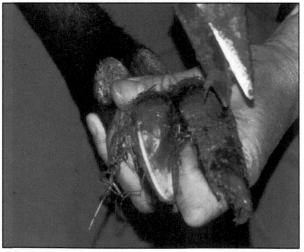

Fig. 9.23 Trimming of an overgrown hoof wall. Note that the wall of the left claw has been trimmed back more severely than is ideal in this goat.

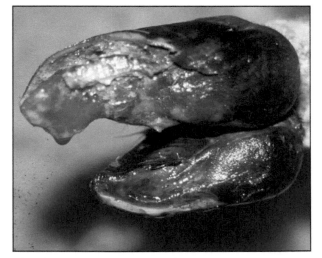

Fig. 9.24 Blood must never be drawn on purpose during foot trimming.

a proportion of the herd. However, there is no set frequency of trimming. If required at all, this will vary from goat to goat and from unit to unit depending on both genetics and environment. In intensively housed goats on deep litter, this may be 3–4 times a year (**Fig. 9.22**), whereas goats kept in drier climates outdoors may never need to have their feet trimmed unless there is a hereditary abnormality of horn growth.

Mild to moderate horn overgrowth does not require trimming if the goat is not lame.

Otherwise, using a pair of sheep foot shears, the wall horn is trimmed to a level just above the sole surface itself (**Fig. 9.23**). Trimming should be as minimal as possible, and blood must never be drawn on purpose (**Fig. 9.24**). Foot trimming equipment is disinfected between animals.

White line disease

White line disease is a condition affecting the junction between the wall and sole horn on the abaxial

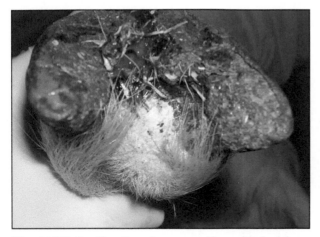

Fig. 9.25 Swollen foot due to a well-established foot abscess.

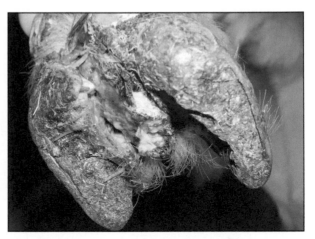

Fig. 9.26 Burst foot abscess, with a tract that leads directly to pedal bone.

solar surface of the foot, whereby the structure becomes weakened and the junction begins to open allowing dirt and gravel to become trapped, causing further separation and eventual pressure on the sensitive laminae causing lameness. The condition is most commonly identified on routine examination and rectified by remedial foot trimming. The condition is more common when the feet are soft and goats are walking along muddy gravel tracks.

Pedal joint abscess

Outbreaks of pedal joint abscess have been encountered in goats, presenting as a sudden onset severe lameness most commonly affecting only one foot (**Fig. 9.3**). The condition presents initially as visible swelling around the top of the hoof, becoming more apparent until the whole foot is affected (**Fig. 9.25**), eventually bursting, leaving a tract into the pedal joint (**Fig. 9.26**). Various treatment regimes have been tried with varying success, and are dependent on the stage the condition has reached before therapy is commenced. In the early stages parenteral antibiosis may be effective. As the condition becomes more visible, and particularly if the abscess has burst, then poulticing and lesion irrigation may be attempted. In severe cases, digit amputation should be considered (**Fig. 9.27**) and can be highly effective in reducing pain and prolonging the productive life of the goat.

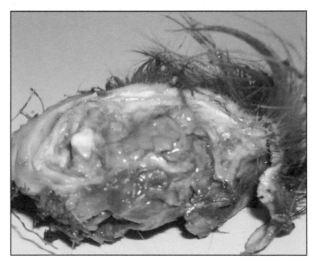

Fig. 9.27 Amputated digit showing suppuration of the pedal joint.

Foreign bodies and foot lameness

These include penetration of the sole by sharp pieces of gravel, thorns or metallic debris, and stones and dried mud becoming trapped between the claws.

Foot and mouth disease

Foot and mouth disease should always be considered as a differential diagnosis if a number of goats become lame simultaneously. (See Chapter 17 for detailed discussion.)

NORMAL STRUCTURE AND FUNCTION

The kidneys in the goat are non-lobulated with a smooth surface, and are about 6–7 cm long by 3.5–5 cm wide. The individual sections of either cortex or medulla are largely fused, resulting in an internal structure similar to the dog. The right kidney lies between the last rib and second lumbar vertebra. The left kidney is pushed over to the right by the rumen and lies more caudal under the 4th to 6th lumbar vertebrae. Similarly, the left ureter initially travels to the right of the midline. The ureters enter the bladder near its neck. The urethra is about 5–6 cm long in the doe, with a 1–1.5 cm long suburethral diverticulum near its caudal end. The buck also has a urethral diverticulum, at the level of the pubic bone. In the male, the urethra ends in the urethral process or filiform appendage, which extends beyond the glans penis (see **Fig. 2.31**, p. 45). An adult goat produces on average 2 litres of urine per day (20–40 ml/kg/day).

CLINICAL EXAMINATION OF THE URINARY TRACT

Clinical assessment

Direct clinical examination of the urinary tract is limited in the goat. Abdominal palpation may reveal pain on palpation in the kidney area, and sometimes an enlarged bladder. Behaviour during urination, such as straining or remaining in a crouched position, and urine flow are important observations. Differential diagnoses for two common presentations, haematuria and haemoglobinuria, are shown in *Table 10.1*. Haemoglobinuria is secondary to haemolytic anaemia, therefore the plasma is discoloured, as well, and the goat may show signs of anaemia.

Ancillary diagnostics
Urinalysis

Obtaining urine is not straightforward in the goat, but worth pursuing. Some females will respond to gentle stroking of the perineal area, taking care not

Table 10.1 **Diseases presenting with haematuria or haemoglobinuria.**

HAEMATURIA	HAEMOGLOBINURIA
Cystitis	Bacillary (*Clostridium haemolyticum*)
Pyelonephritis	Nutritional (brassica species; nitrite/nitrate)
Urolithiasis	Babesiosis, anaplasmosis, theileriosis
Septicaemia (in particular salmonellosis)	Leptospirosis (*Leptospira interrogans* serovar *Pomona*)
Enzootic haematuria (bracken fern toxicity)	Chronic copper poisoning
Renal infarction	Photosensitisation (some cases)
Embolism of renal artery	Post-parturient (phosphorus deficiency, possibly also copper deficiency)
	Water intoxication

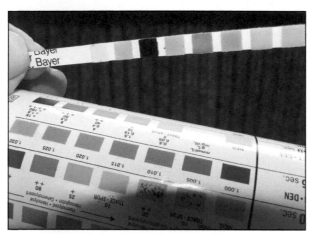

Fig. 10.1 Human urine dipsticks provide for convenient goat-side urinalysis. However, they are not reliable for specific gravity or protein.

appendage, sigmoid flexure and urethral diverticulum make catheterisation impossible.

Urine dipsticks are useful for initial goat-side assessment (**Fig. 10.1**). Their indication of specific gravity is not accurate and, in the alkaline urine of goats, there may be false-positive results for proteinuria. Both these parameters should be established with a refractometer.

Normal urine parameters are: alkaline with a pH of 7.0–8.0; specific gravity of 1.020–1.040 and osmolarity of 800–1,200 mOsm/kg. The urine typically contains low concentrations of sodium, chloride, phosphorus ions, calcium and magnesium, but high concentrations of potassium. A trace of protein is common, as is a small amount of ketones in lactating goats.

Sediment is examined for presence of blood cells, bacteria, cell casts and crystals. The latter are not significant unless present in large numbers; for example, calcium carbonate and triple phosphate crystals are common in normal urine.

Culture is useful to aid choice of antimicrobials and monitor response to treatment.

Changes detectable by urinalysis and their interpretation are shown in *Table 10.2*.

to hold the tail and touching or holding the goat as little as possible. A good proportion will urinate on standing up. Catheterisation, using a bitch catheter, is reasonably easy in the doe, but care must be taken to avoid the urethral diverticulum. The urethral opening lies ventrally at the junction between the vagina and the vestibulum. In the buck, the filiform

Table 10.2 **Abnormalities detected by urinalysis and their interpretation.**

CHANGE SEEN	COMMON CAUSE
pH abnormal	Usually falls with urinary tract disease, but can rise with some bacterial infections. Despite metabolic alkalosis, the urine may be acidic (paradoxic acidosis)
Low specific gravity (<1.015) or osmolarity (<500 mOsm/kg)	If no change despite water deprivation or administering a large quantity of water, indicates renal insufficiency
Proteinuria	Physiological: stress (e.g. transport), pyrexia, heavy lactation. False-positive result with human dipsticks. Otherwise indicates renal involvement
Bacteria – direct counts	<10,000 bacteria/ml = contamination 10,000–100,000 bacteria/ml = questionable relevance >100,000 bacteria/ml = infection
Glycosuria	Diabetes (a rare condition)
Haematuria	Presents as blood clots or discolouration or brown sediment. Sediment examination confirms presence of red blood cells. Usually also positive for haemoglobinuria. Contamination from the reproductive tract must be ruled out in does. See *Table 10.1*
Haemoglobinuria	False-positive results from haemolysed red blood cells, therefore sediment examination is important. See *Table 10.1*
Myoglobinuria	Due to myopathies. Usually concurrent rise in blood muscle enzymes (CK, AST)

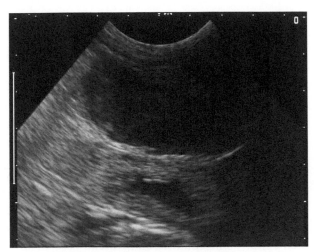

Fig. 10.2 Transabdominal ultrasonogram of a normal urinary bladder in a 10-year-old Pygmy doe. Of note are the thin wall, clear urine (appearing black) and lack of sediment. Ventral to the bladder is a thicker-walled, slightly fluid-filled uterine horn.

Ultrasonography

Ultrasonography is invaluable to assess the urinary tract and is easy to perform transabdominally in the conscious goat. The bladder is assessed for size, wall thickness or neoplasia, and debris or foreign bodies in its lumen (**Fig. 10.2**). The kidneys are both visualised through the right flank and assessed for size, changes in the appearance of the cortex and medulla, hydronephrosis, calculi in the renal pelvis and neoplasia (**Fig. 10.3**).

Radiography

Radiography is most usefully employed in the form of an intravenous urogram, especially to detect congenital malformations of the urinary tract.

Cystoscopy

A paediatric endoscope is required and, because of the males's anatomical features (described earlier), cystoscopy is restricted to the female.

Renal biopsy

Renal biopsy is performed under local anaesthesia through a stab incision, and ideally ultrasound guided. Complications such as haematuria appear to be rare.

Renal function tests

- Serum urea:creatinine ratio. This ratio is increased in renal insufficiency, but because ruminants recycle urea, results are not very clear cut and do not allow differentiation of a prerenal versus renal cause.
- Phenolsulphonphthalein (PSP) excretion. A simplified version entails: inject 0.4 mg/kg of PSP i/v; collect blood into EDTA 30 minutes later and measure concentration. Normal concentration is <50 µg/dl serum. Elevated serum levels indicate decreased tubular action.
- Fractional excretion of electrolytes. There appear to be no validated normal values in the goat, in particular for different feeds or diets.

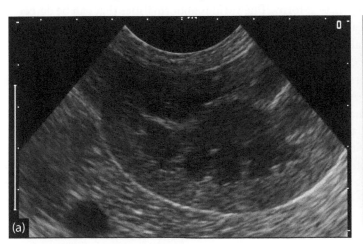
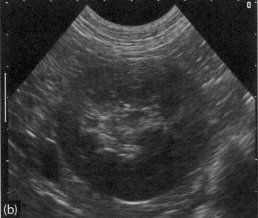

Fig. 10.3 Transabdominal ultrasonogram of a normal kidney in a 10-year-old Pygmy doe. (a) Longitudinal scan; (b) cross-sectional scan. The medulla may appear more echodense than in this case.

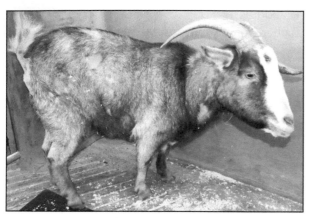

Fig. 10.4 A buck with obstructive urolithiasis, with an arched back indicating abdominal discomfort and a raised tail indicating stranguria.

NON-INFECTIOUS DISEASES

Urethral obstruction caused by urolithiasis

Definition/overview
Obstruction of the urethra is of particular importance in meat and pet goats.

Aetiology
Castrated males are most at risk of urethral obstruction because of a narrower urethra due to lack of testosterone. Uroliths may form in the female goat, but rarely lead to obstruction in their short and relatively wide urethra. Predisposing factors include rations rich in concentrates (≥2.5% of body weight dry matter intake for 2 months or more), alfalfa (high calcium content) or pasture with high levels of silica, oxalate or oestrogens. Urethral obstruction may also be caused by high levels of magnesium in milk replacers, and retinol (vitamin A) deficiency may play a role. A contributing factor is 'nidus formation' – organic material as the core of the calculus; for example, epithelial cells or necrotic tissue after local infection. Diets with low salt content and restricted access to water favour precipitation of solutes.

The types of calculi in ruminants are:

- Clover pasture – calcium carbonate.
- Extensive pasture– silica.
- Meat/fattening ration – phosphates (calcium, magnesium, ammonium).

Clinical presentation
Common sites for the calculus to lodge are the sigmoid flexure or the urethral process. The goat shows abdominal discomfort (e.g. arched back, colic, shortened stride; **Fig. 10.4**). There is dysuria or stranguria, with no or only a few drops of urine produced. Sometimes crystals are present on the preputial hair or the inner thigh. Digital rectal examination reveals pulsation or spasms of the urethra. A distended bladder may be palpable through the abdominal wall in young, thin goats.

Rupture of the urinary bladder or urethra may occur after about 48 hours. This results in sudden relief of discomfort and, in the case of urethral rupture, ventral subcutaneous fluid swelling, cellulitis and possibly toxaemia. Bladder rupture results in uroperitoneum, uraemia, anorexia and depression.

Diagnosis
Signs of colic or dysuria in the male should always prompt investigation for urethral obstruction. Uraemia is present on bloods. A serum phosphate level >2.9 mmol/l is associated with a poor prognosis in cattle. A creatinine concentration in peritoneal fluid 1.5–2 times higher than serum levels indicates uroperitoneum.

Calcium-containing stones (e.g. calcium-oxalate, calcium-carbonate, silicate) can be detected on radiography, but ultrasonography is often easier to perform. The various abnormalities that can be detected on ultrasound, depending on the stage of disease, are a distended bladder or urethra (**Fig. 10.5**), the calculus if lodged in the externally accessible part of the urethra, free peritoneal fluid or subcutaneous fluid accumulation.

Differential diagnosis
Other abdominal problems for colic. For dysuria: prostatitis, cystitis or pyelonephritis. For subcutaneous swelling: ruptured penis, snake bites or haematoma.

Treatment/management/control
Pain, considerable electrolyte disturbances and onset of hydronephrosis by 48 hours (**Fig. 10.6**) mean that prompt treatment is required. In small ruminants,

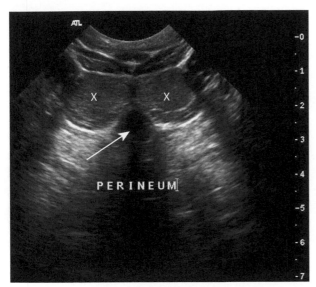

Fig. 10.5 Ultrasonogram showing enlarged diameter of the perineal urethra (arrow) resulting from obstructive urolithiasis. (The image is of an alpaca, hence the small testicles [X].)

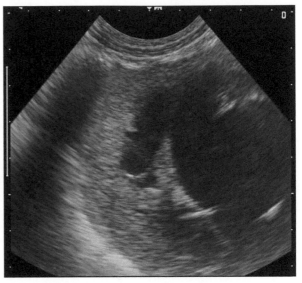

Fig. 10.6 Cross-sectional ultrasonogram showing hydronephrosis in a 12-year-old Pygmy goat.

17–55% long-term recovery after urethrostomy and 88% after cystotomy are reported.

Supportive treatment

The goat should receive intravenous fluids at maintenance rate once urinary output is established, and maximum water intake should be encouraged (including adding salt to the diet – see below). NSAIDs are best avoided for pain relief until normal kidney function is restored. Opioids can be used for analgesia in the meantime (e.g. butorphanol is available under the cascade in the UK). Antibiosis is indicated.

Medical treatment (not indicated if bladder rupture has occurred)

- Passing a urinary catheter in the male goat is impossible because of the urethral process, sigmoid flexure and urethral diverticulum.
- A smooth muscle relaxant (e.g. xylazine, clenbuterol, Buscopan®, acepromazine; **note:** all constitute off-licence use) may be tried. The animal is placed onto concrete or shavings to monitor urine output. Xylazine increases urine output, so if not successful, prompt surgical treatment is required.

- Ultrasound-guided cystocentesis and lavage with Walpole's solution (effective against struvites) has been described, but carries the risk of inducing peritonitis.

Removal of urethral process

This is worthwhile, regardless of any further approach, either to cure or to prevent other calculi becoming lodged at this point. With the goat on its haunches, the penis is exteriorised and the process cut with sharp scissors as close to the glans penis as possible. In entire bucks, breeding capacity is not majorly affected.

Surgical treatment

Urethrotomy or tube cystotomy are the two most commonly used procedures (see below). Both can also be tried if bladder rupture has occurred: they will ensure that pressure within the bladder is kept low while the defect is healing. Urethroscopy and laser lithotripsy, and bladder marsupialisation are other options.

Salvage slaughter

Uraemia is likely present at the time clinical signs are detected, making the animal unfit for human consumption. Euthanasia is, of course, an option.

Prevention and control

- Ensure calcium:phosphorus ratio is at least 1.2:1 in ration.
- Adequate water intake can be helped by adding 4% salt to the ration. Salt also prevents silica calculus formation. Plus basic husbandry of providing readily accessible, clean water.
- Ammonium chloride at 100–200 mg/kg q12h or 0.5–1% of ration dry matter prevents phosphate calculi. **Note:** This salt is bitter and must be mixed with feed or molasses.
  - In fattening kids, 0.5% ammonium chloride may be routinely added to concentrates, plus <1% sodium chloride.
  - In dogs and cats, prolonged use of acidifying agents causes skeletal decalcification. Therefore, continuous use of ammonium chloride may not be appropriate for breeding or pet animals.

Urethrotomy and urethrostomy

Indication

Urethrotomy is a salvage procedure to allow urination while the animal recovers from the effects of urolithiasis, such as uraemia, prior to slaughter.

Preparation and equipment

The tail is tied away and the perineal area clipped and surgically prepared. A small procedure instrument kit is sufficient. A small gauge tomcat urinary catheter is useful if patency is not obvious at the end of surgery. Suture materials: polyglactin 910 (Vicryl®), polyglycolic acid (Dexon™) or polydioxanone (PDS®).

Restraint

Light sedation and either caudal epidural or local infiltration anaesthesia. The patient is placed into sternal recumbency with flexed hind legs and the backend slightly overhanging the edge of the operating table. Alternatively, the patient may be placed into either left or right lateral recumbency, with the uppermost hind leg elevated.

Technical description

A 5–8 cm long skin incision is made midline in the perineum. The centre point of the incision should coincide with the most caudal point of the perineum (i.e. where it begins to slope cranio-ventrally). After incision of the fascia, blunt dissection is used to part the retractor penis muscles. If the penis cannot be visualised, it can be identified on palpation as a firm tubular structure of about small finger thickness. A curved pair of artery forceps is pushed underneath the penis and, using blunt and sharp dissection staying close to the penis, it is freed around its entirety to gain some movability. The penis is cut at a right-angle to its axis near the ventral margin of the skin wound. The aim is to have the stump just ventral to the most caudal point of the perineum to avoid urine scalding, but not too ventral to avoid irritation from hind leg movements.

Using 3–4 metric suture material on a cutting needle, the penile stump is fixed to the skin by a figure-of-eight suture (through skin on one side, then through corpus cavernosum and skin on the other side, then tied off underneath the stump). Great care must be taken not to include the urethra (which lies dorsally in the reflected stump) in this suture. If pressure application is not sufficient to arrest haemorrhage, the dorsal penile artery is ligated. The skin incision is closed in a routine manner. It is not necessary to remove the distal portion of the dissected penis. The urethra may be spatulated over a length of a centimetre or so, suturing the mucosa to the skin. This should be considered if there is marked oedema around the urethra.

An alternative to the above technique, which may provide longer survival, is urethrostomy. The approach is the same, but instead of cutting through the penis, the surgeon dissects onto the urethra and, following its incision lengthwise, sutures it to the skin to create a stoma (**Fig. 10.7**).

Aftercare

Fly-repellent, ointments such as Vaseline® to reduce urinary scalding and the supportive treatment described above.

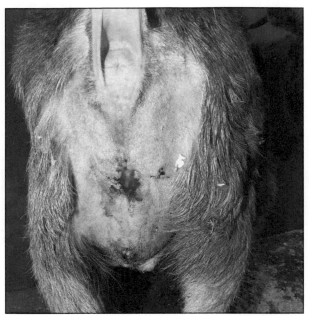

Fig. 10.7 Stoma created by an urethrostomy in a pet wether. The swelling ventral to the stoma resulted from subcutaneous urine pooling after pre-operative urethral rupture.

Potential complications

Stricture, scalding, fly strike, ascending infection. Adhesions from sterile peritonitis if bladder rupture has occurred.

Tube cystotomy

Indication

Tube cystotomy is indicated in patients where reproductive function or long-term survival are desirable, such as a breeding buck or pet animal.

Preparation and equipment

The left flank is clipped and surgically prepared. Required are: a standard instrument kit, Steinman pin, Foley catheter of suitable size (e.g. 14 Fr), zinc oxide tape, tomcat urinary catheter, sterile saline, suture material (polyglactin 910 [Vicryl®], polyglycolic acid [Dexon™] or polydioxanone [PDS®]).

Restraint

GA or lumbosacral epidural anaesthesia, or sedation and local infiltration, with the animal in right lateral recumbency.

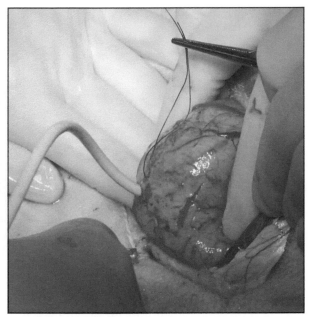

Fig. 10.8 Tube cystotomy. The bladder is exteriorised through a paramedian abdominal incision. After placing a purse-string suture, a Foley catheter is inserted into the bladder.

Technical description

An incision long enough to allow passage of the surgeon's hand is made in the caudoventral left flank, just above and roughly following the knee-fold. If the urinary bladder can be exteriorised, an absorbable purse-string suture is placed, a stab incision made in the centre of this suture into the bladder, and a Foley catheter passed into the ventral bladder, close to the apex (**Fig. 10.8**). If the bladder cannot be exteriorised, a Steinman pin is placed into the Foley catheter, the bladder grasped intra-abdominally with one hand, and the catheter pushed blindly into the ventral bladder.

The cuff of the Foley catheter is inflated with saline and pulled against the bladder wall (**Fig. 10.9**). The catheter end is passed out through a stab incision 2–3 centimetres away from the surgical incision, and secured with a butterfly-tape anchored with skin sutures. The abdominal wound is closed in a routine manner. Using the Foley catheter, the bladder is lavaged several times with sterile saline. Retrograde lavage via a tomcat catheter placed into the distal urethra (after urethral process removal) can also be tried.

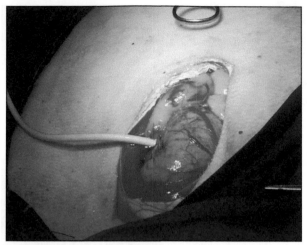

Fig. 10.9 Foley catheter secured in the bladder by inflating the balloon, but catheter not yet passed out through a stab incision a few centimetres away from the abdominal incision and secured with butterfly tapes.

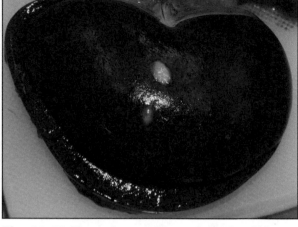

Fig. 10.10 Two infarcts (white nodules) in a kidney after septicaemia.

An alternative is to place a human percutaneous transabdominal catheter, under ultrasound guidance, via a cutaneous stab incision in either the left or right flank.

Aftercare

Continuous urine passage is allowed through the Foley catheter for the first few days. Supportive therapy is given during this time (see earlier). The bladder may be flushed with Walpole's solution (50–200 ml of a 1:10 Walpole:water dilution, retained in the bladder for 30–60 minutes by blocking the catheter). After a few days, the catheter is blocked for trial periods of several hours, and the animal observed for normal urination. Once normal urination has been established for 24–48 hours, the Foley catheter is removed (but not before 7 days post operation).

Potential complications

Peritonitis: either septic from the surgical procedure or sterile from bladder rupture. Non-resolution of urethral obstruction.

Renal insufficiency and failure
Overview

Because causes of renal insufficiency and failure are not restricted to the urinary system, renal function should be considered in a range of clinical conditions.

Aetiology

Pre-renal causes include: reduced cardiac output (e.g. in rumen tympany or congestive heart failure), acute circulatory compromise caused by shock, marked haemorrhage or dehydration, or septicaemia (**Fig. 10.10**); nephrosis. Renal causes include pyelonephritis, interstitial or glomerulonephritis, or amyloidosis. Post-renal causes include obstruction of ureters or the urethra and bladder rupture. Dehydration, or an increased susceptibility to it, is present.

Clinical presentation

In the acute phase, signs include depression and inappetence, reduced rumen activity, tachycardia, colic or abdominal pain, and watery or haemorrhagic diarrhoea. The goat is often recumbent and shows muscle tremors. Polyuria or oliguria is present, and bleeding diathesis may occur (e.g. epistaxis, melena, or bleeding of mucous membranes or at a venepuncture site). Chronic cases show marked weight loss, anorexia, dependent oedema and, in addition to polyuria or oliguria, polydipsia. Marked hypocalcaemia and sodium–potassium imbalance may result in circulatory failure, muscle weakness and nervous signs.

Diagnosis

Metabolic alkalosis and blood electrolyte imbalances are common: increased levels of phosphate, magnesium and sulphate; decreased levels of calcium, sodium, chloride and often potassium (in contrast to non-ruminants). Atypical hypocalcaemia (i.e. in a doe outside the periparturient period) often indicates renal insufficiency.

Goats in terminal failure show hypoproteinaemia and metabolic acidosis.

Differential diagnosis
Other causes of abdominal discomfort, diarrhoea or marked weight loss. For goats in peak lactation, hypocalcaemia.

Treatment/management/control
Specific treatment is given for the underlying cause. Intravenous saline, potentially spiked with potassium (10 mEq/litre of fluids) and calcium. Once urination has been established, furosemide (1–2 mg/kg every 2 hours) or mannitol (0.25–2.0 g/kg as a 20% solution) can be considered. Slaughter is not an option because of the uraemia.

The following serum values have been suggested as a guideline for poor prognosis in cattle: magnesium >3.5 mmol/l, phosphate >2.9 mmol/l, creatinine >130 mmol/l and urea >16.5 mmol/l. Some animals with much higher urea levels (<40 mmol/l) may survive; of particular concern is urea levels remaining elevated despite fluid therapy.

Toxic nephrosis
Overview
A variety of plants or chemicals can cause degenerative changes to the renal tubules.

Aetiology
Some of the poisons that may lead to nephrosis include arsenic, some wood preservatives, mercury, ethylene glycol (antifreeze) and mycotoxins such as ochratoxin A or citrinin. In other species oak (young leaves or buds in spring, acorns in autumn) may be a cause, but goats appear to have some resistance to oak poisoning. Some antibiotics can also induce nephrosis, including: aminoglycosides (e.g. neomycin if given at 10 mg/kg for more than 10 days, or at lower doses in dehydrated animals), oxytetracycline (if long-acting formula accidentally given daily, or one-off high dose rates ≥40 mg/kg) and sulphonamides

(risk of crystalluria if long-acting forms are used, urine is acidified, or animal is dehydrated).

Clinical presentation
Progressive depression, inappetence, poor milk yield and further signs specific to the causative agent.

Diagnosis
Blood analysis shows high urea and creatinine levels.

Differential diagnosis
A wide range of other conditions may cause similar signs, but in particular abdominal catastrophe and septicaemia or toxaemia.

Treatment/management/control
Fluid therapy and diuresis. Prognosis is guarded to poor.

Neoplasia
Lymphosarcoma (**Fig. 10.11**) may affect the kidney as a primary tumour or as metastases of other neoplasia. Kidney tissue-specific tumours include nephroblastoma.

INFECTIOUS DISEASES

Cystitis and pyelonephritis
Overview
Compared with companion animals, cystitis and pyelonephritis are far less often detected clinically in

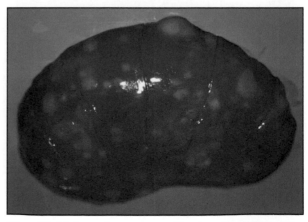

Fig. 10.11 Lymphosarcoma affecting the kidney of a 7-year-old Anglo-Nubian goat.

livestock, but are regularly found at slaughter, with a prevalence of about 10%.

Aetiology

Almost always bacterial, involving both gram-negative (e.g. *Escherichia coli*, *Klebsiella* spp., *Pseudomonas* spp., *Proteus* spp.) and gram-positive (e.g. *Corynebacterium* spp., *Streptococcus* spp.) pathogens. Route of infection is more likely ascending than haematogenous.

Cystitis (**Figs. 10.12, 10.13**) occurs after contamination or trauma of the urinary bladder caused, for example, by dystocia, retained fetal membranes or prolapsed uterus. Urine stasis often facilitates infection, such as pressure in late stage pregnancy, malformation of vagina after dystocia, or inflammation or obstruction of the urethra or ureters. Urolithiasis will also cause cystitis. Pyelonephritis occurs mainly via ascending infection from the lower urinary tract.

Because of their shorter urethra, females are more often affected than males. Both conditions are relatively rare in young animals.

Clinical presentation

Goats present because of frequent urination or malodour being noticed in the milking parlour. Weight loss, acutely reduced milk yield or a suspected gastrointestinal problem are common complaints in cases of pyelonephritis.

Cystitis presents as frequent urination with only small amounts of urine passed, and the animal remaining in the urinating position for some time. There may also be bruxism or other signs of pain when urinating. In very acute cases, there are temporary colic signs, such a kicking at the belly, tail swishing and shifting weight on the back legs. Digital rectal examination may trigger a pain response in acute cases.

The first sign of pyelonephritis often is haematuria in an otherwise healthy animal. There may be a history of episodes of acute pain. Rectal temperature often fluctuates, and milk yield and body condition are reduced.

Diagnosis

Blood and pus are often present macroscopically in the urine, and urine sediment contains erythrocytes and leukocytes. If the kidneys are involved, proteinuria, a urine pH above 8.5 and reduced specific gravity results. Neutrophilia is commonly present on haematology, and raised blood creatinine and urea levels suggest kidney involvement.

Interpretation of culture results must take into account the normal bacterial flora of the vulva (e.g. some *Corynebacterium* spp.).

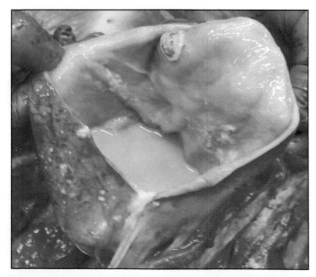

Fig. 10.12 Acute cystitis with purulent urine and mucosal plaques.

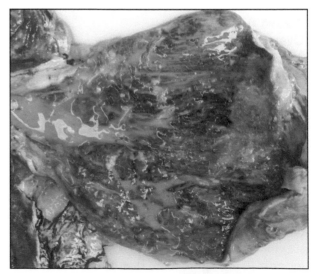

Fig. 10.13 Chronic cystitis with purulent urine and marked mucosal inflammation and bladder wall thickening.

Ultrasonography may show debris within the bladder or renal pelvis and, in chronic cystitis, a thickening of the bladder wall. Kidney enlargement may be detected.

Differential diagnosis

Where colic is caused by a gastrointestinal catastrophe, pain typically persists, faeces may be abnormal in quantity or consistency, and the goat develops shock and toxaemia. Auscultation, abdominal palpation and ultrasonography will aid differentiation.

Urine sediment examination is used to rule out cystitis secondary to urolithiasis.

Enzootic haematuria will also present with a thickened bladder wall, but no pus or bacteria are present in the urine. There is often evidence of anaemia.

Treatment/management/control

Because of the quite varying antimicrobial sensitivities of likely pathogens involved, urine culture is important. Trimethoprim and sulphonamide or ampicillin are useful against *E. coli* and procaine penicillin against *Corynebacterium* spp. While currently not licensed in many countries against urinary tract disease, ceftiofur, enrofloxacin and florfenicol may also be considered. Aminoglycosides, although effective against gram-negative pathogens and mainly excreted renally, should be avoided because of their nephrotoxic potential. Antibiosis must be continued for at least 7 days for cystitis and at least 3 weeks for pyelonephritis. Ideally, cessation of treatment is based on negative urine culture. Repeat culture is advisable, as recurrence is common.

Acidifying the urine will enhance the efficacy of procaine penicillin: monobasic sodium phosphate at 10 g daily or ammonium chloride at 100–200 mg/kg q12h, each orally for 5–7 days.

Prognosis of between 35% and 85% is reported in cattle after prolonged antibiosis. Nephrectomy may be considered in unilateral cases, carrying a prognosis of about 75%.

Control includes good hygiene around kidding and prompt treatment of post-partum disease.

CHAPTER 11

SKIN DISEASES

CLINICAL EXAMINATION OF THE SKIN AND INTEGUMENT

Clinical assessment

Skin disease should be suspected when presented with any of alopecia, erythema, coat staining, skin thickening, crusting, hyperkeratosis, swellings, discharge and excessive grooming or other signs of pruritus. Lesion distribution, depth and characteristics are determined. This may require putting the animal into lateral recumbency to inspect ventral body areas. Hair is parted or clipped where necessary to allow examination.

Historical factors that are of particular interest are number and age affected, current or recent environment, and type of animal (e.g. recently introduced). Because the skin can reflect general health status, a general clinical examination is important, potentially combined with blood analysis and serology. Causes of immune suppression should be considered where only one goat in a group is affected, particularly with a typically contagious disease.

Ancillary diagnostics

First-line diagnostics

Lice and ticks are usually visible with the naked eye, and detection can be made easier in coat brushings. For other ectoparasites, hair plucks can be used to detect lice nits (**Fig. 11.1**) and follicular pathogens such as *Demodex* spp. or dermatophytes. Skin scrapes, using a scalpel blade along the edge of the lesion (or in the interdigital space) until blood is drawn, are particularly useful in mange cases (**Fig. 11.2**). For these methods, the samples are mixed with 20% KOH or paraffin, and examined under a cover slip.

Tape strips are useful to detect ectoparasitic or microbial agents and for cytology: a piece of clear adhesive tape, such as Sellotape®, is pressed onto the lesion, then transferred onto a microscope slide. Impression smears are obtained by pressing

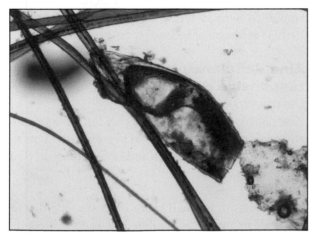

Fig. 11.1 Hair plugs are useful to confirm some ectoparasites. Here, lice nits are present on calf hair. (Image courtesy Aiden Foster.)

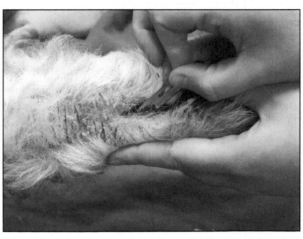

Fig. 11.2 For a skin scrape (here in the interdigital space) a scalpel blade is used, going deep enough to draw blood.

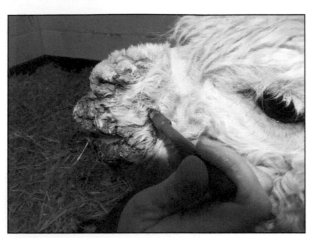

Fig. 11.3 A punch biopsy taken at the edge of a muzzle lesion in an alpaca. Note that no clipping or disinfection was carried out.

a microscope slide directly onto the lesion, and are useful for microbial agents and cytology.

Bacterial and fungal culture
Samples obtained by direct swab, fine needle aspirate or skin biopsy can all be used to isolate infectious agents. Normal commensals need to be taken into consideration when interpreting results.

Biopsy
Biopsy is performed under local anaesthesia, ideally by infiltrating some distance from the biopsy site (e.g. in a square pattern). The biopsy site itself is not clipped; however, surrounding hair may need to be removed to allow accurate positioning of the biopsy. To avoid distortion of histological features, no disinfection is carried out unless the area is particularly dirty. (**Note:** Disinfection will render the sample unsuitable for culture.) A punch biopsy (6–8 mm diameter) is preferable over a wedge biopsy (**Fig. 11.3**). The sample is taken at the leading edge of the lesion, without including normal skin. Multiple samples are useful where the lesion shows variable characteristics or to submit for culture in addition to histopathology.

Ultrasonography
Ultrasonography is useful to investigate swellings, allowing identification of content and the extent of the lesion. Also useful to guide a fine needle aspirate.

NON-INFECTIOUS SKIN DISEASES

Pemphigus foliaceus
Definition/overview
Cases of pemphigus foliaceus (a condition more fully understood in dogs, cats and horses) are occasionally reported in goats.

Aetiology
The condition is considered to be an immune-mediated skin disorder, although the triggers for the autoantibody production are poorly characterised in animals.

Clinical presentation
The main presenting signs include a generalised severe pustular eruption involving most of the body. Pustules are very transient and associated with marked crusting and multifocal alopecia.

Diagnosis
Definitive diagnosis is by histological examination of skin biopsy samples.

Treatment/management/control
Treatment or control of clinical signs is based predominantly on the use of corticosteroid therapy; for example, 1.0 mg/kg prednisolone i/m q12h for 7 days, followed by 1.0 mg/kg q48h for maintenance, tapering the dose further if possible. Regular bathing is useful for removing crust material and may be combined with systemic antibacterial agents where there is evidence of secondary bacterial infection.

Zinc deficiency (zinc-responsive dermatosis)
Definition/overview
Zinc deficiency is probably more common than generally recognised, particularly in pygmy goats. Disease can be associated with skin and/or foot disorders.

Aetiology
Deficiency can occur if there is an absolute dietary shortfall or uptake is inhibited by excessive copper or calcium in the diet (e.g. animals on lucerne/alfalfa diets), or in goats fed excessive dietary levels of oxalates, cadmium, iron or molybdenum. There may be

individual goat variation in the ability to absorb and also to metabolise any zinc ingested. Zinc deficiency is not regarded as a clinical problem of grazing animals in the UK.

Pathophysiology

Zinc is required for the proper function of a wide variety of enzymes. Deficiency signs include loss of appetite and anorexia, reproductive disorders, impairment of the immune system and abnormalities of the skin and coat.

Clinical presentation

The skin is the most common site for signs of deficiency to be identified. These include alopecia, pruritus, hyperkeratosis and crust formation on the back, legs, udder or scrotum, face (particularly around the eyes, nose and mouth), neck and ears (**Fig. 11.4**). Dry scaly skin linked to poor keratin production can also be widespread over the animal's body. Coat quality can be affected in fibre goats.

Diagnosis

The clinical signs are relatively non-specific, and other causes should be eliminated. Blood zinc levels can be estimated using a sample taken into a sodium citrate vacutainer, but correlation between serum and dietary zinc levels may be poor. Skin biopsy may confirm keratin production disorders. A clinical response trial to daily supplementation may also be of benefit, although some goats may respond to zinc supplementation, despite normal plasma and dietary levels.

Differential diagnosis

There are a number of potential contagious and non-contagious causes of such skin lesions, and these need to be eliminated by a structured skin examination, particularly the pygmy goat syndrome in which there are clinical similarities. Zinc deficiency may also be an exacerbating factor in other causes of skin disease.

Treatment/management/control

Zinc is a trace element, and daily requirements are low but should be consistent, as there are no readily available body stores. Presenting drinking water in galvanised containers may be sufficient, as zinc (a component part of the galvanising process) will leach into the water. Supplementation can be achieved by administration of a daily dose of 1 g zinc sulphate either in crushed tablet form or as a drench for 3–4 weeks. Slow release boluses containing zinc and other trace elements marketed for sheep are also available.

Pygmy goat syndrome (syn. seborrhoeic dermatitis)

Overview

Pygmy goat syndrome is a condition confined to the Pygmy goat breed, and is relatively common in the UK.

Aetiology

Appears to have an underlying hereditary basis, which can be an issue because the genetic pool of the breed is relatively limited.

Clinical presentation

Hair loss, and skin flaking and/or crusting seen around the eyes, lips, ears, chin, ventral skin surface and perineal area (**Figs. 11.5, 11.6**).

Diagnosis

Diagnosis is based on elimination of other causes and the breed of goat affected. Skin biopsy may indicate abnormalities of keratin production, a recognised feature of the disease.

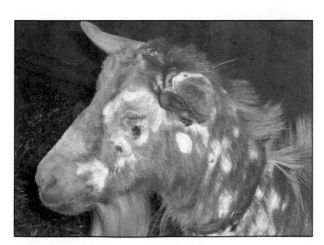

Fig. 11.4 Skin hyperkeratosis. Zinc deficiency was confirmed, with no other aetiology identified.

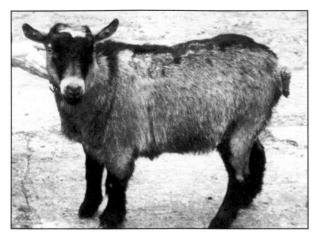

Fig. 11.5 Pygmy goat syndrome – hyperkeratosis.

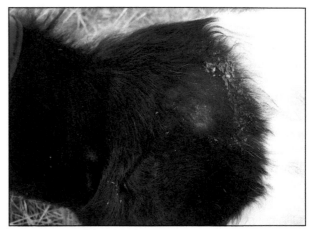

Fig. 11.6 Pygmy goat syndrome – skin flaking, poor keratin production (shoulder region).

Differential diagnosis

Zinc deficiency presents similarly; mange lesions are typically drier.

Treatment/management/control

Treatment may be disappointing as the condition will often recur. Some relief can be given via the topical use of corticosteroid and antibiotic creams, parenteral corticosteroids and antiseptic skin washes. Anecdotally, a selenium sulphide wash has proved beneficial. There are occasional reports of the condition gradually resolving as affected immature goats grow.

Photosensitisation

Overview

Photosensitisation has been occasionally reported in goats.

Aetiology

Primary photosensitisation occurs as a result of the ingestion of photodynamic toxins found in many different plants worldwide, for example St John's Wort (*Hypericum perforatum*). Other potentially photodynamic agents include tetracyclines and sulphonamides. Secondary photosensitisation is linked to liver disease, resulting in a failure to excrete the photodynamic agent phylloerythrin itself, a degradation product of chlorophyll. Any severe liver disease can lead to secondary photosensitisation, including those caused by hepatotoxic plants (e.g. ragwort [*Jacobaea vulgaris*, syn. *Senecio jacobaea*]).

Clinical presentation

Clinical signs are seen most commonly in the thinner coated areas of the body, particularly those covered with white non-pigmented hair. Erythema (**Fig. 11.7**) is followed by superficial skin necrosis and sloughing. In the secondary form there may be additional signs of liver disease such as icterus.

Diagnosis

Diagnosis is based on a history of access to photodynamic plants for the primary form and raised liver enzymes (gGT, GLDH, SDH) for the secondary form.

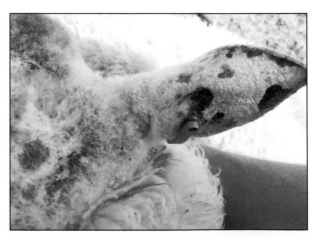

Fig. 11.7 Erythema is seen in the early stage of photosensitisation, particularly on areas with little hair coverage, such as the ear in this sheep. Hypersensitivity to biting midges may present similarly.

Differential diagnosis

Acute bacterial or ectoparasite infection. Skin scrapes and culture to rule out.

Treatment/management/control

Treatment consists of moving affected goats indoors away from sunlight and any potentially toxic plants they may be consuming. Anti-inflammatory and antimicrobial therapy is indicated, plus liver support therapy (like B vitamins, glucose or glucose precursors). Fly repellents are important, and skin emollients may aid local skin recovery. Severely affected cases, particularly those with marked liver damage, carry a poor prognosis.

Physical and toxic causes

Skin lesions can result from a variety of physical or toxic insults. Repeated contact with solid material in the goat's environment (e.g. poorly bedded concrete lying areas or metal bars such as feed rails) can result in hair and skin abrasion and callus formation. Poll lesions may result from head-butting, in particular in bucks. Diarrhoea or prolonged contact with urine may result in scalding along the hind legs. Skin burns result from stable fires, close proximity to heat lamps, clippers overheating during shearing of fibre goats, and contact with strong chemicals. Venom typically also results in skin lesions. Frost bite and toxaemia (especially caused by salmonellosis) may result in necrosis of the ear tips and the coronary band.

The location of the lesions often hints at the cause; for example, foot or nose in chemical burns, head in snake bites or heat lamp burns, neck in metal barrier contact, hocks in poor bedding surface.

Fibre break or loss

Fibre problems range from fibres breaking, either on the animal or during processing, to complete shedding of the fleece. This is of economic importance in fibre breeds, but also as an indicator of suboptimal husbandry or health in other breeds.

Severe stress or acute severe disease (e.g. diarrhoea) are common causes. Goats fed a diet that is limited in energy and/or non-degradable protein often produce finer fibre (less in diameter), but it tends to be more brittle. A good level of nutrition in the pregnant dam may lead to improved fibre yield and quality in her progeny.

Hypotrichosis

Hypotrichosis is occasionally seen as a congenital condition, and may affect one kid only in a litter (**Fig. 11.8**). It is caused by partial or complete absence of hair follicles, resulting in either a very fine coat or no hair at all. Partial anodontia is often present. Prognosis is guarded because of increased susceptibility to infectious disease such as pneumonia.

INFECTIOUS SKIN DISEASES (PARASITIC)

Chorioptic mange
Definition/overview

Chorioptic mange is a common form of mange reported in goats worldwide. Lesions tend to be restricted to the lower limbs and are colloquially referred to as foot mange. The condition can cause widespread problems once established.

Aetiology

Caused by the surface dwelling mite *Chorioptes* spp., which resembles morphologically those seen on cattle. It is likely that all livestock carry *C. bovis*, although *C. texanus* has also been reported in goats.

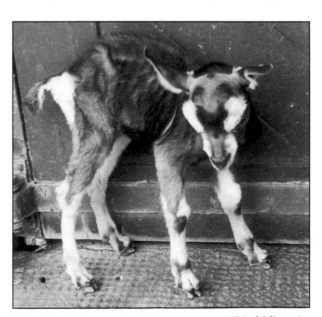

Fig. 11.8 Hypotrichosis in a neonate. This kid's twin was normal in size and coat coverage.

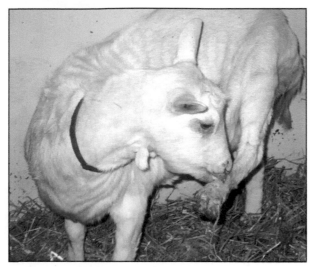

Fig. 11.9 Goat with mange showing self-mutilation, leading to skin damage on her leg and spread of the mange to the head.

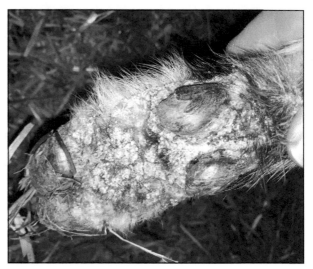

Fig. 11.10 Typical foot lesions associated with chorioptic mange.

Pathophysiology

Lesions are mainly the result of self-inflicted trauma due to the physical presence of the mites (**Fig. 11.9**). This will vary from goat to goat, with some infested individuals showing no or only minimal signs, whereas others may be particularly susceptible to infestation and develop a marked hypersensitivity response, leading to more significant self-trauma.

Clinical presentation

Clinical signs can include intense pruritus, foot stamping, rubbing, scratching and biting and the production of a scaly scab, often fissured and haemorrhaging, ranging in colour between grey and yellow–brown. Lesions are most commonly found on the feet (interdigital space, coronet, accessory digit) and occasionally on the udder, scrotum and tail or around the mouth from nibbling at affected areas (**Figs. 11.10, 11.11**).

Diagnosis

Diagnosis is by identification of the mites on microscopy of skin scrapes, looking for the characteristic short wine glass-shaped pedicels (**Fig. 11.12**). This can sometimes be problematic in severely affected cases in which mites may no longer be present at the lesion site. In such cases, it is worth clipping away normal hair from the margin of the lesion, and then performing a skin scrape at the leading edge of the lesion.

Differential diagnosis

The location of lesions confined to the lower limbs is highly suggestive of chorioptic mange, although there may be a spectrum of severity within an affected group. A full skin work-up will eliminate other ectoparasitic causes.

Treatment/management/control

Management of chorioptic mange can be extremely difficult because these mites can survive off the host for up to 3 weeks in the environment, therefore disposal of potentially infested bedding should be part of any control strategy. It is also important to remember that many infested goats are not severely affected and may even be asymptomatic carriers. As most of the mites will be on the goats, however, it is advisable to treat the whole group with a suitable ectoparasiticide.

A variety of topical agents are applied on an empirical basis, such as topical macrocyclic lactones (MLs), fipronil-based sprays and selenium sulphide shampoos. The absence of a drug licence in many countries and of pharmacokinetic data in goats makes the use of topical MLs (e.g. eprinomectin) problematic. Topical treatments should be pursued

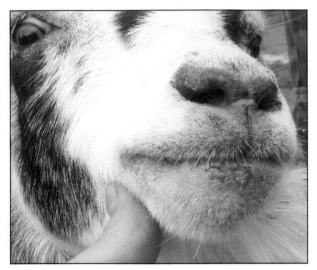

Fig. 11.11 Mouth lesions associated with chorioptic mange self-inflicted trauma.

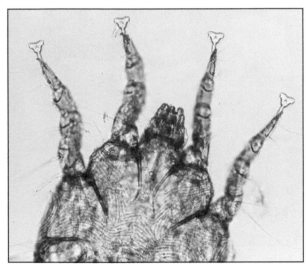

Fig. 11.12 A chorioptic mite under the microscope. Note the pedicle shaped like a wine glass/suction cup. (© Crown Copyright 2017. Used with kind permission of the Animal and Plant Health Agency)

for up to two mite life cycles (i.e. up to 6 weeks, given every 7–14 days). Systemic treatment with MLs has shown limited efficacy for the control of *Chorioptes* mites because of its surface dwelling habit.

Consideration should be given to the use of products in milking goats because of either the long milk withholding periods or restrictions on their use in lactating goats in many countries, and the potential impact on nematode anthelmintic resistance. In a commercial herd, culling severely affected individuals may be part of the control strategy.

Sarcoptic mange

Definition/overview

Sarcoptic mange is a common form of mange reported in goats worldwide. Lesions can be found over most of the body surface, often with intense pruritus. This type of mange, once established, can have a serious impact on goat welfare and productivity.

Aetiology

Sarcoptes scabiei var *caprae*, a burrowing mite and zoonotic pathogen.

Pathophysiology

Once infested, the mites burrow into the horny layer of the skin, where eggs are laid. Hatched larvae migrate to the skin surface, from where they can spread from host to host. Adults die burrowed into the skin, resulting in a significant allergen source and hypersensitivity.

Clinical presentation

Clinical signs include itching and rubbing, redness and papules at the site of infestation, leading to excoriation, scabs and crusts (**Figs. 11.13, 11.14**).

Diagnosis

Although other ectoparasitic causes need to be eliminated, the more widespread distribution of lesions and intense pruritus are characteristic features. A skin scrape may be examined for mites.

Differential diagnosis

A full skin work-up will eliminate other ectoparasitic causes. Scrapie should also be considered (see Chapter 8).

Treatment/management/control

Some control can be achieved by removing and treating individual goats, but when many goats are affected, whole herd treatment may be a better option. Systemic products based on MLs have been the mainstay of treatment for this condition, with

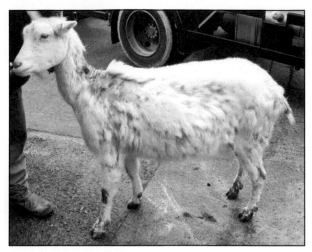

Fig. 11.13 Generalised sarcoptic mange.

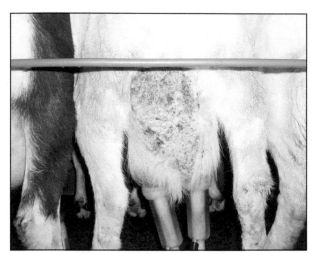

Fig. 11.14 Sarcoptic mange affecting the udder. (Image courtesy Kathy Anzuino.)

at least two treatments 7–14 days apart (see above under chorioptic mange treatment). Many goats will continue to show pruritus after treatment due to the presence of parasite antigen on the skin surface – washing with keratolytic or keratoplastic shampoos 2–3 times a week is often beneficial. Where self-trauma has led to secondary bacterial infection, a 3–5 day course of systemic antibiotic (e.g. a potentiated penicillin) is indicated. Quarantine of incoming goats is important, treating any visibly affected goats before they enter the herd. The condition is extremely contagious and will spread rapidly if it gets into a herd.

Demodectic mange

Definition/overview

Demodectic mange is a sporadic (rather than herd) problem, mainly affecting growing kids, and not of great economic significance.

Aetiology

Demodex caprae, a small cigar-shaped mite.

Pathophysiology

Infection appears to be contracted from the dam as kids are suckling, but lesions are not usually seen until they are around 10–15 months of age. Many infestations are asymptomatic and inapparent. *Demodex* spp. infect the hair follicles, which can become distended with mites, their faeces and sloughed skin together with epithelial cells forming the characteristic nodules.

Clinical presentation

Small lesions (often only detectable by careful palpation) develop principally over the head and neck but also along the neck and over the shoulders. These may enlarge to 1–2 cm diameter, often with a caseous necrotic core in which large numbers of mites can be seen.

Diagnosis

Diagnosis is by demonstration of the typical cigar-shaped mites found when the nodule content is squeezed onto a microscope slide.

Differential diagnosis

The age of goat and appearance of the lesions is fairly characteristic.

Treatment/management/control

There is rarely a need to treat this condition, which is mainly unsightly and therefore a particular problem in show goats. Individual nodules can be excised, or incised with expression of the content. Multiple nodules may respond to systemic ML therapy, but even then nodules may not regress for some time. Most will regress spontaneously in time.

Psoroptic mange

Definition/overview

Psoroptic mange infestation is usually limited to the ear canal and referred to colloquially as ear mange.

Aetiology

Psoroptes cuniculi (syn. *P. caprae*).

Pathophysiology

Mites feed off the exudate and debris in the ear canal, and many infestations are asymptomatic. Susceptible goats, or those carrying heavy infestations, may develop a build-up of scale and wax in the ear canal, and this may extend outwards onto the ear pinna in severe cases.

Clinical presentation

Head shaking and scratching of the ear with the hind feet. Aural haematoma formation is a potential complication.

Diagnosis

Diagnosis is based on clinical signs and the demonstration of typical mites in ear canal wax or scale.

Differential diagnosis

The clinical signs and presence of scale and debris in the ear canal are fairly typical.

Treatment/management/control

If treatment is deemed necessary, then the use of dog/cat ear mite preparations can be useful in individual goats (if drug licensing rules permit). Such preparations are more effective if the ear is cleaned first. If a larger number of goats are to be treated, then systemic MLs have been shown to be effective (see above under chorioptic mange treatment). Any treatment should be repeated 14 days later.

Lice

Definition/overview

Lice are found on goats worldwide, and once established can have both a serious welfare and economic impact, particularly in goats that are kept indoors in large numbers where spread can be rapid.

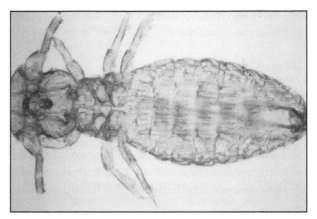

Fig. 11.15 Biting louse *Bovicola limbata.*

Aetiology

Goats can be infested with the blood sucking louse *Linognathus africanus* and *Linognathus stenopsis* and the chewing species *Bovicola (Damalinia) caprae*. Of more significance in fibre producing goats are two species of chewing louse: the red louse, *Bovicola limbata* (**Fig. 11.15**), and the less common *Bovicola crassipes*.

Pathophysiology

It is the feeding behaviour of these two classes of lice that dictates the clinical signs seen.

Clinical presentation

Heavy burdens of sucking lice, particularly in young kids, can cause anaemia, increased susceptibility to other infectious diseases and, in severe cases, may even cause death. Biting lice cause general irritability in goats due to their movement and feeding behaviour resulting in alopecia through self-inflicted trauma. This is a potentially serious issue in Angora goats. The irritation may also result in reduced feed intake, leading to weight loss and reduced milk yield.

Diagnosis

The clinical signs, particularly if many goats are affected, should raise a suspicion of lice. They (or their eggs or 'nits' sticking to hair shafts; **Fig. 11.1**) can often be seen, either with the naked eye or a hand lens, after parting the hair. At least ten areas of the body should be inspected, changing the angle of view onto each area. If just one or two individuals are affected, the louse problem may be secondary to a debilitating disease (e.g. a heavy endoparasite burden).

Differential diagnosis
A full skin work-up will eliminate other ectoparasitic causes and confirm lice as the cause of the anaemia.

Treatment/management/control
Disease is rarely limited to one or two goats, and any treatment regime should include the remainder of the cohort in which disease may be subclinical or developing.

As a general rule, injectable MLs are highly effective against sucking lice, but ineffective against chewing lice. A number of preparations have been used to treat chewing lice including pour-on products, such as cypermethrin or deltamethrin, and sprays or washes with 12.5% amitraz solutions (care in pregnant does). Shearing thick coated goats such as Angoras before treatment is beneficial. The availability of licensed ectoparasiticide products and their potential use in goats will vary from country to country. Blood transfusion should be considered in severely anaemic animals (PCV <0.12 l/l).

Lice infestations are often an indication of other underlying management problems such as overcrowding, concurrent disease or poor nutrition, and any investigation into a louse problem should consider the overall management.

Ticks
Ticks are important ectoparasites of goats, causing disease directly by actively sucking blood in very heavy infestations, and indirectly by spreading disease. Tick species and the diseases they transmit will vary from country to country. In Europe, for

example, the most common species is *Ixodes ricinus* (**Fig. 11.16**), transmitting the following infections between goats and other hosts on which ticks feed such as sheep, cattle and deer:

- Tick-borne fever (see Chapter 2).
- Tick pyaemia – as ticks penetrate the skin, they can under certain circumstances inoculate surface *Staphylococcus aureus*, causing local abscess formation and bacteraemia or pyaemia. This in turn leads to abscess formation in a variety of sites including the vertebral column, joints and internal viscera such as liver.
- Louping ill (see Chapter 8).

Individual ticks can be removed by simple plastic tick removers. Heavy infestations can be treated and controlled by the strategic use of suitable sprays, dips and pour-on products such as amitraz, cypermethrin or deltamethrin.

Flies
Overview
Fly worry, caused by nuisance flies, and blow fly strike (myiasis) are the two main fly-induced disease entities in the UK. Warble fly (*Przhevalskiana silenus*) problems occur outside the UK, including southern Europe.

Aetiology
Biting (stable and horn flies) and non-biting (house, face and head flies) species lead to fly worry. Fly strike may be caused by fly species able to penetrate intact skin (*Lucilia* spp., *Phormia terranovae*), but any fly species can act as opportunist when skin is damaged. Risk factors for fly strike include soiled skin, damp coat, wounds (including surgical) and grazing on pastures containing thistles or other rough vegetation. Grazing animals are more exposed, but marked problems may also be seen in housed goats.

Clinical presentation
Nuisance flies cause three main problems: (1) irritation, leading to reduced feed intake, stress and possibly self-trauma; (2) blood loss causing anaemia (e.g. horn flies may take up to 200 ml blood/day);

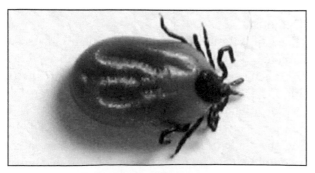

Fig. 11.16 *Ixodes ricinus* tick.

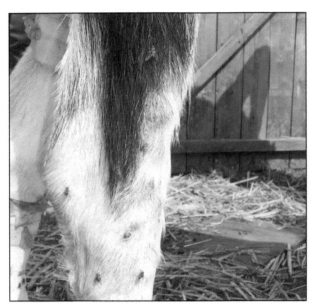

Fig. 11.17 Fly bite dermatitis on the leg.

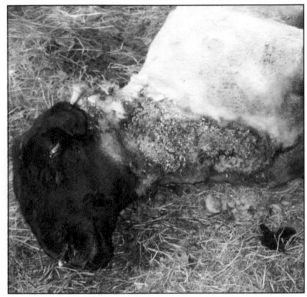

Fig. 11.18 Myiasis (fly strike) on the neck of a ram, that was in toxaemic shock as a result.

and (3) acting as vector (e.g. for mastitis or ocular pathogens). Clinical signs include epiphora and tear scalding. Biting flies are capable of causing superficial skin damage to outright wounds, especially on areas with less coat covering such as the bridge of nose, ears, caudoventral abdomen, udder and teats (**Fig. 11.17**).

Affected goats often show restlessness, stamping of feet and rubbing on housing structures. Staining of the fleece commonly occurs. Fly strike may be anywhere on the body if associated with a wound; otherwise it is commonly found in the perineal area or over the goat's dorsum. It can lead to severe toxaemia, with recumbency, dehydration and shock (**Fig. 11.18**).

Diagnosis
Biting flies are typically found on the legs of affected goats. More than ten biting flies or more than 50 non-biting flies on an animal should prompt intervention. Areas of stained fleece should be examined closely for fly strike, with larvae visible by the naked eye.

Differential diagnosis
Mange will cause crusting lesions and pruritus. Photosensitisation may manifest predominantly in areas with thinner coat.

Treatment/management/control
Treatment of struck goats includes physical removal of larvae, application of a pyrethroid or ivermectin to kill remaining larvae, wound lavage and application of a restorative ointment, and administration of an antibiotic and a NSAID. Goats suffering from toxaemic shock are treated accordingly (including i/v fluids).

Environmental steps in the control of nuisance flies include reducing proximity of goats to fly-favouring features such as trees, water and dung (**Fig. 11.19**). Fly numbers in stables can be reduced by installing fly curtains (to sweep off the majority of flies as goats enter the building), predatory wasps and fly traps. On pasture, pheromone-based traps mounted on fence posts can also be useful.

Control options on the animal include pyrethroids (e.g. permethrin, deltamethrin, pyrethrin and, for organic farms, chrysanthemum extract), either as pour-on or sprays. Impregnated ear tags or tail tapes must be manufactured specifically for goats, as their fleece and skin characteristics are different to cattle (i.e. a cattle product may not disperse as expected). Care must be taken regarding milk withholding periods, and several products are highly toxic to aquatic life (i.e. goats must be kept away from natural watercourses).

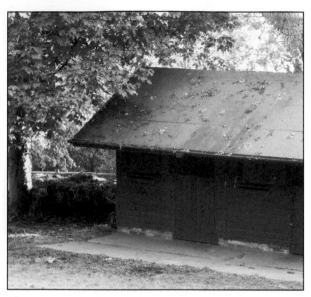

Fig. 11.19 Having the dung heap close to goats' stabling will increase fly worry unnecessarily.

Blowfly strike prevention relies on prompt attention to wounds and diarrhoea, avoiding routine procedures like castration during the fly season and applying fly-repellent ointment to surgical wounds, plus strategic use of topical insect growth regulators (e.g. dicyclanil).

Insect bite reactions
Overview
Insect bite reactions typically affect individual animals, where it can cause marked irritation.

Aetiology
Biting midges (*Culicoides* spp.) are the most common cause.

Clinical presentation
Hair loss, erythema and mild to moderate crusting. Often found on the head, but can be anywhere on the body and is always symmetrical between left and right body sections. Lesions are seasonal, occurring in spring and summer.

Diagnosis
Seasonality and symmetry of lesions are strong indicators. Trial housing may be useful to confirm the diagnosis.

Differential diagnosis
Other ectoparasites, hormonal skin conditions, dermatitis.

Treatment/management/control
Housing at dawn and dusk is labour intensive, but often reduces the effects. If primarily the head is involved, fly masks designed for miniature ponies can be useful. Repellents (e.g. deltamethrin) have variable persistence.

Besnoitiosis
Besnoitia caprae is a coccidian parasite causing oedema and gross thickening of the skin in goats. It has been reported in Africa and the Middle East. The definitive hosts are believed to be domestic cats and wild felids, with transmission to ruminants via faeces. *B. caprae* may be transmitted between ruminants by biting flies. Besnoitiosis is a threat when importing goats from affected countries. After initial pyrexia and painful ventral oedema, the skin hardens and thickens and develops wrinkles and cracks (with the risk of fly strike or secondary bacterial infection). The presence of parasitic cysts in the scleral conjunctiva is suggestive, supported by skin biopsy samples. Treatment is symptomatic, with response to antibiosis limited.

INFECTIOUS SKIN DISEASES (VIRAL/BACTERIAL/FUNGAL)

Contagious pustular dermatitis (syns. orf, contagious ecthyma)
Definition/overview
Contagious pustular dermatitis (CPD) occurs in goats and sheep worldwide, and is a significant zoonotic pathogen.

Aetiology
The cause is an epitheliotropic parapox virus.

Pathophysiology
The virus gains access via superficial skin abrasions whereupon it replicates in proliferating epidermal keratinocytes, resulting in the development of typical lesions. Transmission is by direct contact with an

infected sheep or goat or indirectly from infected scab material in the environment. There may also be asymptomatic carrier animals acting as a source of infection.

Clinical presentation

After a short incubation period, papules appear first, progressing rapidly to form pustules. These in turn become crusted, proliferative and coalescing lesions, which can be extremely painful. They are typically found on the lips, muzzle and in the mouth (**Fig. 11.20**). Lesions may also be found on the udder and teats, a particular problem when does are nursing infected kids. The pain can prevent kids from suckling and these may require bottle or tube feeding. Nursing does with lesions on their udders may abandon their kids.

Diagnosis

The lesions are quite characteristic. Laboratory diagnosis is based on electron microscopy examination of typical scab material.

Differential diagnosis

The most important differential diagnoses are foot and mouth disease (FMD) (see Chapter 17) and goat pox.

Treatment/management/control

Lesions will regress spontaneously over 4–6 weeks, and this will result in natural immunity lasting up to 3 years. There is no specific treatment for this condition, although a number of proprietary preparations are marketed as having a beneficial effect. Antiseptic and antibacterial ointments or sprays applied to the lesions will control secondary infection. If an outbreak develops, it is important to identify any possible underlying risk factors and remove or control them, particularly those causing superficial skin abrasions such as feeding on thistles or brambles. A number of vaccines are available, and these are usually administered via scarification of the superficial epidermis in thin-skinned areas of the body such as the axilla or perineal area (although this latter site is best avoided in does with kids at foot). The vaccine is usually non-attenuated and as such should only be used in herds in which infection is present and control is needed. Its use in a clean, uninfected herd may inadvertently introduce infection. Care should be taken at all times to avoid this zoonotic infection being acquired by those handling infected goats – the skin of the hands and arms is most commonly affected (**Fig. 11.21**).

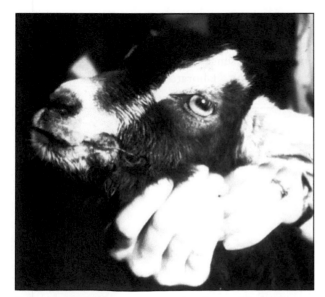

Fig. 11.20 Contagious pustular dermatitis (orf) at the lip commissure.

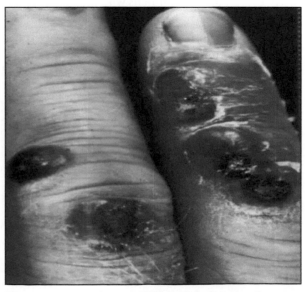

Fig. 11.21 Confirmed CPD (orf) lesions on the fingers of a farm worker.

Goat pox

Definition/overview

Capripox viruses are among the most serious of all animal poxviruses. They cause economic loss by damaging hides and fibre and by forcing the establishment of trade restrictions in response to an outbreak. At the time of writing, goat pox is endemic in Africa north of the Equator, the Middle East, Turkey, Iran, Iraq, Afghanistan, Pakistan, India, Nepal, parts of the People's Republic of China and Bangladesh. It is a scheduled OIE listed disease and as such is subject to strict statutory control measures in each country. The morbidity rate in endemic areas is between 70 and 90% with a mortality rate of 5–10%, approaching 100% in recently imported goats into infected herds.

Aetiology

The goat pox virus is a member of the genus Capripox, which also contains the sheep pox virus. Capripox virus strains are often recognised by how the main target host responds; they cannot be distinguished using routine laboratory tests. The virus is very resistant to desiccation and is capable of surviving in scab material for up to 3 months.

Pathophysiology

Transmission is usually by aerosol after close contact with severely affected animals with ulcerated papules on the mucous membranes of the nose and mouth. Infection may also develop following virus transfer directly through mucous membranes or damaged skin. Indirect transmission via contaminated implements, vehicles or material such as litter or fodder can occur. After a short incubation period, a viraemia develops and the virus is redistributed to the skin, regional lymph nodes, lungs, kidneys and spleen. Virus is then excreted through skin lesions, nasal exudate and milk, with spread being facilitated by close housing.

Clinical presentation

Clinical signs vary from mild to severe, depending on host factors such as age, breed, immune status, and viral strain virulence. In the acute phase, an initial pyrexia is quickly followed by the appearance of skin papules, rhinitis, conjunctivitis and enlargement of all superficial lymph nodes, especially prescapular lymph nodes (**Figs. 11.22, 11.23**). Papules on the eyelids cause blepharitis of varying severity and papules on the mucous membranes of the eyes and nose ulcerate, creating a mucopurulent discharge. Breathing may become laboured and noisy due to pressure on the upper respiratory tract from the swollen retropharyngeal lymph nodes draining developing lung lesions. The mucosae of the mouth, anus and prepuce or vagina become necrotic. If the goat survives this acute phase, papules become necrotic from vascular thrombosis and ischaemic necrosis, forming scabs that may persist for up to 6 weeks.

Diagnosis

Diagnosis is based initially on the clinical signs and the presence of the disease in the locality. Samples for laboratory confirmation include

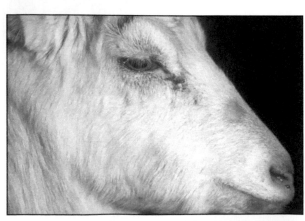

Fig. 11.22 Goat pox. Conjunctivitis and developing facial lesions. (Image courtesy Paul Kitching.)

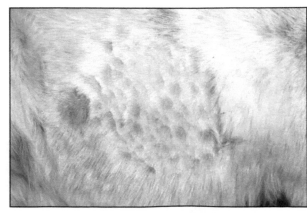

Fig. 11.23 Cutaneous lesions of goat pox. (Image courtesy Paul Kitching.)

vesicular fluid if available, scabs, lymph node aspi-rates, EDTA or heparin blood samples and paired sera. Post-mortem examination findings include skin lesions often extending full thickness into the under-lying musculature. In addition, massively enlarged lymph nodes and typical pox lesions are evident on the mucous membranes of the eyes, mouth, nose, pharynx, trachea, vulva and prepuce. Lung pathol-ogy is often severe and includes well established and extensive pox lesions, focally and uniformly distrib-uted throughout the lungs. Fresh skin, lymph node or lung lesions can be taken for virus isolation.

Differential diagnosis

Includes CPD (orf), insect bites, bluetongue and peste des petits ruminants (PPR).

Treatment/management/control

There is no treatment. As goat pox is an OIE listed disease, it is controlled globally by the implementa-tion of statutory measures designed to keep the virus out of those countries in which it is not found, and eradicating or controlling infection in countries in which it is currently a problem. Confirmation of dis-ease must be reported to the World Organisation for Animal Health (as per the OIE Terrestrial Animal Health Code).

Vaccines are available and are used in infected areas.

Bluetongue

See Chapter 17. Classic signs of bluetongue are a swollen face (oedema of the face, muzzle and ears), with buccal and nasal mucous membrane ulceration.

Peste des petitis ruminants

Goats with PPR can develop lesions and scabs on the lips in the early stages (see Chapter 5).

Foot and mouth disease

FMD vesicles, which rupture and produce scabs, can develop on the visible mucous membranes of the lips and nose and the coronary band (see Chapter 17).

Aujeszky's disease (syn. pseudorabies)

Goats with Aujeszky's disease can develop a severe pruritus (see Chapter 8).

Staphylococcal dermatitis/folliculitis

Definition/overview

Staphylococcal skin infections are relatively com-mon in goats, and may be either primary or second-ary to some other skin insult.

Aetiology

Staphylococcus aureus is most commonly associated with the condition, although *Staphylococcus inter-medius* and *Staphylococcus hyicus* are also seen. The recently recognised pathogen *S. aureus* subsp. *anaero-bius* has been associated with the condition referred to as Morel's disease, which is described later in this chapter.

Pathophysiology

The resulting dermatitis is referred to as a folliculi-tis, where infection involves hair follicles, or impe-tigo (or non-follicular), which is a more superficial condition. The primary lesion is a papule, develop-ing into a pustule, which in turn may burst, liberat-ing pus and leading to superficial scab formation, or coalesce to form larger lesions.

Clinical presentation

Multiple small impetigo lesions may develop on the thin skin of the udder and teats (colloquially referred to as udder impetigo (**Fig. 11.24**). These can be easily spread during milking and, if con-centrated around the teat end, may predispose

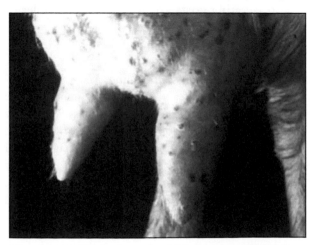

Fig. 11.24 'Udder impetigo'. Multiple small 'acne'-like lesions associated with *Staphyloccocus aureus*. Bacteria around the teat end pose a mastitis risk.

to staphylococcal mastitis. Some goats appear to be more susceptible to infection and may develop multiple lesions, which may be superficial and only identified by palpation (important in show goats), or be more severe, leading to focal areas of hair loss. Lesions can be found initially on the skin of the ventral abdomen, inguinal and axillary areas, but may become more widespread. Secondary staphylococcal infection can develop as a result of other skin disorders, such as mange.

Diagnosis
Diagnosis is based on bacterial culture of swabs, which will confirm staphylococcal infection, but this must be interpreted in the context of the lesions identified, as staphylococci are common skin commensals in healthy goats.

Differential diagnosis
Includes fly bites (**Fig. 11.17**), *Dermatophilus congolensis* infection, demodectic mange and ringworm.

Treatment/management/control
Many cases are self-limiting. If treatment is deemed necessary, shampooing with antibacterial washes can be beneficial, with parenteral antibiosis in more severe cases. Care should be taken to prevent mastitis during the milking process, particularly avoiding any action (such as udder washing) that may spread infection from the udder surface to the teat end if lactating goats are affected on the udder or teat skin.

Malassezia
Malassezia organisms, including *Malassezia pachydermatis* and *Malassezia slooffiae*, are opportunistic pathogens producing scaling, dry or less commonly greasy seborrhoea, alopecia and crusting lesions, often involving most of the body. Diagnosis of Malassezia dermatitis in goats can be made by cytological examination of skin impression smears. Topical antifungal therapy using chlorhexidine and miconazole shampoo or selenium sulphide is suggested, soaking animals for 10 minutes, twice weekly for 3 weeks. Any predisposing or underlying disease will also need treating.

Mycotic dermatitis (syns. dermatophilosis, streptothricosis)
Definition/overview
Mycotic dermatitis is a common skin condition in goats in many countries, and it can also affect both sheep and cattle.

Aetiology
Dermatophilus congolensis, an environmental actinomycete-forming motile zoospore that can invade the skin.

Pathophysiology
The organism gains access to the skin via superficial abrasions or bites, and is most common following excessive wetting of the coat or when goats are kept in a warm humid environment. Secondary bacterial infection can develop.

Clinical presentation
There are raised 'paint brush' tufts of hair or scabs that appear over the body surface, including ears, face, limbs, scrotum and perineal area. In severe cases lesions may coalesce and cover a large area of the dorsum of the back. They are generally non-pruritic. The crusty lesions are easily knocked or peeled off, and leave raised, circular granulating lesions beneath. Focal alopecia is a further sequela to long-standing infection.

Diagnosis
Diagnosis is based on clinical signs and laboratory examination of hair and scab material.

Differential diagnosis
Although the lesions are fairly characteristic, they can be confused with ringworm, CPD (orf: if confined to the face) or staphylococcal dermatitis.

Treatment/management/control
Treatment of individual goats with broad-spectrum antibiotics, combined with housing away from environmental moisture, is usually successful. Brushing and combing out scab material, combined with controlling other exacerbating factors such as concurrent ectoparasitism, will improve the goat's appearance.

Ringworm (syn. dermatophytosis)

Definition/overview

Ringworm is a fungal skin condition affecting most animal species worldwide, with cross species infections occurring. It is also an important zoonotic risk to anyone handling infected goats.

Aetiology

A number of dermatophyte species have been isolated from cases of ringworm in goats, including both *Trichophyton* and *Microsporum* spp.

Pathophysiology

Infection can be acquired from an infected goat or, in theory, from direct or indirect contact with another infected animal species, both livestock and companion. Lesions tend to develop more in goats that are ill-thrifty or debilitated through concurrent disease.

Clinical presentation

Lesions in goats may present as the typical annular lesions seen in other species, but they can also be more diffuse, consisting of areas of alopecia, skin scaling and crust formation. Moist eczematous lesions can also develop (**Fig. 11.25**). Lesions can be found mainly over the head, neck and limbs.

Diagnosis

Laboratory examination of scab, scale and hair plucks will confirm a diagnosis of ringworm, and culture techniques can also identify the species involved,

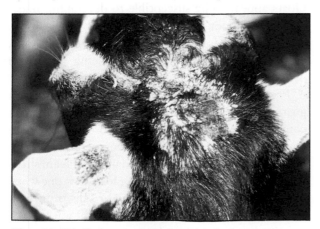

Fig. 11.25 Crusty moist dermatitis lesions – confirmed as ringworm (*T. mentagrophytes*).

which may be useful for epidemiological investigation into zoonotic links.

Differential diagnosis

Dermatophilus sp. and staphylococcal infection are the primary differential diagnoses.

Treatment/management/control

Most cases will regress spontaneously, particularly if any underlying problems related to management, nutrition or concurrent disease are addressed. Treatment includes topical administration of enilconazole or natamycin, repeated depending on response. Oral use of griseofulvin is effective, but has been banned for use in food producing animals in many countries. All in-contact goats should be treated and a thorough cleaning and disinfection programme applied to the housing environment to inactivate resistant spores on fixtures and fittings.

CUTANEOUS SWELLINGS

Caseous lymphadenitis

CLA produces swellings associated with superficial lymph nodes (see Chapter 7).

Morel's disease

Morel's disease is caused by *Staphylococcus aureus* subsp. *anaerobius*. It is a disease identified in both goats and sheep and is a differential diagnosis for CLA in those countries in which infection has been confirmed. Superficial abscesses are located near major lymph nodes, most commonly the cranial cervical, subiliac, parotid and mandibular nodes. Abscesses can be very large and debilitating.

Lymphoma

Lymphoma causes lymph node enlargement and is discussed in Chapter 7.

Neoplasia

The most common cutaneous tumours in the goat are:

- Papilloma (warts) – usually small and self-limiting, found on the head, neck and occasionally on the skin of the udder and teats.

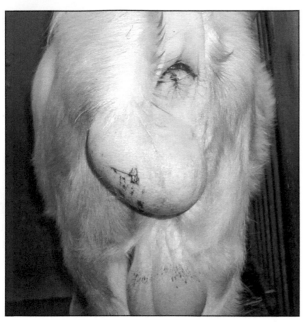

Fig. 11.26 Perineal mass in an entire 2-year-old Saanen buck.

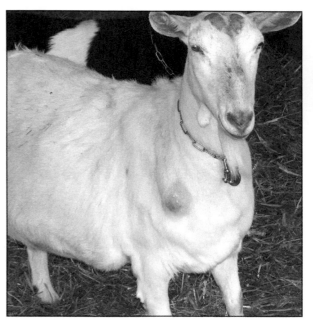

Fig. 11.27 Injection site abscess in front of the shoulder.

- Carcinoma – can occur over the head and neck, perineal area (**Fig. 11.26**) and skin covering the udder, but also at other sites. White goats (or goats with areas of white hair) kept in sunny climates may be particularly susceptible.
- Melanoma – has been reported to develop most commonly involving the perineal area and earlobes.

These tumours can be identified initially by their appearance and confirmed by examination of biopsy samples. Management will depend on location, size and tumour type, with metastasising tumours carrying a poor prognosis.

Thymus enlargement

Swelling of the skin over the lower part of the neck in kids may be an indication of thymus enlargement (see Chapter 7). The condition should not be confused with goitre involving the thyroid gland.

Haematoma

Sporadic haematoma formation can occur (mainly in housed goats) as a result of a traumatic insult resulting in rupture of subcutaneous blood vessels and haemorrhage into the subcutaneous tissue. If several goats develop these lesions, then the investigation should focus either on the goat's environment, identifying sites of potential injury, particularly in their daily movement routes (e.g. a projecting gate hinge), or alternatively at identifying an underlying clotting disorder.

Injection site abscesses

Goats appear to be susceptible to developing injection site reactions (ISRs) or abscesses (**Fig. 11.27**). If the swelling is close to a superficial lymph node, CLA must be ruled out prior to lancing and lavage of the abscess.

Prevention relies on carrying out injections in goats with dry fleece and away from obvious skin contamination, using the correct dose, ensuring the needle is in the target tissue (subcutaneous not intradermal; deep intramuscular) and using a clean, sharp needle (i.e. frequently discarding for a new one when treating a larger group). In show or sale animals, it may be possible to place the injection at a less obvious site (e.g. the axilla) where a product is known to have an ISR risk.

SURGERY OF SKIN ADNEXA

Disbudding

Indication

Disbudding is currently routinely performed in many herds in the UK in order to avoid horn-induced injuries to handlers and during hierarchical fighting, and to allow higher stocking densities. In the UK the procedure can only be undertaken by a veterinary surgeon. Several countries have banned routine disbudding, and sentiment towards its routine use is starting to change in the UK.

Preparation and equipment

Ideally performed in 2–4 day-old kids, and no older than 7 days. A disbudding iron with a large enough diameter to encompass the entire horn bud is required. (**Note:** Disbudding heads designed for young calves are usually too narrow in diameter.)

Restraint

Options for anaesthesia are (see Chapter 18 for further details): (1) cornual block, taking care not to exceed the toxic dose of local anaesthetic (maximum total dose across both sides is 3 ml of 1% lidocaine for a 5 kg kid); (2) injectable general anaesthesia (GA); and (3) inhalation GA using a face mask. GA is recommended by the UK's Royal College of Veterinary Surgeons.

(**Note:** Oxygen supports combustion: the disbudding iron must be ignited outside and only brought close to the kid after shutting off the anaesthetic machine).

Technical description

Apply iron for 3–4 seconds at a time with even pressure until the horn-growing tissue is destroyed (**Fig. 11.28**). It is not necessary to 'scoop out' the bud, and no attempt should be made to do this. Kids have a much thinner skull than calves and care must be taken not to overheat the meninges and brain (see **Fig. 8.9**).

Aftercare

Administration of NSAIDs is recommended. Fly repellent should be used depending on the time of year and country.

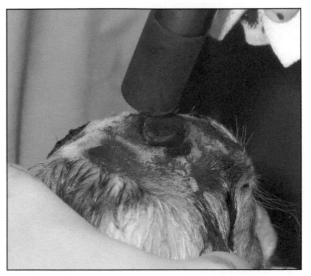

Fig. 11.28 **A wide-diameter disbudding iron is applied for a few seconds at a time until an obvious rim forms and the surrounding skin has become detached from the horn bud.**

Potential complications

Common complications include horn-growing tissue not removed, resulting in re-growth; death under anaesthesia (especially if xylazine is used); and meningoencephalitis as a result of prolonged iron application. Clinical signs typical of encephalitis develop after 2–3 days, usually followed by death.

Dehorning

Indication

Dehorning of an adult goat is a very invasive procedure, resulting in opening of the sinuses, with a relatively long wound healing period. It should, therefore, not be undertaken lightly. However, undue aggression in a horned goat against other goats or humans, or fracture of the horn, may require dehorning (**Fig. 11.29**).

For an in-growing horn, it is usually sufficient to regularly (every 6–12 months) cut a few centimetres off the horn tip with fetotomy wire (**Fig. 11.30**), rather than fully dehorn the animal.

Preparation and equipment

The goat is starved and preoperative antibiosis and NSAIDs given. The site is clipped and surgically prepared. A standard surgical kit, plus either a sterile hacksaw or sterile fetotomy wire, is required.

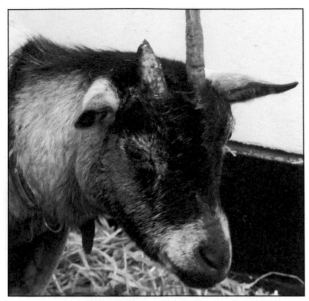

Fig. 11.29 Trauma may warrant removal of the injured horn.

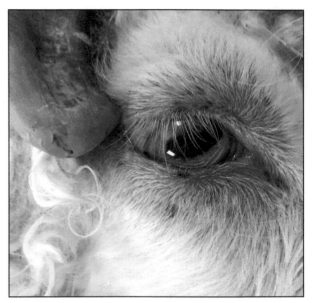

Fig. 11.30 An in-growing horn is addressed by removing the distal section with a fetotomy wire. (Image courtesy Nichol Fisher.)

Restraint

GA is recommended, because the procedure will lead to bleeding into the sinuses, potentially causing stress to a sedated only animal through smell and obstruction of nasal passages. In addition, a cornual block is applied (see Chapter 18).

Technical description

For bilateral dehorning, a figure-of-eight incision is made at a distance of 8–10 mm around both horn bases (i.e. a circular incision around each horn base with an incision connecting the two circles at the poll; **Fig. 11.31**). The skin is undermined for 1–2 cm along the entire incision. The horns are sawed off flush with the skull. A hacksaw gives better control of the cutting angle compared with using a fetotomy wire. To facilitate placement of the saw, the bulk of the horn may have to be removed first a few centimetres above the skull (**Figs. 11.32, 11.33**).

The incision is closed with interrupted horizontal mattress sutures, using a 3.5 to 4 metric non-absorbable suture material (e.g. Prolene®). Closure can be facilitated by making a relief incision caudal to each horn base, but full apposition may not be achievable (**Fig. 11.34**).

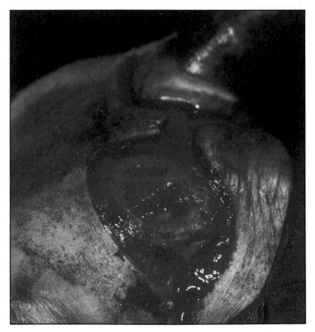

Fig. 11.31 For bilateral dehorning, a figure-of-eight incision is made about 1 cm away from the horn base (photo taken after removal of left horn).

Aftercare

A tight figure-of-eight bandage is placed around the head either side of the ears, starting with a non-adherent wound dressing (e.g. Melolin) and taking

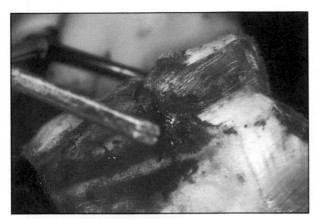

Fig. 11.32 The horn is cut close to the skull. To facilitate a good angle for this, the bulk of the horn was removed first in this goat (lateral view, with the goat's nose to the left-hand side).

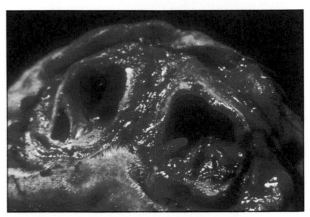

Fig. 11.33 View into the opened sinuses after dehorning.

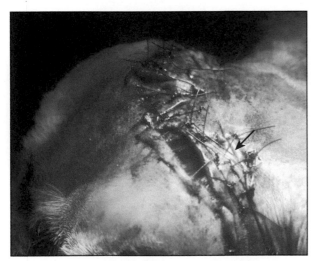

Fig. 11.34 The wound edges are apposed as closely as possible, using relieve incisions where necessary (arrow).

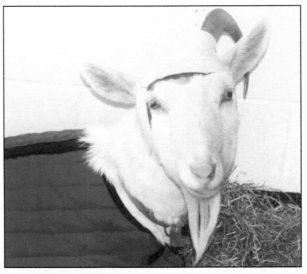

Fig. 11.35 A tight figure-of-eight bandage applied after unilateral dehorning to aid haemostasis and provide wound protection. The bandage was cut out around the eye.

care not to encroach onto the eyes (**Fig. 11.35**). The bandage is first replaced after 3 days, and then again after 7 days. Occasionally, a fourth bandage is required. Sutures are removed after 12–14 days. Postoperative analgesia is provided.

Potential complications
Sinusitis and wound breakdown or prolonged wound healing.

NORMAL STRUCTURE AND FUNCTION

In goats, the udder consists of two glands (or halves), with each half culminating in a teat with a single and very narrow streak canal. Milk production in the mammary gland is by the physiological process of apocrine secretion, unlike the cow in which the process is merocrine secretion. One major implication of this difference is its effect on the milk somatic cell count (SCC), typically being higher in goats and less correlated with udder infection.

CLINICAL EXAMINATION OF THE UDDER

The most common disorder of the udder is mastitis, which, if acute, can result in systemic signs of toxaemia such as pyrexia. Visual examination of the udder may reveal disparity in size between the two halves (**Fig. 12.1**), and skin discolouration (**Fig. 12.2**). This is followed by palpation of the udder for pain, swelling, oedema, firmness or nodular abnormalities. The teats are visually examined and palpated, particularly the teat end for trauma or other lesions. Milk is drawn from the udder and examined grossly for clots, pus, blood or abnormal colour and consistency (**Fig. 12.3**).

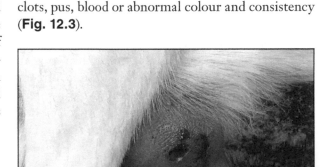

Fig. 12.2 Early gangrenous mastitis, with marked discolouration of the overlying udder skin.

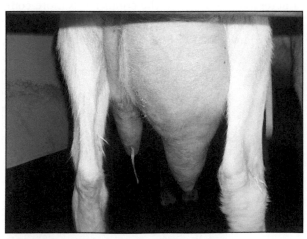

Fig. 12.1 Udder induration and asymmetry (left half affected) associated with caprine arthritis encephalitis.

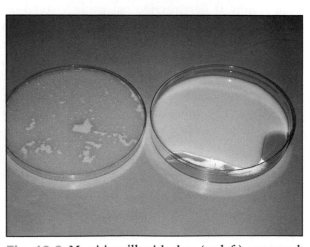

Fig. 12.3 Mastitic milk with clots (on left) compared with normal milk secretion (on right).

Sampling for culture

Any sample for laboratory examination must be taken aseptically to avoid contamination. Loose dirt, bedding or hair is manually brushed off the udder and teats. Dirty teats are washed and dried. Several streams of milk are discarded from each teat that is to be sampled. Ideally, pre-milking teat disinfectant is applied for 30 seconds, followed by drying off using individual paper towels. Using a gloved hand, the teat end is thoroughly scrubbed with 70% alcohol, using several pieces of cotton wool or gauze until no dirt is visible on the swab. A stream of milk is directed into a sterile container held at a 45 degree angle, taking care not to contaminate the inside of the lid. When sampling from both teats, the order of cleaning is furthest away teat to nearest, followed by sampling in a nearest to furthest away order, thereby avoiding touching cleaned teats prior to sampling. Post-milking teat disinfectant is applied to sampled teats. The sample is kept cool until submission.

Ultrasonography

Ultrasonography can be useful in examining the udder, particularly for deep seated chronic pathology such as abscesses or fibrous scar tissue. The normal udder will display a relatively uniform mix of hyperechogenic parenchyma and anechogenic alveoli and milk. Lesions will show up as hyperechogenic delineated areas. Teat ultrasonography is best carried out using a stand-off (e.g. a plastic cup filled with water or contact gel) to avoid distortion of any features. Four distinct layers can usually be identified: (1) anechoic milk in the lumen of the teat; (2) a moderately echodense, thin mucosal layer; (3) a mid-echodense thick layer of connective tissue and muscle; and (4) hyperechoic outer skin.

NON-INFECTIOUS DISEASES

Trauma
Traumatic damage to the udder
The inquisitive nature of goats makes them vulnerable to traumatic injury, and the udder and teats can be damaged by horns, barbed wire or crush injuries.

Teat biting
Teat end damage can also occur as a result of the recognised vice of teat biting (**Fig. 12.4**). This is a behavioural abnormality, seen particularly in adult dairy goats, in which one or more goats in a group start biting the teats of other goats. Careful observation is required to identify the culprits, which should be culled or removed. Injuries can be severe and predispose to mastitis.

Neoplasia

Neoplasia affecting the udder lactiferous tissue has been occasionally recorded. An adenocarcinoma of the udder of a lactating Saanen doe is shown (**Fig. 12.5**). The tissue was firm and nodular on palpation, had ulcerated through the lower skin surface and metastasised to the local lymphatic system, but without evidence of further metastatic spread.

Enlarged pendulous udder

An enlarged pendulous udder can be a problem particularly in elderly goats, in which slackening of the suspensory ligaments are often the underlying problem (**Fig. 12.6**). A hormonal aetiology, such as ovarian abnormalities or pyometra, should be ruled out. In pet goats, a mastectomy may be considered.

Maiden milkers

It is not uncommon for non-bred females to come into milk, and this precocious milking may well be a hereditary trait, since the condition is more common in those breeds and lines known for their heavy milk production. The exact cause remains unknown,

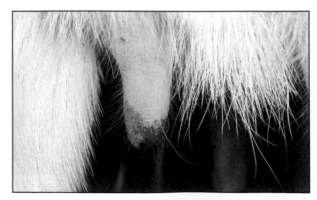

Fig. 12.4 Trauma caused by teat biting –
a recognised vice.

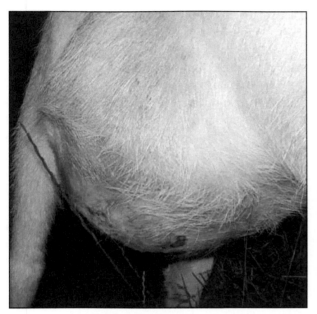

Fig. 12.5 Udder adenocarcinoma. Note the ulcerative change on the surface (blue oxytetracycline spray applied to skin).

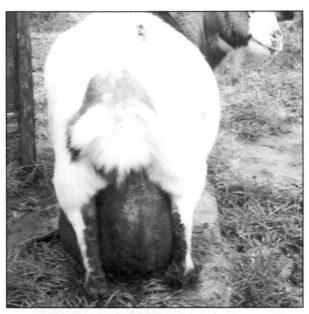

Fig. 12.6 Enlarged pendulous udder. Mastectomy may be an option.

and as such, there is no specific treatment that can guarantee success. It is important where possible not to start milking these goats, as more milk will be produced once the pressure has been relieved, and the teat seal will have been broken, predisposing to mastitis. Milk should only be removed if the goat is in pain or discomfort, when the udder should be completely stripped out under strict hygienic conditions and teat disinfectant used afterwards. If desired, a normal lactation will ensue with regular milking, and the milk will be suitable for human consumption.

Various hormonal treatments have been tried with limited success. Reducing any concentrate or cereal in the diet and feeding only good quality hay may help, but water must never be withheld on welfare grounds. In older goats with a heavy pendulous lactating udder, mastectomy is a final option to consider.

Post-partum agalactia

There are several potential reasons for a dam to not have any milk:

- Severe oedema, in which case an anti-inflammatory drug may help.

- Disruption of the milk let-down stimulus (can be stress- or pain-related), in which case an injection with oxytocin may help (2–5 IU).
- Nutritional problems (i.e. energy balance not sufficient to support milk production).
- Acute mastitis or other causes of pain, in which case NSAIDs may help; udder fibrosis from infection during previous lactation or the dry period.
- Premature kidding, in which case continued stimulation may help; and hormone imbalances.
- The teat may not be patent because of stenosis or obstruction, in which case surgery may help.

Effects on milk stimulation of products such as domperidone or herbal products are ambiguous. The kids of affected goats must receive colostrum from an alternative source to ensure passive transfer.

Induction of lactation

Inducing lactation has been investigated to reduce the risk to the dam associated with kidding and the number of surplus kids. It can be achieved using a combination of hormones and mammary gland stimulation. An example protocol is: (a) 17-beta oestradiol (0.25–0.5 mg/kg i/m) plus progesterone (0.75–1.25 mg/kg i/m) either daily for 7 days or every other day over 14 days; (b) combined with predniso-lone (0.4 mg/kg i/m) or dexamethasone (10 mg/day) for 3 consecutive days anytime between days 14 and 20; (c) reserpine (1 mg/day i/m) may be added every other day between days 12 and 20; (d) the mammary gland is massaged from days 5–7 or the goat is machine milked from day 20.

Peak yield tends to be much lower compared with naturally induced lactation (around 55%), and subsequent pregnancy rates are often poor, as well.

INFECTIOUS DISEASES

Contagious agalactia
Definition/overview
Contagious agalactia affects both goats and sheep, and is one of the most serious mycoplasma diseases of small ruminants worldwide after contagious caprine pleuropneumonia. It occurs in many countries including parts of southern Europe, Asia and Africa, in which its economic importance can be considerable due to dramatic falls in milk yield. It is an OIE listed disease, and as such is notifiable or reportable to the relevant authorities and is subject to statutory controls.

Aetiology
Although *Mycoplasma agalactiae* is often considered the classic agent, *Mycoplasma mycoides* subsp. *mycoides* (large colony type) and *Mycoplasma capricolum* subsp. *capricolum* can produce similar clinical pictures.

Pathophysiology
Despite its descriptive term, it is essentially a disease syndrome involving multiple organs including the udder and articular and ocular tissues. The main sources of infection include ocular and nasal secretions, faeces and milk. Contaminated milking equipment, milking utensils and the milker's hands can all transmit new infection. After infection is acquired, a bacteraemia develops, followed by progressive localisation in lungs, lymph nodes, eyes, mammary glands, joints and tendons. Udder infection leads to atrophy and agalactia. Goats suffering from mastitis can spread disease to kids through colostrum or milk. If goats and sheep are kept together, cross species transmission can also occur.

Clinical presentation
Early signs include inappetence and depression, followed by the development of agalactia and a change in milk secretion, which is initially watery then becomes progressively thicker and more purulent. Other clinical features that may accompany the udder changes include keratoconjunctivitis and arthritis. However, young goats, males and some females may only show non-specific signs, such as depression, pyrexia, keratoconjunctivitis and arthritis, with no evidence of mastitis. Udder atrophy and agalactia is a significant feature, which can be permanent. Mortality rates of up to 20% have been recorded, and morbidity in infected herds can be very high, with repetitive waves of apparent resolution and subsequent breakdown due to chronically infected individuals.

Diagnosis
The clinical signs are fairly characteristic, in particular the combination of mastitis and other signs. Diagnosis is confirmed by laboratory examination of milk samples. Specialist culture techniques are being replaced by molecular testing such as the denaturing gradient gel electrophoresis test, which can be undertaken on milk, body fluid, tissue samples or cultures to identify the *Mycoplasma* spp. involved. In cases of contagious agalactia presenting with non-mastitis signs, paired serology in individuals may be of benefit, and serology is a useful screening tool.

Differential diagnosis
Other causes of mastitis need to be eliminated by laboratory examination of milk samples.

Treatment/management/control
Treatment of infected goats, using antimicrobials such as tetracyclines, tiamulin, erythromycin, florfenicol or fluoroquinolones (where permitted), will alleviate the clinical signs, but recovered goats will often become carriers and pose a particular problem if the disease is to be eradicated. Live attenuated and inactivated vaccines are available and are used as a control measure in endemically infected areas. Unless the goat is from a herd in a heavily infected area, however, statutory control measures including slaughter of all known infected goats is the usual route taken.

Most cases and outbreaks of contagious agalactia result from the purchase of infected goats or sheep. A ban on imports from known infected areas is applied by many disease-free countries, or, alternatively, laboratory testing of purchased goats is a pre-import requirement. In those countries in which the disease is a local problem, a sound biosecurity protocol should be in place to test goats and sheep on the premises of origin (where possible), and test again on arrival after being placed in suitable quarantine facilities.

Mastitis

Definition/overview

Mastitis is a broad, overarching term for any inflammation of the udder tissue in association with changes in the appearance of the milk secretion.

Aetiology

There are many species of bacteria, mycoplasma, fungi, algae and yeasts that have been isolated from clinical cases of mastitis. Some may be involved in outbreaks of mastitis, such as *Staphylococcus aureus* (the most common cause of mastitis in dairy herds spreading from goat to goat), whereas others may be sporadic and environmental in origin such as *Escherichia coli*. Mastitis may also be a clinical presentation in systemic diseases such as caprine arthritis encephalitis (CAE). Any mastitis investigation should include identification of the causative organism or underlying syndrome.

Pathophysiology

This will vary from pathogen to pathogen.

Staphylococcus aureus

Staphylococcus aureus is a contagious mastitis pathogen and can be found in the udder tissue as a chronic infection, or residing on the skin of the udder or teats, spreading between goats predominantly during the milking process. The organism can colonise teat lesions such as cuts, abrasions or skin lesions resulting from, for example, sarcoptic mange. Mastitis will develop mainly as a result of transfer of infection between goats during mechanical or hand milking. *S. aureus* can produce a potent necrotoxin, causing severe udder tissue damage and gangrenous change.

Coagulase-negative staphylococci

Coagulase-negative staphylococci are the most commonly isolated udder organism in many goat milk bacteriology surveys. Opinions vary as to their pathological significance. Some reports state that they are non-pathogenic even commensal in the udder, whereas others believe that they are potentially pathogenic if no other causative agent is identified. A high herd prevalence may be linked to reduced milk production, and a possible indication of a suboptimal milking regime.

Corynebacterium pseudotuberculosis and *Trueperella pyogenes*

These two organisms are both opportunistic pathogens, potentially colonising teat and teat end lesions, and gaining access to udder tissue if there is heavy infection around the teat end and/or damage to the sphincter. *C. pseudotuberculosis* is the causative organism of caseous lymphadenitis (see Chapter 7).

Escherichia coli and *Pseudomonas aeruginosa*

These are environmental organisms potentially gaining access to the udder as a result of heavy contamination of the udder and teat end from goats lying in wet dirty conditions, or being milked when the udder itself is dirty. *E. coli* can produce a potent toxin, resulting in severe tissue damage and gangrenous change.

Tuberculosis

Mastitis associated mainly with *Mycobacterium bovis* (and only rarely with other mycobacterial organisms such as *Mycobacterium avium*) has been recorded in goats. In new *M. bovis* cases, there is most often spread either directly from infected cattle or goats, or indirectly via infected wildlife, particularly in areas with a high bovine tuberculosis incidence. Udder disease occurs as a sequela to dissemination of either respiratory or alimentary infection to a number of systemic sites, including also the lungs and associated lymph nodes, and the liver and spleen.

Mycoplasma spp.

See contagious agalactia earlier in this chapter.

Caprine arthritis encephalitis

One of the manifestations of CAE seen in infected herds is an interstitial mastitis resulting in atrophy and induration of the affected udder half (**Fig. 12.1**). Even in the absence of clinical disease, milk from CAE-positive does will contain high levels of cell-associated CAE virus, making milk and colostrum one of the main routes of dissemination (see Chapter 9 for more details).

Clinical presentation

The clinical signs of mastitis will vary (depending mainly on the organism involved) from peracute gangrenous mastitis, to mild mastitis with little change or subclinical mastitis with no change to the gross appearance of the milk secretion.

In gangrenous mastitis caused predominantly by *S. aureus* and *E. coli*, affected goats show a rapid onset of severe dullness, depression and inappetence. Initial pyrexia gives way to subnormal temperatures due to systemic shock. The affected part of the udder becomes cold to the touch and progressively purple to black in colour, usually with a clear line of demarcation, and serum may ooze from the skin surface (**Fig. 12.2**). This gangrenous tissue may eventually slough (**Fig. 12.7**). The milk

becomes watery and dark in colour due to secretory tissue cell necrosis, and gas may be stripped from the teat end.

In acute bacterial mastitis, signs can range from severe with systemic involvement (grade 3), to udder and milk changes (grade 2), to milk changes only (grade 1). Affected goats are often inappetent and pyrexic. The udder may be firm, oedematous and painful, and milk drawn from the affected half will be of an abnormal appearance, such as watery, thick or discoloured, and may contain clots.

In chronic mastitis, the udder will be firm and often nodular when palpated. The nodules represent chronic suppurative areas associated with *S. aureus* or *T. pyogenes* infection, effectively walled off by tissue fibrosis (**Fig. 12.8**). The associated milk secretion may be abnormal or unremarkable.

Other clinical signs may be apparent in individual goats or within the goat cohort if udder infection is a manifestation of a more complex disease. In CAE, for example, lameness and joint enlargement are most commonly reported in addition to udder changes (see above). In contagious agalactia, arthritis and severe keratoconjunctivitis are other associated clinical signs in both adults and kids (see above).

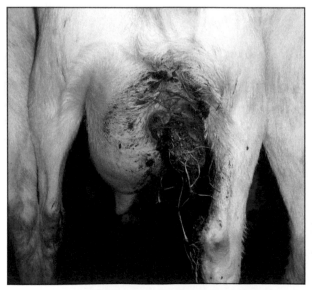

Fig. 12.7 Advanced gangrenous mastitis with sloughing. (Image courtesy Kathy Anzuino.)

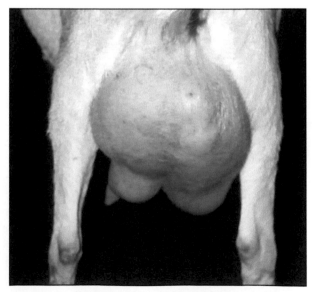

Fig. 12.8 Marked udder fibrosis associated with chronic mastitis.

Diagnosis

Clinical mastitis

In clinical cases of mastitis, changes in milk and/ or the udder will be present. Aseptically taken milk samples should be submitted for laboratory examination. The majority of the bacterial pathogens will grow on blood agar and MacConkey agar, and can be differentiated by colony morphology, Gram staining and other confirmatory tests. Laboratory isolation of *Mycoplasma* spp. is more problematic (see Contagious agalactia).

In tuberculosis infection, culture is difficult but acid-fast organisms may be identified in a spun milk sediment, and a holistic approach is required based on the herd profile supported by the single intradermal comparative cervical skin test. If CAE is suspected, milk examination is of limited value. The CAE status can be confirmed by an ELISA test on blood, but emphasis must be placed on herd status as not all CAE-positive goats produce a hard udder or seroconvert. Histopathology of udder tissue may aid a diagnosis, either by biopsy or at post-mortem examination.

Subclinical mastitis

There are several ancillary tests available for confirming subclinical mastitis or monitoring milk quality, both in individual goats and for use on bulk milk samples from goat herds.

In dairy cows, the SCC is widely used as an indicator of udder infection. In the healthy bovine udder the SCC is made up predominantly of epithelial cells. In response to inflammation, white blood cells enter the udder tissue and milk to combat infection and the SCC rises, giving good correlation with the infection status of the udder. In the goat, however, during the process of apocrine milk secretion, small portions of the cytoplasm of the epithelial cells lining the glandular structure are pinched off and appear in the milk, before degenerating and releasing the milk secretion. These cytoplasmic portions are similar in size to leucocytes and are the main reason why SCC values for both individual and bulk milk samples are considerably higher in goats, and thus of more limited value for mastitis monitoring, and can easily lead to a false-positive result that a goat's udder is infected. As an example, in a UK government study of 2,800 milk samples taken on four commercial dairy goat units, the average individual somatic cell count was 1,258,000 cells/ml. In samples that yielded no significant bacterial growth it was 1,080,000 cells/ml and in those samples in which there was significant bacterial growth suggesting udder infection it was 2,053,000 cells/ml, with some individual samples considerably higher. Applying cattle interpretation values to the California mastitis test (CMT; **Fig. 12.9**) will undoubtedly lead to false-positive results, although a modified CMT has been developed with goat-specific figures for individual CMT scores. The conventional CMT can also be of benefit in excluding a diagnosis of mastitis if negative. To further complicate the picture, there is a breed difference in SCC values and also a seasonal variation linked to stage of lactation, daily yield and onset of oestrus.

The following guidelines may be useful to assess udder health in goats:

- Classifying a CMT score of 0 or 1 = uninfected gland (versus score of 2 or 3 = infected gland); has a specificity of around 80% and negative predictive value of about 85%.

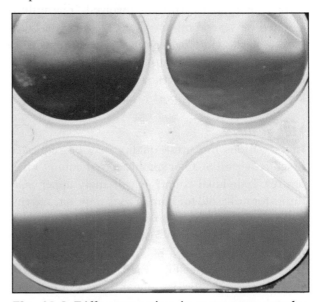

Fig. 12.9 **Different reactions in cow quarter samples to the California mastitis test: strong positive top left, moderately positive top right, and normal milk (no reaction) bottom row. Interpretation of such reactions is more difficult in goats because of their different milk secretion process.**

- Classifying a SCC <500,000/ml = uninfected; identifies about 60% of glands correctly, with a negative predictive value of 90%.
- Using a SCC >1,500,000/ml at peak lactation as an indicator of *S. aureus* infection has a reasonable sensitivity and specificity percentage (80–90%).
- The bulk milk SCC should gradually decrease in the first 6 months of the herd's milking period (if block-kidding).

Current studies have not found a consensus on what parameters and cut-offs constitute an intramammary infection in goats. However, when investigating a potential subclinical mastitis problem, the guidelines above may be of help. Bulk milk somatic cell counts can also used as an indication of milk quality as it leaves the farm, and thresholds/targets applied will vary from country to country (see Milk quality, later).

Milk conductivity testing is increasingly being carried out in many commercial dairy goat herds, with sensors placed at each milking unit in the parlour. Care should be taken in interpreting results, taking other factors into consideration.

Culturing a bulk milk sample is a useful first indicator of potential pathogens involved. The milk is agitated for several minutes before a sample is taken with a sterile ladle or pipette and transferred into a sterile container. Because bacterial counts are as important as type of pathogen, the sample must be kept cool during transport to the laboratory.

Milk quality

Investigations into milk quality may be requested based either on SCC or total bacterial count (TBC) figures. Individual countries will apply upper SCC limits for milk sold for human consumption, and this will vary from country to country with <1,000,000 cells/ml a typical figure. Less is known about the overall significance of TBC figures in goats, but the starting point must always be to identify potential sources of the bacteria counted. Levels of environmental organisms, such as *E. coli*, may rise if goats are kept in dirty conditions with faecal contamination of the udder and teats during milking. The second source comprises the udder pathogens such as *S. aureus* and non-pathogenic/commensal organisms such as coagulase-negative staphylococci. The third category comprises the thermoduric organisms that survive the normal machine, pipework and tank cleaning process. Checks should also be made on the bulk tank cooling to ensure refrigeration temperatures are being met.

Differential diagnosis

Udder trauma or neoplasia may present with pain and swelling, but milk culture will be negative. In those more complex conditions, such as CAE, contagious agalactia and tuberculosis, the combination of the clinical presentation, post-mortem findings, laboratory test results and morbidity and mortality figures will aid the diagnosis.

Treatment

The choice of antibiotics, both parenteral and intramammary, should be based on culture results, ideally from the particular case, but as a minimum from previous herd samples. Availability of licensed products will vary greatly from country to country, and country-specific bans on particular agents (such as fluoroquinolones) must be taken into account. In the UK, a minimum withholding period of 7 days must be observed for milk under the 'prescribing cascade regulations' for any product used off-licence (e.g. any intramammary preparation).

Acute mastitis

Treatment of clinical mastitis depends on the severity and chronicity. For acute grade 1 or 2 mastitis, intramammary antibiosis is usually sufficient. Product groups to consider are cloxacillin, clavulanic acid preparations, cephalosporins, macrolides and tetracyclines. The distribution within the udder or, for systemic administration, into the udder must be taken into account.

For grade 3 mastitis (i.e. causing systemic illness), treatment consists of NSAIDs, intramammary and systemic antibiosis, fluid therapy and nursing care. Frequent stripping of the affected gland is advisable, if necessary facilitated by administration of 2–5 IU oxytocin.

Gangrenous mastitis

These cases carry a poor prognosis, and if tissue necrosis is advanced, immediate euthanasia on humane grounds should be considered. In valuable or pet goats treatment may be attempted with i/v antibiotics such as: oxytetracycline 10 mg/kg q12–24h; where available, ampicillin 3 mg/kg q8–12h; where culture and sensitivity indicates ceftiofur 1–2 mg/kg q12h or cefquinome 1–2 mg/kg q12h. NSAIDs provide important supportive therapy (e.g. flunixin meglumine 2 mg/kg i/v q12–24h; carprofen 1.4 mg/kg i/v or meloxicam 0.5 mg/kg i/v q48h). Affected goats should be kept warm and hydrated. Teat amputation may be indicated in the acute stage of gangrenous mastitis, followed by partial or complete mastectomy depending on the residual udder damage present if the goat survives.

Chronic or recurrent cases

Prolonged antibiosis may be required for chronic or recurrent cases (observing prolonged milk withholding periods as necessary), but carries the risk of inducing fungal or yeast mastitis. Other options include selective drying-off of the affected gland or early drying off (with or without systemic antibiosis in addition to use of intramammary dry cow therapy). Culling should be considered if a doe has multiple episodes of either clinical mastitis or raised SCC, especially if caused by contagious pathogens, such as *Staphylococcus* spp.

Dry goat therapy

Dry goat therapy is not as widely adopted in goats as in the dairy cow sector, not least because there are few, if any, intramammary products licensed for use in goats. Indications include an intractable or persistent mastitis in individual goats or a herd problem. A positive effect on the SCC in the subsequent lactation has been shown. The general recommendation is to use half the contents of a dry cow tube. However, great care must be taken when inserting an intramammary tube into the teat of a goat because of the much reduced diameter of the sphincter, which can easily become damaged. The procedure must be carried out using strict asepsis. The routine use of dry goat therapy is particularly problematic if goats kid early. Enquiries should be made with the manufacturer about suitable milk withholding times, and antibiotic residue testing carried out prior to the milk entering the bulk tank.

The benefits of using teat sealants, either alone or in combination with intramammary antibiotics, are as yet not fully established in goats.

Management/control

The major factors in the prevention and control of ordinary bacterial mastitis are a sound milking regime, a well maintained machine and a clean stress free environment:

- Milking goats should be kept in a clean, well-ventilated, dry environment, free from condensation, on bedding that is regularly topped up (**Fig. 12.10**). Bedding material should be stored under cover to ensure it is dry when being used.
- They should be fed a good wholesome diet that eliminates any change away from the normal dry pelleted faeces they normally produce.

In the parlour:

- Gloves should be worn, and regularly disinfected, to eliminate spread of infection between goats.

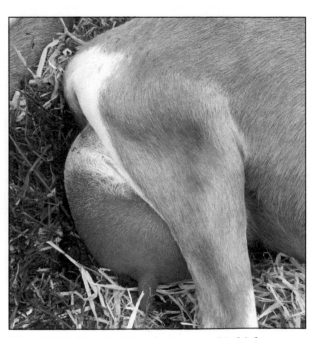

Fig. 12.10 Poor bedding hygiene in this high-yielding goat's pen.

- Teats should only be washed if they are visibly dirty. If they are washed, they should be dried with individual disposable paper towels.
- Pre-milking teat disinfection should be considered to control environmental mastitis where this is a problem.
- Each goat should be checked for mastitis at every milking. This may be by udder palpation, by drawing milk from each half into a strip cup, or by the use of in-line filters or electrical conductivity meters. This procedure is, inadvisably, often omitted in high throughput parlours.
- Post-milking teat disinfection should be used routinely, but as a minimum in herds with a known mastitis problem.
- Prompt recognition and treatment of new clinical cases, and culling of chronic cases, is essential. Some mechanism for identifying affected goats, such as spray marking or leg tapes, should be in place.
- Known infected goats should be segregated where possible and milked last, using either dedicated clusters and dump buckets or thorough flushing and disinfection of clusters and milk lines.

- Ideally, after milking goats are encouraged to stand for 30 minutes to allow teat sphincter closure, for example by having fresh feed available.

The milking machine can impact on the incidence of mastitis in a number of ways:

- Spread of infection between goats via contaminated liners.
- Defective pulsation rates or excessive vacuum levels at the teat end can cause damage to the sphincter, allowing bacteria to enter (**Fig. 12.11a**).
- Rapid fluctuations in vacuum level at the teat end can lead to 'teat end impacts' in which potentially infected milk droplets can be driven back up into the udder. This is particularly important if infected milk from a previous goat remains in the cluster, and this is a potential mechanism for spread of the CAE virus.
- Over-milking can cause teat end damage (**Fig. 12.11b**) and may result from insufficient stimulation of milk let-down at the start of milking or delayed cluster removal at the end of milking.

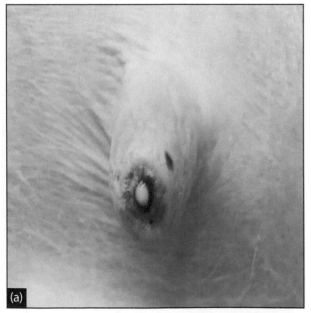
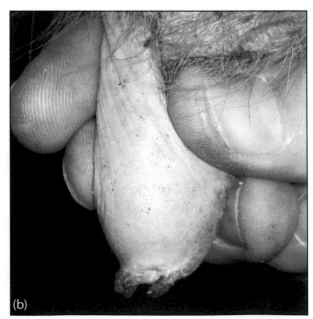

(a)   (b)

Fig. 12.11 Teat end damage should prompt investigation into plant function, liner quality and over-milking. (a) Acute damage, and (b) hyperkeratosis as a result of recurrent insult to the teat end (both images are cow teats).

Milking machines must be designed and calibrated specifically for milking goats as operating parameters are different to those employed for dairy cows (**Fig. 12.12**). In the UK, the following parameters have been suggested:

- Vacuum levels 37–38 kPa.
- Pulsation speed 90–120 ppm.
- Pulsation ratio of 50% (50:50).

Vacuum levels should be checked at the start of every milking session and pulsation rates should be assessed on a weekly basis. This can be done easily by inserting a thumb into an activated teat cup and counting the number of times the liner collapses on the thumb every 60 seconds. The service requirements of a milking machine will depend greatly on the number of hours the machine operates. Generally, the plant will require some service input from a dairy engineer every 750 operating hours. For a plant milking and washing 5 hours each day, this equates to a service every 150 days (5 months). If the plant is operating for 8 hours each day, the service interval will fall to 94 days or three monthly. Rubber liners require changing after milking 2,500 animals. Silicone liners require changing after approximately 5,000 milkings. Liners that go beyond their normal life expectancy will result in increased liner slip and teat discolouration, be less effectively cleaned and therefore harbour pathogens, and milk slower.

Tuberculosis management/control
See Chapter 17.

Caprine arthritis encephalitis management/control
See Chapter 9.

Udder impetigo (syn. staphylococcal folliculitis of the udder)
See Chapter 11.

SURGERY OF THE MAMMARY GLAND

Supernumerary teat removal
Indication
Supernumerary teat removal is carried out either for cosmetic reasons or because the surplus teat is likely to interfere with cluster attachment (**Fig. 12.13**). As this is an inherited abnormality and may result in disqualification in show goats, there is often an ethical dilemma as to whether removal should be done.

Preparation and equipment
Antiseptic, haemostats, sharp scissors or scalpel blade.

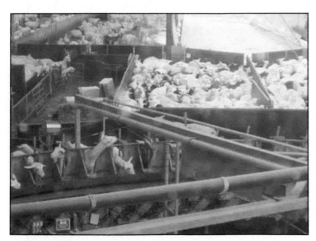

Fig. 12.12 **A purpose built commercial rotary parlour for milking goats. Regular plant maintenance is important for mastitis control, including exchanging any rubber ware and liners.**

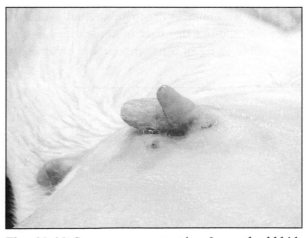

Fig. 12.13 **Supernumerary teat in a 3-month-old kid (in dorsal recumbency).**

Restraint

In the UK, there are currently no guidelines for the removal of such teats in goats, but in cattle this procedure must be carried out under local anaesthesia and by a veterinary surgeon if the animal is 3 months of age or older.

Technical description

After application of an antiseptic, the teat is grasped with haemostats as close to its base as possible and crushed. After moving the haemostats slightly closer to the teat end, and using either sharp scissors or a scalpel blade, the teat is cut close to its base. Haemostasis is usually achieved by applying pressure with a gauze swab for several minutes.

Aftercare

Topical antibiotic spray. Clean, dry environment. Monitoring by owner for bleeding or infection.

Potential complications

Supernumerary teats occasionally have associated glandular tissue, potentially leading to mastitis once the goat starts lactating. A supernumerary teat close to the main teat may have a connection to the teat sinus. Where it is difficult to differentiate between the proper and the supernumerary teat, the removal is best delayed or the decision on which teat to remove left to the owner.

There are a number of other potentially inherited teat abnormalities that have been identified, including double or fused teats, an example of which are

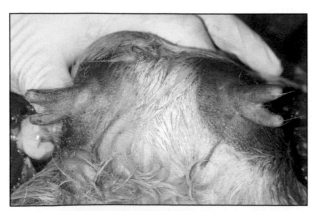

Fig. 12.14 Bilateral congenital 'fishtail' teats.

the so-called 'fishtail' teats (**Fig. 12.14**). These can be removed at birth, although problems can occasionally develop later when the doe comes into milk, potentially resulting in mastitis. Culling may be a better option.

Teat surgery

Indication

Teat surgery may be necessary because of obstruction of the teat canal or lacerations of the teat. Occasionally, amputation of the teat is indicated as a salvage procedure to manage severe purulent or gangrenous mastitis or severe teat trauma. Teat fistulae may be congenital or secondary to trauma.

Lacerations should be viewed as any acute wound and attended to as soon as possible (**Fig. 12.15**). Chronic lesions and fistulae are best dealt with during the dry period if they do not interfere with normal teat drainage. (**Note:** Mastitis risk is heightened in such glands.)

Preparation and equipment

A clean environment is essential. A tourniquet (e.g. rubber band), teat bandage and spray, teat cannula, fine gauge polydioxanone (PDS®) on a round bodied and cutting needle and a small procedure instrument kit are required. For obstructions, various instruments may be useful, including a Hudson teat probe, teat spiral, Barrett's papillotome and a McLeans knife.

Restraint

Sedation to facilitate lateral recumbency, with the uppermost hind leg tied out. For procedures involving the teat wall, anaesthesia is achieved via intravenous regional anaesthesia or a ring block, using local anaesthetic without adrenaline (epinephrine). For anaesthesia of the teat canal, 2–3 ml of local anaesthetic is infused into the canal and distributed by massage.

Technical description

Small obstructive lesions can often be removed via the streak canal, using teat instruments. Larger obstructive lesions may require surgical opening of the teat canal.

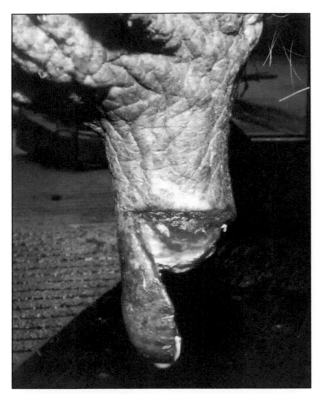

Fig. 12.15 Horizontal laceration, leading to substantial detachment of the distal teat in a cow. Such injuries should be treated like any other wound, aiming to preserve as much tissue as possible.

For surgical procedures, a rubber band is placed at the base as a tourniquet. Teat lacerations are prepared like any wound with pressure lavage, debridement and, if presentation is delayed, freshening of the wound edges using a scalpel blade. Full-thickness wounds (i.e. breeching the teat canal) are ideally repaired in three layers: the mucosal lining using simple interrupted or continuous sutures (round bodied needle), the connective tissue and muscle layer using vertical mattress sutures (cutting needle), and the skin using simple interrupted sutures (cutting needle).

Aftercare

Intramammary and systemic antimicrobials and NSAIDs. The teat is bandaged with purpose made tape and spray, and the bandage possibly anchored proximally with a suture. A self-retaining teat cannula is inserted for several days, and the plug removed 3–4 times a day to allow drainage.

Post-milking teat dip or spray is applied after each such 'milking'. Sutures are removed after 10–14 days if non-absorbable material was used.

Potential complications

Mastitis, stenosis of teat canal, breakdown of suture line and sinus formation are the main problems.

Mastectomy
Indication

Mastectomy is indicated to address udder changes caused by gangrenous mastitis, non-healing wounds, inappropriate lactation syndrome (pseudolactation) in pet goats or neoplasia.

Preparation and equipment

If possible, the procedure is delayed until the udder is undergoing involution. A large instrument kit with good number of haemostats, suture material for vessel ligation and skin sutures, and a Penrose drain are required.

Restraint

General anaesthesia is preferred as surgery time can be unpredictable. Alternatives include sedation combined with high epidural anaesthesia. For total mastectomy, the goat is placed into dorsal recumbency. For unilateral mastectomy, lateral recumbency with the affected gland uppermost and the upper hind leg tied out may be used.

Technical description

During the incision to expose the gland, as much healthy skin as possible is preserved to maintain a skin flap large enough to cover the defect. Blunt dissection is used to separate the skin from the mammary tissue. The mammary gland is then freed *en bloc* from its attachments. Haemorrhage is controlled immediately by tying off any vessels, ideally prior to cutting through them. Some of the main vessels include the internal and external pudendal and superficial epigastric ones, and their course varies from goat to goat. However, multiple other vessels will be present, especially if the gland is still producing milk. Great care must be taken not to incise into the glandular tissue, as resulting milk leakage will greatly obscure the surgical field and contaminate the site. Dead space is reduced as much as possible with interrupted sutures. One or several Penrose drains are placed prior to routine skin closure.

Aftercare

Parenteral antibiosis for a minimum of 5 days, NSAIDs and nursing care in a clean environment.

Depending on the season, fly repellent. The Penrose drain is removed after 48–72 hours.

Potential complications

Marked blood loss if haemorrhage control proves difficult and wound breakdown are the main complications. Overall, prognosis is reasonable in goats not systemically ill at the time of surgery.

THE EYE

NORMAL STRUCTURE AND FUNCTION

The palpebral conjunctiva lines the inside of the eyelids and the bulbar conjunctiva overlies the sclera, together forming the conjunctival sac. A fold of conjunctiva in the medial canthus forms the nictitating membrane (syn. third eyelid). It contains an anchor-shaped cartilage.

About 90% of corneal depth is formed by the stroma, covered by the outer epithelium consisting of several cell layers and the innermost Descemet's membrane. The anterior chamber, containing aqueous humour, and the posterior chamber, containing vitreous humour, are demarcated by the pupil, which is formed by the iris, lens and ciliary body. The iris is mid-brown in colour in most breeds. When constricted, the pupil adopts a rectangular shape, becoming more rounded when dilated (**Fig. 13.1**).

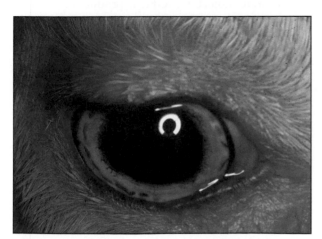

Fig. 13.1 Normal eye of a goat, with the pupil dilated. The iris has the typical mid-brown colour of many breeds. The downward curvature of the upper eyelid is not unusual.

The eye background shows the optic disc, the tapetum lucidum (roughly a horizontal strip just above the optic disc), the tapetum nigrum and loosely arranged vessels. The tapetum lucidum and width of the retina supports good night vision. As in other prey animals, goats have a wide field of vision but limited perception of depth. They can see blue, purple and green well.

The tear apparatus consists of the lacrimal gland and a dorsal and ventral lacrimal puncta with associated small ducts. These combine and drain via the lacrimal sac into the nasolacrimal duct, which ends in the ventral corner of the nostril at the mucosal–skin border.

Cranial nerves of interest are shown in *Table 13.1*.

CLINICAL EXAMINATION OF THE EYE

The examiner's hands should be clean and ideally gloved. Equipment for a basic eye examination includes: pen or head torch, haemostats, cotton buds, fluorescein and an ophthalmoscope. To reduce pain during examination or manipulation of the eye, topical anaesthetic is applied (e.g. lidocaine hydrochloride, tetracaine hydrochloride, amethocaine hydrochloride; **note:** none are licensed for veterinary use in the UK.) An auriculopalpebral block is useful if blepharospasm is severe (see Chapter 18). Dilating the pupil with 2–4 drops of atropine sulphate aids examination of the eye background; however, the goat must be kept out of bright light for several hours until the effect has worn off.

The conjunctival sac should always be explored for foreign bodies (see below).

Ocular swabs can be obtained effectively with human interdental brushes. A smear is prepared with Romanowsky stain (e.g. Diff-Quik®) for cytology. Swabs for culture must be harvested prior to application

Table 13.1 **Cranial nerves involved in eye sensation, movement and reflexes, and vision.**

NUMBER	NAME	FUNCTION
II	Optic	Vision
III	Oculomotor	Pupil constriction, eye movement (ventral and ventral oblique, dorsal, medial)
IV	Trochlear	Eye movement (dorsal oblique)
V	Trigeminal	Sensory to orbit, cornea and eyelids including medial canthus
VI	Abducens	Eye movement (lateral, retraction), third eyelid protrusion
VII	Facial	Motor supply to eyelids (auriculopalpebral branch). Facial expression

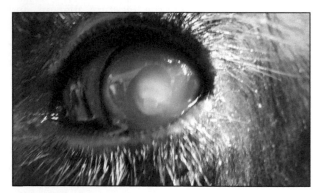

Fig. 13.2 Neovascularisation in response to a melting corneal ulcer in a bovine.

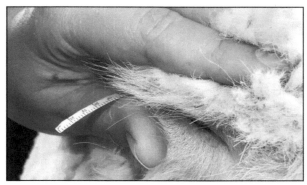

Fig. 13.3 A Schirmer tear test strip placed in the conjunctival sac of an alpaca. The test is read by measuring the advancement of the blue discolouration on the strip after 1 minute.

of any medication or prolonged examination, and both bacterial and fungal culture should be carried out.

The position of the eye in the orbit may be altered by ocular pathology, but also by hydration status and body condition (with reduced retrobulbar fat in thin animals).

Damage to the corneal epithelium can be highlighted using fluorescein strips or drops placed into the conjunctival sac. Patency of the nasolacrimal duct can also be established. The stain should appear at the corresponding nostril within 5–10 minutes.

Neovascularisation indicates pathology and can be used to roughly age the lesion. It tends to start 3–4 days after the ocular insult, and vessels advance about 1 mm per day (**Fig. 13.2**).

Further diagnostics
Schirmer tear test, intraocular pressure, ophthalmoscopy
Normal parameters for more advanced examination include:

- A Schirmer tear test reading of ≥18 mm (adults) or ≥14 mm (kids less than 1 month old) after 1 minute indicates good tear production (**Fig. 13.3**).
- Normal intraocular pressure (IOP, in mm Hg) is reported as 19–20 in adults and 15–16 in young kids using Schiotz tonometry, with lower IOP values of 9–11 reported for a TonoPen™ (**Fig. 13.4**).
- A white aqueous flare when examining the anterior chamber with an ophthalmoscope indicates debris. For direct ophthalmoscopy, the fundus will typically be in focus at a setting of –1 to –2.

Ultrasonography
Corneal oedema is often marked in goats with ocular disease, preventing visual assessment of deeper structures. Ultrasonography allows examination of external and internal structures and aids detection of inflammation, neoplasia, abnormal structures

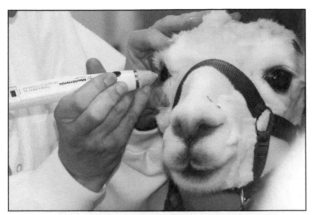

Fig. 13.4 Measuring intraocular pressure (IOP) with a TonoPen™ in an alpaca. IOP values of 9–11 have been reported in normal goats using this instrument.

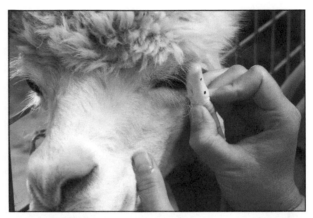

Fig. 13.5 Placing an ultrasound probe directly onto the globe is well tolerated by animals with the aid of topical anaesthesia.

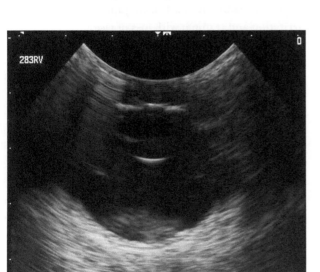

Fig. 13.6 Ultrasonogram of a normal eye, highlighting some of the structures that can be assessed such as anterior and posterior chamber, thickness of sclera and iris, lens position and periocular tissues. The apparent debris in the posterior chamber in this image is an artefact.

and material and disruption of normal features. After applying a topical anaesthetic and coupling gel, a linear or curved probe (7.5–12 MHz) is placed either directly onto the globe or onto the eyelid (**Figs. 13.5, 13.6**). The procedure is well tolerated.

FIRST AID FOR OCULAR TRAUMA

To prevent further injury or self-trauma, the goat's head is cross-tied with the aid of two halters.

Owners should never attempt to force a swollen or painful eye open. Disinfectants must not be used in or around the eye. A cold towel or wrapped ice pack can be gently applied if the ocular region suffered blunt trauma or bruising. Owners may attempt to flush out a foreign body that is not embedded in tissue and is causing only minor irritation. The lower eyelid is gently pulled down and lukewarm, clean water poured in a steady stream onto the eye for up to 15 minutes, periodically checking whether the foreign body has gone. Chemical contamination of the eye needs to receive immediate flushing (note that trauma is more severe with alkaline fluids than acidic). Eyelid tears, just like other wounds, have the best chance of healing and restoring normal contour and function if they receive veterinary attention within 6 hours. An owner should never cut off any eyelid fragments.

NON-INFECTIOUS DISEASE

Entropion
Overview
Entropion is inward rolling of the eyelid. This may be uni- or bilateral and affect the lower or upper eyelids.

Aetiology
A genetic predisposition exists, with some breeds or individual bucks producing affected offspring.

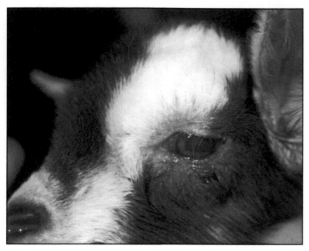

Fig. 13.7 Epiphora caused by entropion affecting the lower eyelid.

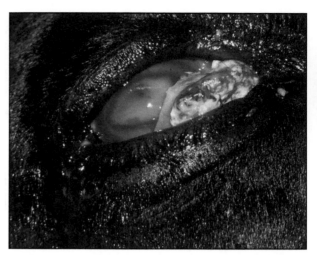

Fig. 13.8 A neglected conjunctival foreign body in a bovine, leading to marked conjunctival and corneal irritation and trauma, with loss of vision.

Clinical presentation

The condition is present at birth or develops within 24 hours post partum. Entropion is acutely painful, leading to blepharospasm and epiphora (**Fig. 13.7**). If left untreated, corneal ulceration follows within 24–48 hours.

Diagnosis

Kids should be inspected for entropion within 24 hours of birth. The abnormal contour is obvious on visual inspection.

Differential diagnosis

An ocular foreign body will present similarly. Infectious keratoconjunctivitis (IKC) (see below) is rare in neonates.

Treatment/management/control

Measures that cause temporary eversion are usually sufficient. This may be achieved by: (a) placing a pair of haemostats parallel to the affected eyelid as close to its margin as possible and pinching the eyelid skin for 20–30 seconds; this procedure is repeated every few hours over the next 24 hours; or (b) injecting 0.5 ml of a non-irritant drug (penicillin, lidocaine, water for injection) s/c into the eyelid to form a subconjunctival bleb. A single treatment is often enough, but may be repeated at 12–24 hours if required.

Surgical treatment is rarely required, but is an option if the entropion is severe and persistent

(using the same technique as in dogs). Several days of topical antibiotic is required in addition if corneal ulceration has occurred.

Bucks producing affected offspring should be removed from the breeding pool.

Foreign bodies
Overview

Conjunctival sac foreign bodies (FBs) are a common ocular problem, leading to marked irritation and potentially corneal ulceration. Sharp FBs may also be found lodged in the sclera or cornea. These may lead to loss of vision.

Aetiology

Grass seeds are commonly involved, either caused by animals grazing long mature pasture or feeding hay from racks above head height. Using straw blowers to top up bedding can also lead to ocular FBs.

Clinical presentation

Typical signs are blepharospasm and epiphora. Conjunctival FBs often cause localised corneal opacity or ulceration (**Fig. 13.8**). Embedded FBs may lead to stromal abscess formation.

Diagnosis

Topical anaesthetic greatly aids examination. For conjunctival FBs, digital pressure is used on either

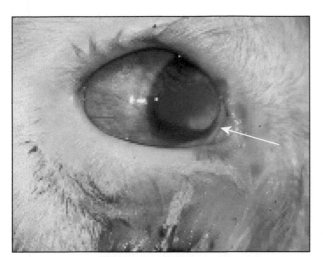

Fig. 13.9 Stromal abscess in the ventral cornea (arrow), causing epiphora and neovascularisation.

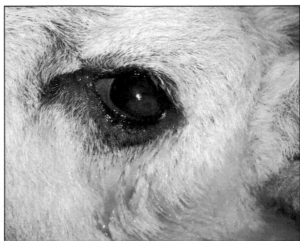

Fig. 13.10 Corneal ulceration secondary to entropion in a 2-day-old lamb. Infectious keratoconjunctivitis ('pink eye') would appear similar, but with the ulcer in the centre of the cornea.

the upper or lower eyelid to gently push the eyeball into its socket. The opposite eyelid is everted and the corresponding conjunctival sac visually examined. A moistened cotton bud can be passed through the conjunctival sac to dislodge any FB. A cotton bud or pair of fine haemostats is used to lift the third eyelid to allow examination behind it.

An ophthalmoscope or magnifying lens may be required to detect small embedded FBs.

Differential diagnosis

In cases with IKC, the ulcer is almost always placed centrally, whereas the corneal changes caused by FB are often more peripheral.

Treatment/management/control

The FB is removed either manually or flushed out (using clean water). If the cornea is damaged, a course of topical or systemic antibiosis and a NSAID is indicated.

FBs embedded in the sclera or cornea should be treated as ocular emergencies and receive prompt attention. Heavy sedation or general anaesthesia (GA) is advisable to allow removal without the risk of further trauma if the patient moves during the procedure. If the FB has created a large defect, this is sutured.

Prevention involves placing hay racks at a suitable height. Goats should be moved out of the housing prior to using a straw blower.

Corneal ulceration and stromal abscessation

Overview

The pain element with ulceration, and the risk of loss of vision with both conditions, means prompt and assertive intervention is required.

Aetiology

Ulcers may result from physical trauma or infectious processes. A stromal abscess is caused either by infection becoming trapped underneath the epithelium when an ulcer heals, or by pathogen or foreign body deposition into the stroma secondary to a corneal puncture.

Clinical presentation

Blepharospasm, photophobia, epiphora and localised or generalised corneal oedema are typically present with ulceration, but often less marked with stromal abscessation. The latter present as single or multiple yellowish deposits in the cornea (**Fig. 13.9**). Corneal neovascularisation is common in both conditions (**Fig. 13.9**).

Diagnosis

The surface of the eye is viewed from different angles, including the sky-line view, to detect any defects (**Figs. 13.2, 13.10**). Fluorescein staining

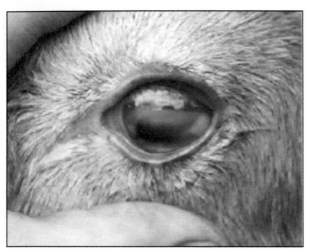

Fig. 13.11 Fluorescein staining highlighting a corneal defect near the lateral canthus.

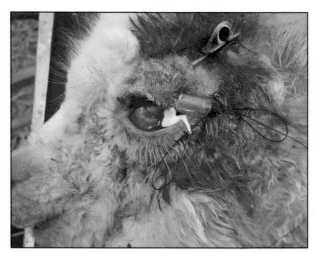

Fig. 13.12 Third eyelid flap and subpalpebral lavage system to address a full-thickness corneal ulcer in an alpaca cria. The white substance near the lateral canthus is ointment.

highlights any epithelial damage (**Fig. 13.11**). Stain underrunning the epithelium indicates poor healing, with newly formed epithelium not becoming tightly attached to the underlying stroma.

Bacterial and fungal cultures should be performed for progressive or non-healing ulcers. Culture or cytology of a corneal swab is not useful for a stromal abscess, as the pathology affects deeper structures.

Differential diagnosis
Acute physical trauma to the cornea may present similarly. Hypopyon involves the ventral anterior chamber, rather than the stroma.

Treatment/management/control
Treatment of ulcers up to 50% corneal depth consists of topical or subconjunctival antimicrobials. Collagenase inhibitors, such as autogenous serum, 0.2% calcium-EDTA or tetracycline, are a useful adjunct (apply a few drops 4–8 times per day). Topical or subconjunctival NSAIDs should be considered to provide analgesia. To prevent iris adhesions, 1% atropine sulphate drops may be applied twice a day (see Note, p. 293). An uncomplicated ulcer will heal within 5–7 days.

If the ulcer is more than 50% in depth or progressive, surgical procedures such as a tarsorrhaphy (see p. 293) or a third eyelid flap are carried out additionally

to provide corneal protection (**Fig. 13.12**). Advanced techniques include conjunctival grafts or flaps and keratectomy. Healing typically takes 2–6 weeks.

In non-healing ulcers (as indicated by stain underrunning the epithelium), under topical anaesthesia a dry sterile cotton bud is used in a rubbing motion to remove any loose epithelium. This is followed by antibiosis and a corneal protection technique plus, potentially, a grid keratotomy.

For a stromal abscess, because the epithelium tends to be intact, antimicrobials need to be administered parentally. A superficial abscess may benefit from debridement, using a dry sterile cotton bud rubbed vigorously over the area under topical anaesthesia. A 4–6-week healing period should be expected, and healing is indicated by the abscess changing from a yellowish to a white colour and corneal vessels disappearing. If severe uveitis develops, surgical intervention such as a keratectomy is indicated.

Neoplasia
Overview
There are few reports of ocular neoplasia in goats and the likely incidence is unknown.

Aetiology
Reported types include squamous cell carcinoma (SCC) and lymphoma. Usually mature animals

are affected. The role of viral agents (e.g. papilloma-virus) and genetics in the aetiology of SCC remains unclear.

Clinical presentation

Common sites for SCC are the eyelids and the junction between the sclera and the cornea. From early white nodules, the tumour progresses to proliferative nodular lesions, often pink in colour.

Lymphoma may affect any lymphatic tissue in and around the orbit (**Fig. 13.13**). Keratitis is often marked and a degree of facial asymmetry may be present.

Both SCC and lymphoma can affect intraorbital tissues, leading to exophthalmos or changes to the normal eye axis (**Fig. 13.14**).

Regional lymph nodes should always be assessed for metastasis. If present, rejection at the abattoir is likely and prognosis is poor.

Diagnosis

Biopsy is the most reliable method. Neoplastic cells can sometimes be detected on impression smears.

Differential diagnosis

For early SCC eyelid lesions, scar formation after trauma. Other causes of severe keratitis need to be ruled out for lymphoma.

Treatment/management/control

Surgical excision may be possible for relatively discreet lesions affecting the conjunctiva, cornea or third eyelid. A margin of 2 mm into healthy tissue should be aimed for. Excising lesions on the upper or lower eyelid should only be undertaken if the eyelid contour and function can be maintained. Excision can be performed under sedation and local anaesthetic blocks (see Chapter 18), but GA is preferable.

Enucleation is the best option for extensive lesions or those affecting the eyelids or orbital tissues. Adjunct treatments such as cryosurgery, radiotherapy or chemotherapy are useful in valuable pedigree or pet goats.

The recurrence rate is unknown in the goat. In cattle, recurrence of SCC befalls one in three patients after surgical excision.

INFECTIOUS DISEASE

Infectious keratoconjunctivitis (syn. pink eye)

Definition/overview

IKC is a contagious disease affecting goats (and sheep) and is common in many countries. Disease can vary from mild to severe, one or both eyes can be infected and morbidity, particularly in housed goats, can be very high.

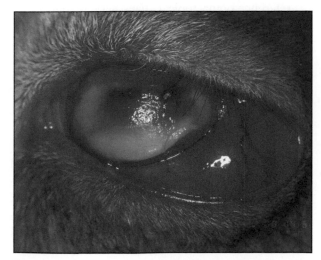

Fig. 13.13 Ocular lymphoma affecting the cornea and conjunctiva.

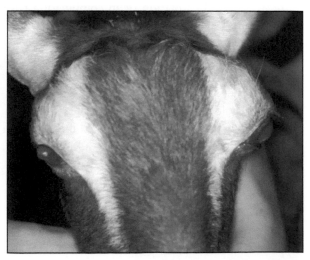

Fig. 13.14 Exophthalmos caused by ocular lymphoma on the left-hand side in a 9-year-old Toggenburg.

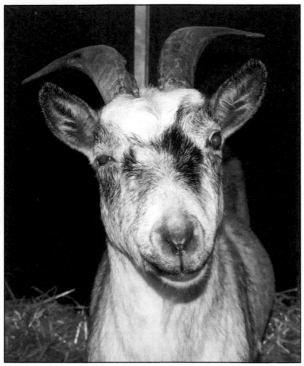

Fig. 13.15 Blepharospasm affecting the right eye. This typically indicates ocular pathology and the goat should be examined promptly.

Aetiology

Mycoplasma conjunctivae is most commonly associated with disease in goats and sheep in those countries in which laboratory testing has been undertaken. A number of other organisms capable of causing clinical disease in isolation or in combination with other agents have been incriminated. These include *Chlamydophila pecorum*, *Moraxella* spp., *Listeria monocytogenes* and other *Mycoplasma* spp. such as *M. agalactiae* (contagious agalactia) and *M. arginini*.

Pathophysiology

Infection is spread from one goat to another via a number of routes including flies and direct contact, particularly when housed and fed in close contact with each other or with infected sheep.

Clinical presentation

Clinical signs include conjunctivitis with marked hyperaemia, excessive lacrimation and blepharospasm (**Fig. 13.15**). This is followed by corneal opacity and vascularisation and corneal ulceration, which may result in rupture of the eye. Even following healing and remission, the cornea may remain 'cloudy' for many weeks. Outbreaks can occur and care should be taken to observe both eyes when examining groups of affected goats as the vision impaired eye will invariably be facing away from the observer.

Diagnosis

Diagnosis is based mainly on clinical signs and several animals being affected. Swabs taken from affected eyes can be submitted for denaturing gradient gel electrophoresis testing to confirm infection with *M. conjunctivae*.

Differential diagnosis

Includes entropion in young kids, an ocular foreign body or keratoconjunctivitis associated with listeriosis. Cobalt deficiency can lead to excessive lacrimation.

Treatment/management/control

There are a number of treatment regimes that have been tried, including:

- Use of dedicated antibiotic-containing ophthalmic ointments administered q4h to q48h (depending on the product).
- Subconjunctival antibiotic injection. The head of the animal is rotated to expose as much sclera as possible. Using an episcleral vessel as the reference point, topical anaesthetic is applied with a cotton bud to the scleral conjunctiva. A 23–25 gauge needle is inserted under the conjunctiva and advanced for a few millimetres parallel to the eye ball (see Chapter 1, p. 18).
- Parenteral antibiosis (at full BW dose) has also been shown to be effective, including long-acting tetracyclines, macrolides or fluorfenicol.

Severely affected goats should be isolated and kept in subdued lighting because of the marked photophobia that occurs. If there is marked ulceration, the cornea can be protected by the use of a tarsorrhaphy, third eyelid flap or a conjunctival pedical flap. For extensive damage, or where full-thickness ulceration has resulted in prolapse of the Descemet's membrane, enucleation should be considered.

Uveitis and iritis

Overview

Inflammation of the iris and its surrounding tissues is occasionally seen in goats.

Aetiology

Listeria monocytogenes uveitis is linked to silage feeding, in particular big bale silage where fermentation is often suboptimal, leading to an insufficient drop in pH and survival of this pathogen. Trauma to the cornea appears to be a prerequisite, and the condition is limited to times of silage feeding. *Mycoplasma* spp., *Chlamydophila psittaci* and *Toxoplasma gondii* may also cause uveitis, presenting either with just ocular signs or also with signs of systemic disease (including abortion).

Clinical presentation

Blepharospasm, epiphora, photophobia and conjunctivitis are seen. Closer examination of the eye shows opacity of the anterior chamber in addition to corneal oedema and typical folds in the iris.

Diagnosis

The swelling and undulation of the iris are typical. History of feeding silage supports the diagnosis.

Differential diagnosis

IKC is the main differential, but typically leads to corneal ulceration without uveitis.

Treatment/management/control

Oxytetracycline or penicillin are administered, together with dexamethasone (or a NSAID in pregnant females). These are ideally given as a subconjunctival injection, otherwise topically or systemically. Atropine sulphate 1% applied twice daily is thought to reduce the risk of iris adhesions forming (**Fig. 13.16**) and to provide some analgesia by reducing ciliary spasms. (**Note:** Not licensed in food producing animals and may possibly negatively affect gastrointestinal tract motility.) Healing typically takes 2 weeks.

Prevention relies on avoiding any feed presentation that leads to the goats burying their head into silage. Additionally, good silage production to achieve a low pH, little soil contamination and few aerobic pockets.

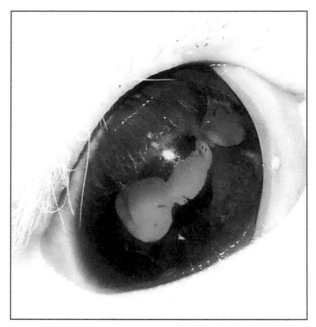

Fig. 13.16 Synechia (adhesion of iris) secondary to uveitis in a lamb.

OCULAR SURGERY

Tarsorrhaphy

Tarsorrhaphy is a useful first-line option to support corneal healing. The eyelids are sutured together with a single horizontal mattress suture using 4–6 metric suture material on a cutting needle. Ideally, the suture is tied with a single knot and shoelace bow, rather than a series of knots. This allows periodic release of the suture to monitor progress and apply topical medication.

Third eyelid flap

A third eyelid flap is also employed to aid corneal healing and is beneficial because of the close contact that is established between cornea and conjunctiva. 3–3.5 metric suture material on a cutting needle is placed through the upper eyelid close to the lateral canthus (in direction skin to conjunctiva), then, with a good-sized bite, through the external conjunctiva overlying the third eyelid, and fed out through the upper eyelid again (direction conjunctiva to skin). The free ends are passed through a stent (e.g. a button or short piece of tubing) and tied off. A shoelace bow is useful to allow periodic release to monitor progress and apply medication (**Fig. 13.12**).

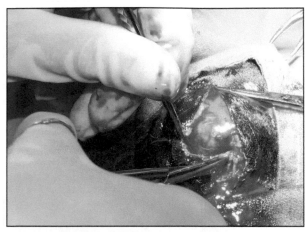

Fig. 13.17 After incising the skin close to the eyelid margin, blunt and sharp dissection are used to free the eyeball.

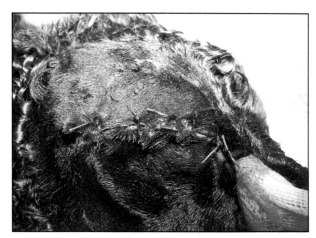

Fig. 13.18 Wound closed, leaving an opening near the medial canthus for drainage. In this case, the orbit was packed with a gauze swab.

Conjunctival pedicle flap

A conjunctival pedicle flap is performed under GA. A club-shaped piece of bulbar conjunctiva is freed (leaving the 'stalk' attached) and secured over the corneal ulcer with multiple single interrupted sutures, using absorbable fine gauge suture material. Ophthalmic instruments and magnifying lenses are required to perform this procedure.

Enucleation

Indication

Any condition where vision is unlikely to be retained or restored or pain remains uncontrolled, including physical trauma (e.g. fighting injury) and non-healing corneal ulceration. Also ocular neoplasia, either as stand-alone treatment or to debulk prior to chemotherapy or radiotherapy.

Preparation and equipment

Preoperative antibiosis (e.g. potentiated penicillin) and a NSAID. The ocular area is clipped and scrubbed. A standard surgical kit is required. A pair of haemostats with right-angle jaws is useful for clamping the optic vessels in the depth of the orbit.

Restraint

Lateral recumbency under light sedation combined with a retrobulbar block or a Petersen plus auriculo-palpebral block (see Chapter 18), or under GA.

Technical description

The transconjunctival approach may be used in goats under GA. More tissue is retained, resulting in a better cosmetic appearance and the procedure is as in dogs or cats. The transpalpebral approach is preferable if the procedure is performed under local anaesthesia, especially if any vision is left in the eye or where neoplasia makes more substantial tissue removal desirable. For this, the eyelids are sutured together with 1–2 horizontal mattress sutures. Using a scalpel blade, the eyelid skin is incised all the way around, as close to the eyelid margin as possible without leaving any cilia behind. The skin is undermined to the level of the bony orbit. Using a combination of blunt and sharp dissection, the eyeball is freed from attaching muscles and connective tissue (**Fig. 13.17**). Care must be taken not to apply excessive traction on the eyeball, as this may traumatise the optic chiasm, leading to blindness in the opposite eye. Equally, excessive inward pressure must be avoided, as this may lead to bradycardia. Once connections have been broken down to the depth of the orbit, a haemostat is applied to the optic nerve and its adjacent blood vessels. The eyeball is removed and the stump ligated. An alternative for haemostasis is to remove the eyeball and pack the cavity with a large single gauze swab or a gauze bandage. Otherwise, packing is not usually required in the goat. The wound edges are closed in a routine manner, leaving a 5–7 mm opening near the medial canthus for drainage (**Fig. 13.18**).

Aftercare

Antibiosis and analgesia are continued for several days and, if necessary, fly repellent applied. If packing was used, this is removed, ideally gradually over several days from 24 hours postoperatively, or all at once after 72 hours. Skin sutures are removed after 10–14 days.

If vision was lost suddenly, the goat should be handled and guided gently until it becomes accustomed to unilateral vision.

Potential complications

Excessive haemorrhage, infection of the orbit and surrounding tissues, fly strike, wound breakdown and, in the case of neoplasia, recurrence. Blindness in the remaining eye if excessive traction was applied to the eyeball during surgery.

SYSTEMIC DISEASES AFFECTING THE EYE

Ocular lesions may be caused by systemic disease. This should be considered in particular where lesions are bilateral and the animal shows, or has a history of, other abnormalities such as pyrexia. There may also be a mix of clinical signs in a group of goats.

Examples include:

- Hypopyon secondary to septicaemia, in particular in neonates.
- Conjunctivitis in conjunction with respiratory tract infection.
- Diseases affecting the ability to blink often lead to a dry eye keratitis (e.g. tetanus, or facial paralysis caused by trauma or listeriosis).
- Injected conjunctivae are often seen with endotoxaemia.
- Hyphaema secondary to bleeding disorders.
- Uveitis caused by *Mycoplasma* spp., *Chlamydophila psittaci*, *Toxoplasma gondii*.

Some systemic causes of true or apparent blindness include:

- Pregnancy toxaemia.
- Cerebrocortical necrosis or polioencephalomalacia.
- Listeriosis.
- Space-occupying lesion such as a brain abscess.
- Brainstem lesions caused by caseous lymphadenitis.
- Neurological disorders of the eye (see Chapter 8).
- Toxicities (e.g. lead).

THE EAR

CLINICAL EXAMINATION OF THE EAR

The ear lobe is examined for any lacerations or other trauma and swellings (e.g. insect sting or haematoma). The skin of the external ear lobe is inspected for any lesions (such as mange, sunburn, necrosis, infection or abscess, lacerations). Of interest on the internal ear lobe are signs of inflammation, crusting or deposits of debris (e.g. wax). Notice is taken of any unusual smell or discharge emanating from the ear canal. A small animal otoscope is used to examine the ear canal, with the head of the goat well restrained.

Also of interest is the position of the ears and their muscular tone. If abnormal, this may indicate a neurological defect, such as facial paralysis, or systemic disease such as tetanus.

NON-INFECTIOUS DISEASE

Ear lacerations

Common causes include trauma from the goat's environment (e.g. barbed wire fencing, protruding nails) and ear tags becoming caught and torn out (**Fig. 13.19**). Typically, these are allowed to heal by secondary intention, after cleaning the wound and administering a course of antimicrobials (e.g. potentiated penicillin) and a NSAID. In show animals, surgical repair to achieve optimum cosmetic results is an option. This is best carried out under GA. After thorough cleaning, the wound edges are freshened up and sutured together using a simple interrupted pattern. The ear is bandaged to the head for 7–10 days.

These lacerations pose a considerable welfare concern, and every care should be taken to reduce their occurrence; for example, by choosing well-fitting ear tags and appropriate types of fencing and removing any injury risks from the environment.

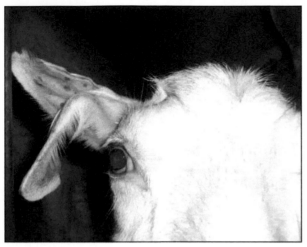

Fig. 13.19 Laceration caused by an ear tag catching in the environment and tearing out.

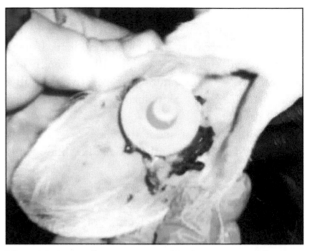

Fig. 13.20 Inflammation and infection around an ear tag.

Tagging injuries

Incorrectly placed ear tags may lead to haemorrhage, infection (**Fig. 13.20**) with potentially secondary fly strike, and chronic inflammation with tissue hyperplasia or distortion ('cauliflower ear'). These problems are entirely avoidable by adopting a good ear tagging technique. Treatment is as for any other acute or chronic injury: pressure or ligation to control haemorrhage, and cleaning, lavage, tissue debridement and antibiosis to deal with infection, combined with a NSAID to address inflammation.

Ear tagging technique

Ears should be visibly clean and dry. Housing the goats for 12–24 hours beforehand facilitates this. Tags are placed into the ventral half of the ear, not more than one-third of the way from the base of the ear, and through the ear cartilage (**Fig. 13.21**). Blood vessels are easily visible and must be avoided. The correct applicator for each particular type of tag must be used. Good head restraint is essential, and periods of fly activity should be avoided.

The male part is always inserted from the back of the ear, and application of an antiseptic or sterile lubricant (e.g. K-Y® Jelly) onto the male part reduces trauma and infection risk. When placing loop tags in kids, the thickness of a pencil is left between the edge of the ear and the tag loop, to allow for growth.

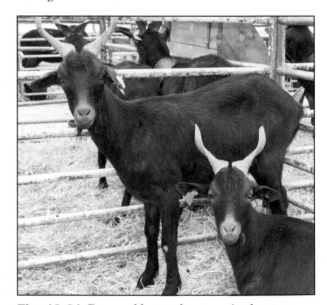

Fig. 13.21 Reasonable tag placement in the goat lying down. The tag in the standing goat has been placed too far away from the ear base, leading to drooping of the ear.

Equally, growth should be allowed for in goatlings. Animals are checked 1 week after application for inflammation or infection, which is dealt with as necessary.

Aural haematoma

Overview

Aural haematoma is typically seen in individual goats.

Aetiology

In most cases caused by irritation of the ear by mange mites (see Otitis, below), grass seeds or other foreign bodies, leading to repeated and forceful headshaking or rubbing. Occasionally caused by direct trauma, including bite wounds.

Clinical presentation

Noticeable swelling of the ear lobe, which is soft and fluctuant on palpation.

Diagnosis

Palpation findings are usually sufficient. Ultrasonography may be used to confirm a haematoma (accumulation of echolucent fluid), as well as a fine needle aspirate (observing strict asepsis; **Fig. 13.22**).

Differential diagnosis

Severe inflammation causing oedema, or ear abscess; the swelling will feel firm and a pain response is likely. Ultrasonography shows echodense tissue swelling or purulent material.

Treatment/management/control

Small haematomas that do not induce further head-shaking typically do not require any treatment. Marked haematomas should be treated to avoid ear lobe distortion caused by fibrosis, and this can be addressed in three ways. For all three ways, a sterile swab is placed into the ear canal prior to

commencing disinfection, and after the procedure the ear is tightly bandaged to the head to prevent movement:

1 Fluid aspiration. A scrupulously aseptic technique is essential. Under mild sedation, the goat's head is restrained well and anaesthetic gel applied to the point of needle entry (internal surface of lobe). A 16 g hypodermic, or 18–20 g butterfly, needle is inserted, the fluid drained and the cavity flushed with sterile saline. In non-pregnant goats, this may be followed by injecting dexamethasone into the cavity (0.2–0.4 mg diluted to about 1 ml total volume, q24h for up to 5 days).
2 Surgical drainage under GA. The serum and any blood clots are removed through either a single incision or multiple smaller incisions. Several mattress sutures (possibly with suture buttons) are placed through the ear lobe, parallel to the lobe edge and any vessels, to reduce any dead space.
3 Cannula drainage. The owner needs to be able to provide good nursing care and a very clean environment for this technique. After drainage and lavage as above, a bovine disposable teat cannula is placed through the incision. The plug-end is positioned to lie distally once the goat is standing. The plug is removed 2–3 times each day to allow drainage. Because of the risk of ascending infection, a course of antibiosis is advisable.

The underlying cause (e.g. ear mites) must be addressed to avoid recurrence.

INFECTIOUS DISEASE

Otitis

Overview

Otitis is possibly less often recognised than in companion animals because the prevailing husbandry of goats limits owner's observations.

Aetiology

In the UK, *Psoroptes ovis* is the main pathogen involved in otitis externa. In other countries, *Raillietia caprae* is commonly found in the ear canal of goats, and

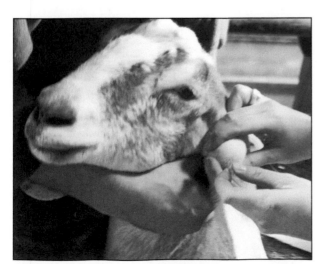

Fig. 13.22 Fine needle aspiration of an ear swelling.

Psoroptes cuniculi has been reported. All age groups may be affected. *Malassezia* spp. are normal commensals, but occasionally cause otitis externa.

Corynebacterium pseudotuberculosis and *Mycoplasma* spp. have been isolated from goats with otitis media.

Clinical presentation

Otitis externa: a large proportion of goats in a group may have subclinical infection. The presence of wax, purulent material, crusts and malodour indicates clinical disease. Headshaking, rubbing against fencing and scratching the ear with the hind leg are commonly seen.

Otitis media or interna: a head tilt towards the affected side and other neurological signs are common, in particular vestibular syndrome or, if infection has spread, signs associated with brainstem lesions or meningoencephalitis.

Diagnosis

Microscopic identification of mites, either from direct ear swabs or ear flushings. Identification of vast numbers of yeasts on tape strips suggests *Malassezia* spp.

Advanced diagnostic imaging is required to confirm otitis media or interna.

Differential diagnosis

For otitis externa: secondary infection after ear trauma. A number of infectious skin diseases can manifest as lesions affecting the ears. These include dermatophilosis, psoroptic mange, sarcoptic mange and ringworm (see Chapter 11).

For otitis media/interna: fascial paralysis and brainstem lesions, and other causes of vestibular syndrome.

Treatment/management/control

For mites, ivermectin is effective (0.2 mg/kg s/c every 7–10 days for 2–3 treatments). Using an acidifying ear flush (e.g. MalAcetic) may be sufficient for *Malassezia*. Otherwise, topical antifungal drugs (e.g. miconazole or clotrimazole), combined with antibiotics and steroids, are indicated, but are not licensed in goats in the UK.

Aggressive systemic antibiosis can be tried for acute otitis media. In non-responsive or chronic cases, the treatment options described for dogs may be considered (myringotomy, bulla osteotomy or total ear canal ablation). If *C. pseudotuberculosis* is involved, deeper CNS structures are often also infected, therefore prognosis is poor.

Ear tip necrosis

Conditions causing severe vasoconstriction or damage to the capillary epithelium may lead to necrosis of the ear tips. Examples include salmonellosis, ergot poisoning, snake venom and frost bite. Once the damage has occurred, it cannot be reversed. However, any secondary bacterial infection should be addressed.

METABOLIC DISORDERS

Hypocalcaemia (syns. milk fever, eclampsia, parturient paresis)

Definition/overview

Unlike dairy cows, in which clinical hypocalcaemia is a relatively common occurrence, true clinical disease is more unusual in periparturient goats, although subclinical manifestation may be more common and can be easily overlooked.

Aetiology

Hypocalcaemia is associated with a decrease in blood calcium levels in the periparturient period (including late pregnancy).

Pathophysiology

Blood calcium levels are kept under tight homeostatic control via parathyroid hormone, 1,25-dihydrocholecalciferol and calcitonin. As kidding becomes imminent, and lactogenesis commences, there is a sudden demand for both calcium and phosphorus. Fetal growth in late pregnancy also increases calcium demands. This is normally offset by an increased absorption of calcium from the intestinal tract or mobilisation from skeletal reserves. If there is any delay in maintaining this homeostasis, hypocalcaemia will develop, with clinical signs being dependent on the degree of hypocalcaemia present.

Clinical presentation

Clinical signs are confined to the periparturient period and initially include a decrease in appetite, lethargy, unsteady gait, muscle tremors (especially of the shoulder muscles), mild bloat and constipation. Uterine inertia may be a feature during parturition. As clinical signs progress, affected goats may become recumbent and unable to rise within a few hours (**Fig. 14.1**). Respiration is often shallow and fast, and the pulse is weak and fast. Mental depression follows, with death within 6–12 hours if not treated.

Secondary hypocalcaemia may also be a feature of some toxaemic conditions such as toxic mastitis or enterotoxaemia.

Diagnosis

Diagnosis is based on the clinical signs, stage of pregnancy, response to treatment and the demonstration of hypocalcaemia (normal reference range 2.3–2.9 mmol/l) in ante- or post-mortem blood. Calcium levels in cerebrospinal fluid (CSF) or vitreous humour can be used in does found dead. Vitreous humour levels reflect plasma iodised calcium, which is about two-thirds of total plasma calcium, and a level <1 mmol/l is suggestive of disease.

Differential diagnosis

Includes pregnancy toxaemia, toxic mastitis, enterotoxaemia, uterine rupture and internal haemorrhage associated with dystocia, metritis and rumen acidosis.

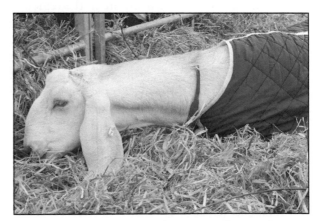

Fig. 14.1 Recumbency and unresponsiveness is seen with hypocalcaemia, but also with pregnancy toxaemia (if the doe is in late pregnancy).

Atypical hypocalcaemia (i.e. outside the periparturient period) may be associated with renal disease.

Treatment/management/control

The condition will usually respond quickly to therapy by slow i/v injection of 50–80 ml 20% calcium borogluconate. Injection must be stopped if cardiac dysrhythmia develops. An additional 100 ml of 20% calcium borogluconate with magnesium mixture is given s/c.

The condition is often clinically indistinguishable from pregnancy toxaemia, and appropriate treatment for this should also be given, if presented with a pregnant doe.

Supplementary milk should be given to any kids until the doe has recovered.

Hypocalcaemia is usually sporadic and unpredictable and as such is still poorly understood. If cases escalate, initial investigation involves identifying any recent underlying stress factors or dietary changes that may be relevant, and noting the diet fed during the dry period. Dietary calcium levels should be kept low (suggested target of 6.6 g/head/day) in the dry period to stimulate bone mobilisation, combined with adequate magnesium and phosphorus levels. To facilitate this, forages with low potassium levels should be considered, such as straw and whole crop or maize silage. Grass (fresh or as hay or silage) from mature older pastures with little manure or potash fertiliser application may also be suitable. During lactation, calcium requirements are in the region of 21 g/head/day for dairy goats. By extrapolation from the dietary management of hypocalcaemia in dairy cows, aiming for a negative cation–anion balance [= (Na + K) - (Cl + S)] by acidifying the dry period diet may be worth considering. Strategic sampling of the herd for calcium levels gives an indication of the risk and presence of subclinical disease.

Hypomagnesaemia (syns. grass tetany, grass staggers)
Definition/overview

Hypomagnesaemia is another relatively rare condition in goats compared with cattle due predominantly to the differences in feeding behaviour (browsing versus grazing). The condition can occur when goats are confined to an area of lush grazing and their normal browsing behaviour is impeded. Reduced feed intake during harsh weather or management procedures can also trigger disease.

Aetiology

Clinical disease is associated with a decrease in blood magnesium levels. It is associated with improved pastures, typically in spring, but also in mild, wet autumns. It may also be seen in goats grazing winter cereals. High dietary levels of potassium and protein, or low levels of calcium, may predispose to the condition.

Pathophysiology

Magnesium is essential for normal neuromuscular function. There is no physiologically relevant storage of magnesium in adult animals, so daily access to magnesium is required. Young animals can store and mobilise magnesium to a degree and are less susceptible.

Clinical presentation

In its classical acute form, the disease will present as hyperexcitability, muscle tremors, incoordination, twitching of facial muscles and rapid ear movement, progressing to recumbency, convulsions and death within 1–4 hours if not treated.

Diagnosis

Diagnosis is based on clinical signs, grazing history and demonstration of low serum magnesium levels in acute cases (normal reference range 0.8–1.3 mmol/l). In a goat found dead, magnesium levels stay stable for 24 hours in aqueous humour, with levels <0.33 mmol/l suggestive of disease in sheep. Levels in vitreous humour stay stable for 48 hours, and <0.65 mmol/l is suggestive of disease. Care must be taken not to aspirate the iris during humour harvest.

Differential diagnosis

Includes lead poisoning and nervous acetonaemia. Also hypocalcaemia, but this progresses less rapidly and hyperaesthesia is rare.

Treatment/management/control

Fifty ml of a 20% calcium borogluconate and magnesium solution is given slowly i/v, plus 100 ml of 25% magnesium sulphate s/c. In advanced cases, i/v magnesium may be required to prevent death. However, this may cause cardiac dysrhythmia and medullary depression leading to respiratory failure, therefore it is a last measure and the client must be warned accordingly. The animal should be in a quiet, dark environment with minimal stimuli. Sedation with xylazine HCl (0.01 mg/kg), butorphanol or barbiturates may be beneficial.

In general terms, if goats are allowed to follow their normal browsing behaviour when outdoors, or are confined on a ration of conserved forage, the condition is unlikely to occur. There are limited data available on dietary magnesium requirements of goats. Supplementation options include: magnesium oxide (7 g daily or 14 g every other day by mouth); a magnesium bolus (lasts about 1 month); foliar spraying, adding to drinking water, or enriched fertiliser. The provision of a simple salt lick may be useful in reducing serum potassium levels, thus stabilising magnesium absorption from the gut. For outdoor animals, turn-out or stress in inclement weather should be avoided, and shelter and supplementary feed considered during harsh weather periods. Strategic sampling of the herd for magnesium levels gives an indication of risk.

Pregnancy toxaemia

Definition/overview

Goats are potentially susceptible to the generic condition referred to as ketosis, either in the last 6 weeks of pregnancy, in which it is referred to as 'pregnancy toxaemia', or during early lactation when it is referred to as 'lactational ketosis' (see later). The condition is most commonly seen in goats carrying multiple fetuses in the last trimester. It tends to be a problem only in goats being managed intensively or overfed as pets, and is rarely encountered in extensive management systems with does carrying a single fetus.

Aetiology

Typically the result of longer-term undernourishment, combined with an acute lack of energy. The pregnant doe roughly requires an additional 80% of her own glucose requirements for every fetus she carries. In late pregnancy, appetite is reduced because of uterine enlargement and reduced rumen capacity. In overfat does, this is exacerbated by body fat laid down in the abdominal cavity – a specific trait in goats. A ration of suitable energy density is therefore required. The acute lack of food intake can be caused by cold inclement weather, inadequate trough space, increased demand due to lack of shelter, gathering for management procedures without provision of feed, sudden change of feed and stress.

Pathophysiology

In late gestation, the liver increases gluconeogenesis to facilitate glucose availability to the fetuses. Where the ration does not provide enough energy, mobilisation of fat stores is increased. If this is excessive, the Kreb's cycle becomes overwhelmed and ketone bodies are formed.

This increased fat mobilisation can progressively overwhelm the liver's capacity and result in hepatic lipidosis (see **Fig. 14.3**) with subsequent impairment of function. The brain is affected by the hypoglycaemia and hyperketonaemia, resulting in an encephalopathy.

Clinical presentation

Clinical signs typically appear from 48 hours after the triggering factor. Inappetence, initially refusing concentrate, rapidly leads to anorexia. The affected goat is lethargic and spends increasing amounts of time lying down. Often finding it difficult to rise in late pregnancy, some does will adopt a dog-sitting posture (**Fig. 14.2**). There is marked weight loss.

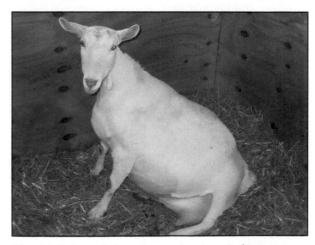

Fig. 14.2 Dog-sitting posture that goats in late pregnancy complicated by pregnancy toxaemia may adopt.

In the advanced stages, nervous signs may develop including apparent blindness, twitching of muzzle and lips, head pressing, coma and death within 2–3 days if untreated. Deterioration may be more rapid if fetal death and putrefaction develops. Affected goats may have an increased susceptibility to prolapses and dystocia, a higher kid mortality and a subsequent poorer lactation.

Diagnosis

The condition should be suspected in late-pregnancy does carrying multiple fetuses showing the clinical signs described. Elevated blood ketone levels, particularly beta-hydroxybutyrate (BHB; normal reference range <1.2 mmol/l), and ketonuria support the diagnosis. Plasma glucose levels are low in early disease, but become more variable in advanced cases. Evidence of renal failure and metabolic acidosis may be seen in advanced or terminal stages. At post-mortem examination, the liver is enlarged with a rounded margin and a yellow–orange discolouration, and the adrenal glands may be enlarged. Due to fat infiltration, small portions of liver may float in water. A BHB level >2.5 mmol/l in aqueous humour or >0.5 mmol/l in CSF supports the diagnosis.

Differential diagnosis

Includes hypocalcaemia, enterotoxaemia and septicaemia or toxaemia secondary to fetal death. If nervous signs have developed, listeriosis, cerebrocortical necrosis and louping ill.

Treatment/management/control

Intervention must be early and aggressive. In the early stages (inappetence only), propylene glycol and other glucose precursor products, given orally and dosing at the manufacturer's recommended dose, can be beneficial. Some commercial products also contain B vitamin complex constituents such as choline, which supports the liver to metabolise and clear mobilised fat. It is important to entice the goat to eat by offering good quality hay, green forages, herbal and non-toxic leaves, palatable concentrates (e.g. sugar beet pulp, maize flakes) and potentially sprinkling molasses onto feeds.

More severe cases that refuse to feed or have become recumbent benefit from i/v glucose (100 ml of 40% glucose or 50% dextrose), plus B vitamins, oral propylene glycol and good quality feed. Administration of oral electrolyte solutions (alkaline and containing bicarbonate or bicarbonate precursors) has been found beneficial in ewes. In valuable goats, i/v fluids should be considered. Hypocalcaemia is often clinically indistinguishable and may be present concurrently, therefore calcium borogluconate should be given. Insulin has been used (20–40 units of zinc protamine insulin i/m twice 48 hours apart). Bovine somatotropin has been used successfully, but is not commercially available in the UK. Anabolic steroids are banned in the UK.

Induction of parturition, with or without subsequent caesarean section, should be considered to stop the glucose drain by the fetuses, but must be done early in the course of the disease to have any value. If the fetuses are still alive, dexamethasone is the drug of choice: it stimulates lung surfactant and gluconeogenesis. Otherwise, prostaglandin-F 2 alpha is given. Kids more than 1 week preterm have a low chance of survival, but the dam's life may be saved.

Prognosis is guarded. Inability to stand, continued disinterest in food and rising blood urea levels indicate poor prognosis.

Prevention is based on the following:

- Develop a planned breeding programme, such that individual kidding dates are known and dry goat feeding can be planned accordingly.
- Use regular body condition scoring (see Chapter 1). (**Note:** Weight loss in overfat animals must never be attempted in the last trimester of pregnancy.)
- Scan for number of fetuses and feed accordingly. Manage doelings and adult goats separately and allow for continued growths in doelings when calculating rations.
- During the early dry period, feed a ration of low energy density *ad libitum* to maintain maximum rumen capacity without overfeeding.

- Increase energy density of the ration in the last 6–8 weeks of pregnancy to allow for fetal demands and reduced dry matter intake.
- Provide adequate trough space and always have feed available and easily accessible. For outdoor goats, provide shelter to decrease energy demands for thermoregulation.
- Periodically monitor energy status in the dry doe group with a metabolic profile (BHB, non-esterified fatty acids, triglyceride, glucose levels).

Lactational ketosis (syn. acetonaemia) and fatty liver complex

Definition/overview

Lactational ketosis can be a problem in does bred for high milk production, developing in the first few weeks post kidding. In severe cases, fatty liver infiltration (**Fig. 14.3**) can be substantial, resulting in profound liver damage.

Aetiology/ pathophysiology

Most does, particularly those bred for high milk yields, suffer a mild acetonaemia in early lactation. The increase in dry matter intake lags behind increase in milk yield (and with it energy demand) until about 6–8 weeks post kidding, resulting in a negative energy balance (NEB) in early lactation. This inevitably results in fat mobilisation which, if excessive, can lead to fatty infiltration and degenerative liver change. Overfat does may show a marked drop in appetite post kidding, and are therefore particularly at risk. This scenario is referred to as primary ketosis. Secondary ketosis occurs when some underlying condition, such as lameness or mastitis, suppresses appetite, resulting in a NEB and triggering fat mobilisation.

Clinical presentation

Inappetence, leading to complete anorexia as the condition develops. Affected goats may be ataxic, develop gastrointestinal atony and constipation, and the milk yield will be reduced. The nervous form presents with neurological signs such as blindness, head pressing, sham-chewing and convulsions. Concurrent hypocalcaemia or hypomagnesaemia may also be a feature.

Diagnosis

Diagnosis is based on the clinical signs and stage of lactation. Ketones may be detected on the goat's breath. Blood samples will demonstrate high levels of ketones and BHB, and low glucose with evidence of liver damage (raised GLDH, AST, gGT and bile acids). Ketonuria is present.

Differential diagnosis

Other causes of weight loss and reduced milk yield should be eliminated, such as parasitic gastroenteritis, fluke, haemonchosis and Johne's disease. For reduced appetite, also mastitis and urogenital tract infection.

Treatment/management/control

Treatment follows the principles outlined under pregnancy toxaemia earlier in this chapter. Prevention is based on ensuring goats do not kid down in overfat condition and paying attention to feeding in the dry, transitional and early lactation period. The aim during the dry period is to keep rumen capacity and dry matter intake at its maximum (adjusting energy density in the early dry period to avoid excessive weight gain). Three weeks prior to kidding, the components of the lactational diet should be introduced to allow rumen microbes to adjust. After kidding, steps to increase dry matter intake include: feeding best quality forage available (e.g. first cut silage), providing sufficient trough space, reducing competition and bullying,

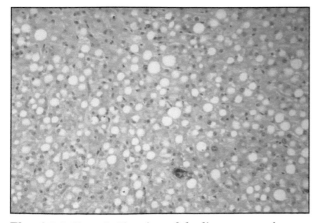

Fig. 14.3 Fatty infiltration of the liver as seen in advanced pregnancy toxaemia/hepatic lipidosis.

removing stale feed at least every 24 hours, ensuring easy access to feed including regularly pushing feed up, preventing rumen acidosis (e.g. by feeding a total mixed ration) and monitoring actual feed intake (**Figs. 14.4, 14.5**).

Metabolic acidosis

Resulting from a primary rumen acidosis, systemic metabolic acidosis can result in lethargy, anorexia, abdominal pain and teeth grinding, subnormal temperature, a fast weak pulse and death if untreated. (See Chapter 5.)

Floppy kid syndrome

Floppy kid syndrome is a metabolic acidosis without diarrhoea or dehydration, affecting kids typically between 7 and 14 days of life (range 3 days to 4 weeks). Herd morbidity of between 30 and 50% is most commonly reported, although in outbreaks described in North America morbidity did approach 100%. Mortality in unrecognised and untreated outbreaks can be high. (See Chapter 4.)

Swelling disease in Angora goats
(See Chapter 7.)

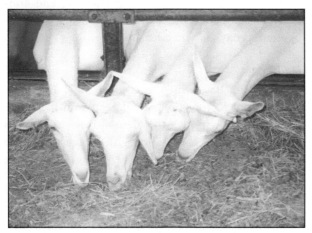

Fig. 14.4 Feed management to maximise dry matter intake could be improved in this herd. The ration is not provided truly *ad libitum*, with obvious competition. Sorting of the total mixed ration has taken place (although this cannot always be avoided with goats); the goats cannot easily reach because of the high feed barrier and feed not being pushed up regularly. A positive aspect is the use of a feed platform (versus troughs), making removal of stale or leftover feed easy for farm staff.

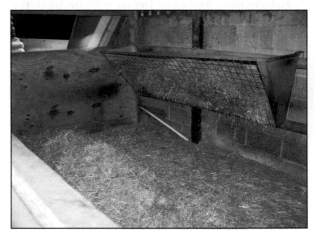

Fig. 14.5 A poorly positioned hayrack. Being at the back of the pen makes access difficult for staff. In this case, this had led to stale and partially mouldy hay being present.

TRACE ELEMENT AND VITAMIN DISORDERS

TRACE ELEMENTS

In goats, copper, selenium, cobalt, iodine and zinc have all been associated with deficiency disorders affecting health and productivity. Deficiencies are more likely to be encountered in grazing goats, goats fed forage only diets or goats fed home grown feed products – all in the absence of any mineral or trace element supplementation (**Fig. 15.1**). Deficiencies are far less likely in goats fed a balanced ration, including commercial feeds such as concentrates. The browsing behaviour of goats, leading to consumption of not only herbage but also mature plants, shrubs and trees, may make them less susceptible to deficiency than grazing cattle and sheep.

The potential for deficiency-related clinical signs to develop will depend on the duration and degree of inadequate mineral intake. There are four stages that occur in the progression from inadequate intake to the development of clinical disease:

1 Depletion. There is loss of mineral from storage sites such as the liver, but levels in the circulating blood are within the reference interval.
2 Deficiency. During this phase, the circulating blood levels fall.
3 Dysfunction. As levels continue to fall, trace element-dependent enzyme systems involved in metabolism begin to fail and body functions become impaired. At this stage the goat will be showing no clinical signs.
4 Disease. The metabolic dysfunction gradually leads to detectable clinical abnormalities.

Mineral deficiencies can either be primary and associated simply with an insufficient supply in the diet, or secondary, when the dietary level is adequate but other factors limit availability and uptake. There are marked geographical differences within each country in soil and herbage trace element availability. In some areas outright deficiencies may be the significant feature, in others it is an excess of antagonistic inhibitors (such as other trace elements) that causes the problem. The animals' drinking water as a source of such antagonists must be considered (e.g. water sulphate levels above 500 ppm are thought to cause meaningful interference).

For supplementation, the following general aspects are of interest. The organic form of minerals (complexed chelates) generally has the highest bioavailability. Free access minerals (mineral licks, mineral buckets; **Fig. 15.2**) are convenient, but have the disadvantage that intake is voluntary, such that some individual goats may consume an excessive (and potentially toxic) amount, whereas others may

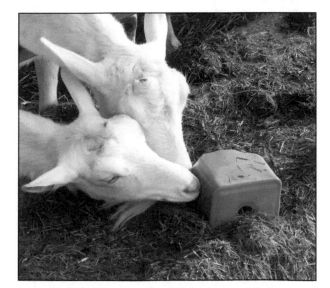

Fig. 15.1 Rock salt and salt licks are useful dietary additions, but are no substitute for a balanced mineral and vitamin supplement.

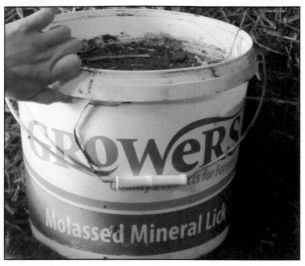

Fig. 15.2 Self-help mineral licks are convenient for the stockperson, but intake can be highly variable from goat to goat.

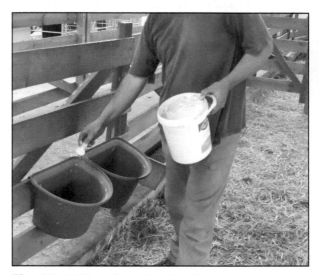

Fig. 15.3 Mineral powder should not just be sprinkled onto feed; because of the bitter taste, animals will sort and avoid.

take nothing. Minerals typically have a bitter taste and animals will avoid eating them if they can. To overcome this and make the mineral powder stick and prevent sorting, top-dressing of pasture should be done while it is still wet with dew. If a mineral mix is to be added directly to a feed, the feed itself must be moist or be molassed (**Fig. 15.3**).

When supplementing via the drinking water, there must be no alternative source of water and animals must be monitored for sufficient intake.

Copper deficiency

Definition/overview

Both primary and secondary copper deficiency can occur. A number of differing clinical presentations have been attributed wholly or in part to copper deficiency in older goats, but many remain unproven. Angoras and other fibre breeds appear to be more susceptible than dairy breeds.

Aetiology

Simple copper deficiency due to lack in the goat's diet can occur, but the majority of cases are secondary and linked to copper uptake antagonists. The predominant ones are molybdenum, sulphur and iron. Molybdenum, for example, reacts with sulphur in the rumen to form thiomolybdate, which irreversibly binds copper and prevents its absorption.

Pathophysiology

Once absorbed, the liver is the main storage site of body copper reserves. The majority of circulating copper is bound to the acute phase protein ceruloplasmin. Other circulating copper is bound to erythrocytes, and the remainder is free albumin-bound copper. Clinical signs of copper deficiency will only occur after liver stores have been exhausted. Blood copper levels begin to fall, followed by a gradual reduction of available copper in body tissues. Copper plays an essential role in a number of metabolic and developmental functions, but is specifically involved in myelination, osteogenesis, haematopoiesis, hair pigmentation and daily growth, thus defining the main clinical presentations.

Clinical presentation

Deficiency during fetal development can lead to congenital swayback in newborn kids or delayed swayback developing between 1 week and several months after birth (**Fig. 15.4**). In the congenital form, kids are abnormal at birth, with weakness and in most an inability to rise. Fine muscle tremors, abnormal head movements and vocalisation are features. Signs secondary to the inability to nurse properly may develop. In the delayed form, sometimes referred to as enzootic ataxia, kids are born normally, but develop a progressive paresis that

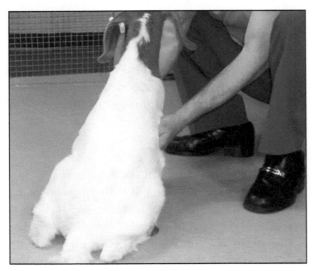

Fig. 15.4 Delayed swayback in a 4-week-old Boer kid.

may vary in onset from 1 week to several months after birth, and from days to weeks in progression. Paresis and ataxia are usually noticed in the hind legs first, and are always bilateral. Affected kids can initially support their weight, but slowly become paralysed. Some may adopt a dog-sitting position or drag themselves along with their front legs.

Other clinical signs in an affected herd are less well defined, but may involve various age groups and include ill thrift, anaemia, loss of hair pigmentation (often visible around the eyes), poor fibre quality, diarrhoea, osteoporosis and spontaneous bone fractures (although these skeletal abnormalities are complex and often involve many other co-existing mineral or metabolic abnormalities). The extent of copper deficiency-induced progressive ataxia and subfertility, as reported in other species, is unclear in goats.

Diagnosis

The time of onset and clinical signs exhibited are fairly characteristic of swayback. A blood copper assay may be useful, although this can be within the reference interval, even in confirmed cases, if supplementation has been given after the myelin damage has occurred. Liver copper assay at post-mortem examination (PME), coupled with the characteristic gross pathology of cerebral cavitation and histological evidence of myelin abnormalities of the

central nervous system, will confirm the diagnosis. Herd copper status is best determined by liver assay, either from cull or dead goats, or by liver biopsy (see Chapter 5). Blood sampling a minimum of six goats is an alternative, but results must be interpreted with caution. Subnormal levels indicate deficiency, but normal levels may represent anything from depleted to adequate to toxic status (as the body will aim to keep blood levels stable). Diagnostic laboratories may employ a variety of test procedures for blood copper assay, each with the aim of identifying total blood copper and the percentage of available copper. Interpretation of results should always be based on each laboratory's own reference interval.

Differential diagnosis

For congenital swayback includes hydrocephalus, border disease, hypoglycaemia and hypothermia. For delayed swayback consider spinal abscess, vertebral trauma, muscular dystrophy, caprine arthritis encephalitis (CAE), floppy kid syndrome and listeriosis.

Treatment/management/control

Although goats are susceptible to copper deficiency, it is important to emphasise that they are also susceptible to a dietary excess leading to copper toxicity (see Chapter 16). Therefore, the decision to supplement should always be based on liver assay results. If deemed necessary, there are a variety of commercially available copper supplements, including injectable preparations, such as calcium copper edetate, and oral products such as copper oxide in gelatine capsules or soluble glass boluses containing copper, for slow release. Products should indicate that they are 'suitable for sheep or goats'.

Management of both congenital and delayed swayback cases is focussed on nursing; however, prognosis is very guarded as demyelination occurred *in utero* and response to copper administration is often poor. Newborn kids may need artificial feeding if they are unable to suckle. In the delayed form, ensuring easy or assisted access at all times to feed and water is paramount. Prevention relies on sufficient copper levels in the pregnant doe. A dietary copper level of 8 mg/kg dry matter total ration has been suggested for goats. Copper supplemented compound feeds are available, some of which may need veterinary prescribing.

Selenium/tocopherol (vitamin E) deficiency (syns. nutritional muscular dystrophy, white muscle disease)

Aetiology

Selenium deficiency can occur where goats are on selenium deficient pasture or fed a diet grown on selenium deficient soil, without supplementation. Tocopherol (vitamin E) is synthesised by plants and levels are typically more than adequate in green pasture and conserved forages (**Fig. 15.5**). As a result, tocopherol deficiency tends to occur in goats that are housed and fed poor quality forage such as straw or poorly conserved grass products, with inadequate supplementation. There is considerable overlap between selenium and tocopherol deficiency; clinical signs are largely similar and a dietary excess of one can compensate for a dietary deficiency of the other.

Pathophysiology

During selenium and/or tocopherol deficiency, a failure to protect against cell damage leads to cell membrane damage and cell necrosis. Cells with the highest rate of oxidative metabolism are most susceptible to damage, particularly in skeletal, cardiac and respiratory musculature.

Selenium deficiency has also been shown to have an adverse effect on caprine neutrophil function, which may impact on an immune response to concurrent disease.

Clinical presentation

The predominant clinical presentation of selenium/tocopherol deficiency is white muscle disease (syn. nutritional muscular dystrophy). It is most commonly seen in growing kids, from a few days to 6 months of age. Clinical signs can present in a number of ways, depending on the muscle group(s) affected and the severity of the insult, and in a clinical outbreak, many differing manifestations may be seen. Some kids may simply be found dead due to damage to cardiac muscle. Others may be found recumbent and unable to rise or displaying a stiff legged gait. They are usually alert and aware of their surroundings and will often vocalise. If there is severe muscle damage, myoglobinuria may be present. The immediate history may identify a sudden period of activity as an initiating factor, such as turnout, being driven or transported. Other clinical signs may include dyspnoea, coughing and signs of pulmonary oedema if the cardiac muscle or diaphragm is involved. Stillborn kids may be born to deficient dams. The role of selenium deficiency in retained fetal membrane or cystic ovarian disease in ruminants remains debatable.

Diagnosis

The clinical signs and recent history of increased exercise are highly suspicious. For selenium deficiency, the standard confirmatory laboratory test is measurement of blood glutathione peroxidase (GSH-Px; a selenium containing enzyme). As erythrocyte GSH-Px levels depend on selenium concentrations during erythropoiesis, any GSH-Px result indicates the selenium status 2–4 months ago. In clinical outbreaks, the GSH-Px and tocopherol levels are usually both low. Blood levels of the muscle specific enzyme creatinine kinase are often markedly elevated (>20,000 IU/ml) and can be used to establish the degree of muscle damage.

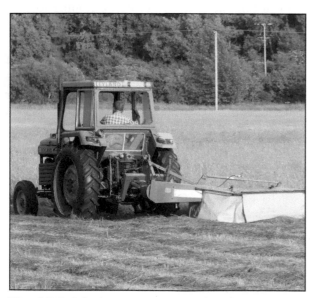

Fig. 15.5 Selenium content of fresh and conserved grass depends on soil levels. Tocopherol content depends on good harvesting and conservation technique.

At PME, in the cardiac form there will be evidence of white to grey discolouration of the myocardial tissue extending into deeper tissue (**Fig. 15.6**). This is often accompanied by evidence of congestive heart failure such as ascites, hydrothorax, pericardial effusion, pulmonary oedema and a swollen liver. The main muscle masses affected are those of the legs, but a detailed examination of diaphragm and intercostal muscles should be undertaken. In affected muscles, changes are usually bilateral and normally present as pale or chalky changes within the muscle belly and areas of haemorrhage alongside unchanged muscle tissue (**Fig. 15.7**). Confirmation can be undertaken by histological examination of affected muscle tissue (showing a hyaline degenerative change), coupled with assay of liver selenium and tocopherol levels, or by blood sampling live cohort goats.

Differential diagnosis
Other causes of recumbency include trauma, delayed swayback, the neurological presentation of CAE and floppy kid syndrome. Sudden death in young kids can occur as a result of colisepticaemia, enterotoxaemia, congenital cardiac abnormalities, trauma or misadventure.

Treatment/management/control
Treatment success depends on the severity of any muscle damage that has occurred. In the early stages, the parenteral administration of a proprietary selenium and tocopherol combi-preparation can result in an improvement over a 24-hour period. Nursing is essential for more severely affected kids, ensuring that they have access to adequate feed and water, and that they are on a surface (e.g. a straw bedded area) that will reduce the risk of pressure necrosis if recumbent. Goats that fail to respond after 48 hours carry a guarded prognosis. Control is based on adequate selenium and tocopherol supplementation, particularly in those units on which the condition has been encountered previously and in pregnant does during the later stages of pregnancy. This can be either via in-feed trace element and vitamin supplementation or by the strategic administration of proprietary oral or injectable supplements. Long term, incorporating selenium into fertiliser prills is the most economical way, and for tocopherol ensuring good grass harvesting and conservation methods.

Cobalt deficiency
Definition/overview
Cobalt deficiency is reported in ruminants worldwide, being a particular problem in sheep and, to a lesser extent, in goats. Cobalt is a component of cyanocobalamin (vitamin B12), which is synthesised by the rumen microflora. This production cycle is reduced if the supply of cobalt is deficient, resulting in cyanocobalamin deficiency.

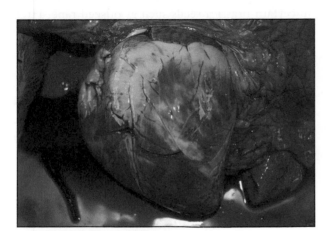

Fig. 15.6 White muscle disease (muscular dystrophy) changes in myocardial tissue (specimen: calf). (© Crown Copyright 2017. Used with kind permission of the Animal and Plant Health Agency.)

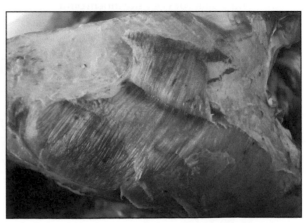

Fig. 15.7 White muscle disease (muscular dystrophy) changes in upper hind leg musculature (specimen: calf). (© Crown Copyright 2017. Used with kind permission of the Animal and Plant Health Agency.)

Aetiology

Cyanocobalamin itself is required as a co-enzyme to methylmalonyl-CoA mutase in the metabolic pathways associated with the Krebs cycle, resulting in the non-specific clinical signs described below. One further specific manifestation of cobalt deficiency is 'ovine white liver disease' (OWLD), which is occasionally reported in goats.

Pathophysiology

OWLD is an indirect sequela to cobalt/cyanocobalamin deficiency, as the dependent co-enzyme deficiency reduces the goat's ability to convert propionic acid to glucose via succinate in the liver. This leads to a build-up of methylmalonyl-CoA, which in turn is converted to branched-chain fatty acids that accumulate in hepatocytes, causing the characteristic pale, swollen and friable fatty liver.

Clinical presentation

The clinical signs with both uncomplicated cobalt deficiency and OWLD are non-specific and include chronic ill thrift or poor growth rates, anaemia, submandibular oedema, reduced milk production, and poor coat quality in fibre goats.

Diagnosis

In live goats, cobalt deficiency is confirmed by serum cyanocobalamin (vitamin B12) assay. Other clinical pathology features include hypoalbuminaemia and a macrocytic, normochromic anaemia. At PME, carcases are pale and in poor or emaciated condition. In OWLD, the liver shows widespread fatty change confirmed by histopathological examination and liver cyanocobalamin assay.

Differential diagnosis

There are many causes of ill thrift and anaemia to consider including parasitic gastroenteritis, haemonchosis, liver fluke, Johne's disease, insufficient dietary protein or energy and poor weaning management.

Treatment/management/control

Treatment is by oral or injectable preparations containing cyanocobalamin or cobalt. Long-term prevention in known deficient areas is based on the use of slow release, sheep-sized rumen boluses (often containing other trace elements, therefore take care to avoid oversupplementation) or providing additional cobalt in the ration. Daily cobalt requirements of 0.25–0.4 mg per adult goat have been suggested.

Iodine deficiency
(See also Chapter 4.)

Definition/overview

Iodine deficiency is a worldwide problem that leads to the development of an enlarged thyroid gland at birth: congenital goitre. This must be distinguished from thymic enlargement (see Chapter 7), which can also cause throat swelling in young kids. A deficiency of circulating iodine in pregnant does may result in abortion, stillbirth or the birth of weak kids. There may be a breed susceptibility to the condition in, for example, Boer and Angora goats.

Aetiology

Primary deficiency can be caused by a straightforward shortage of iodine in the diet or feedstuff grown in iodine deficient geographical regions. Secondary iodine deficiency is linked to the feeding of plants that contain goitrogens, or compounds that interfere with the uptake of iodine from the diet or with its metabolism in the formation of thyroxine. Plants of the Brassica family, including rape and kale, contain the goitrogen thiocyanate, and thiouracil is found in certain brassica seeds such as oilseed rape. High levels of calcium in drinking water may also reduce iodine uptake.

Pathophysiology

Iodine is essential as a constituent of the thyroid hormones T3 (triiodothyronine) and T4 (thyroxine). Approximately 80% of the body's iodine is found in the thyroid gland.

Clinical presentation

In severe congenital goitre, the thyroid gland may be palpable in the upper part of the neck overlying the larynx. Affected kids are typically stillborn or born weak and premature, resulting in unwillingness to stand and suckle. Blindness has occasionally been reported, as well as coat thinning. Some affected kids, however, may show very few clinical signs. In adults reproductive performance may be decreased, including abortion.

Diagnosis

In live goats, T4 levels reflect the thyroid and overall iodine status, and can be very high in kids affected with congenital goitre. Plasma inorganic iodine measures short-term daily iodine intake, and is thus susceptible to sudden changes in dietary intake. The two tests used in tandem can be useful in herd investigations. At PME, the thyroid gland may be visibly enlarged and should be dissected free from any fat and connective tissue and weighed. The normal goat kid thyroid weight is around 2 grams (in cattle, the figure quoted is 0.03% of total calf weight). Thyroid total iodine concentration (<1,200 mg/kg dry matter of tissue indicates a deficiency) and histological evidence of thyroid hyperplasia confirms the diagnosis.

Differential diagnosis

Other causes of stillbirth (such as dystocia) and weak or premature neonates (including abortive agents).

Treatment/management/control

Treatment of clinically affected kids is typically unrewarding. However, prompt supplementation of does still pregnant should be started.

Management is based at ensuring a regular daily intake of iodine in those areas or on those units in which there is a known deficiency. This can be achieved by a number of methods, including intraruminal sheep-sized boluses, iodised salt licks (care: intakes can be more haphazard) and top dressing feed or pasture with iodised salts (potassium or sodium iodide). For individual pregnant goats, potassium iodide can be given 2 months and 2 weeks prior to kidding at a dose rate of 10 ml/20 kg BW of a mixture containing 20 g in one litre of water. There is a lack of information on whether painting tincture of iodine onto pregnant does is as effective as it is in cattle (the animal licking off the iodine during grooming).

Zinc deficiency

See Chapter 11.

VITAMINS

The four stages leading to clinical signs of deficiency outlined at the start of this chapter can also be applied to vitamin deficiency.

Retinol (vitamin A) deficiency

Definition/overview

True retinol deficiency is not commonly reported in goats, but has been linked experimentally to a range of non-specific clinical signs.

Aetiology

The dietary precursor to retinol is beta-carotene, which is usually abundant in green leaved plants and grasses and well preserved and stored forages. Deficiencies are most likely to occur in arid or semi-arid locations where green grazing is limited, or when goats are supplemented with poor old forage or with mostly cereal grains (which are low in carotene). Colostrum is a rich source of retinol, so deficiencies are unlikely to occur until animals are older (unless colostrum deprived).

Clinical presentation

Inappetence, weight loss and a general unthrifty appearance have been linked experimentally to deficiency. The retinal degeneration-associated blindness recognised in calves is not considered to be a problem in goats.

Diagnosis

Feeding evaluation and history, and by serum or liver retinol assay.

Differential diagnosis

Signs are non-specific, and other causes should be considered before retinol deficiency is incriminated.

Treatment/management/control

Deficiency should not occur in goats fed a well-balanced ration based on good quality forage. Dietary supplementation may be employed if deficiency is identified.

Thiamine (vitamin B1) deficiency

See Chapter 8 under Cerebrocortical necrosis.

Cyanocobalamin (vitamin B12) deficiency

See Cobalt above.

Calciferol (vitamin D) deficiency

See Chapter 9 (Rickets and Osteodystrophy of mature bone).

Tocopherol (vitamin E) deficiency

See under Selenium above. Swelling disease of Angora goats has been linked to this deficiency (see Chapter 7).

CHAPTER 16

POISONING AND TOXICITIES

INTRODUCTION

Due to their browsing and naturally inquisitive behaviour, goats could consume a wide variety of potentially toxic plants, shrubs and trees present in their environment. However, they can apparently ingest small quantities of such material without any ill effects. This may be due to their browsing activity (avoiding ingestion of large quantities by moving from one food source to another) and to the 'protective' environment in the rumen. Goats may also have evolved and developed a natural tolerance, although this is unproven. A hungry goat confined to an area of limited grazing with toxic plant material present is most at risk. Care must also be taken to avoid incorporation of poisonous plants into conserved forages, which may mask any disagreeable taste and/or prevent the animal from avoiding the material (**Fig. 16.1**).

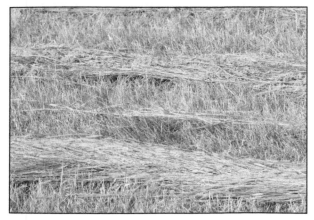

Fig. 16.1 **Ragwort is a classic example of harmful inclusion in hay. The fresh plant is bitter and typically avoided by animals. However, drying makes the plant sweet tasting.**

Poisoning can also occur after ingestion of a range of chemical agents found in their environment or used therapeutically or prophylactically, including excess dietary minerals and some pharmacological products. Poisonous gases that are potentially present in the goat's environment include nitrous fumes from silage clamps and carbon monoxide or dioxide. The burning of poisonous plants can produce toxic fumes, for example oleander.

GENERAL APPROACH

The difficulty when dealing with a suspected poisoning lies in having to consider the vast number of potential toxins while being faced with the urgency to start specific treatment. The four cornerstones of the investigation are circumstantial evidence (toxin present and signs of ingestion), considering all clinical signs both in the patient and the rest of the group, clinical pathology, and post-mortem examination (PME) (*Tables 16.1–16.4*). Useful samples for toxin isolation include feed, blood, urine, stomach contents, hair, bone, aqueous or vitreous humour, and liver and kidney tissue (obtained by biopsy in the live patient).

Treatment concepts include removing the goat from its current environment and feed source to limit further exposure. Elimination of the toxin may be hastened by the use of purgatives or diuresis. Further toxin absorption may be reduced by force-feeding fibre, energy and proteins, or by rumenotomy. Initial treatment is symptomatic and supportive (e.g. fluid therapy, sedation, respiratory support) until identification of the toxin allows the use of the specific antidote where one is available.

The Veterinary Poisons Information Service offers worldwide 24-hour emergency advice on a subscription basis.

Table 16.1 Abnormal urine colour.

POISON	COLOUR	MECHANISM	COMMENTS
Chlorate, copper, kale, rape	Pink (on standing) Dark brown (freshly collected/voided urine)	Haemoglobinuria	Due to excess haemolysis; prehepatic or haemolytic jaundice
Phenols, creosote	Dark green		Differential diagnosis: bilirubin in standing sample
Chlorate, bracken fern, lupins	Pink	Haematuria	Kidney/renal tract damage
Phenothiazine	Red		On exposure to air
Acorns	Black brown		
Phenacetin, aromatic nitro compounds	Bright yellow	Excretion of metabolites	
Hepatotoxins	Red–gold colour of froth on shaking	Biliuria	Excessive excretion due to obstructive or hepatic jaundice

Table 16.2 Abnormal blood colour.

POISON	COLOUR	MECHANISM
Nitrate/nitrite, copper, sodium chlorate	Chocolate brown	Methaemoglobin
Nitrous fumes (e.g. silage clamp)	Light brown	Methaemoglobin
Cyanide	Cherry red	Cytochrome oxidase inhibition
Carbon monoxide	Bright red	Co-haemoglobin
Carbon dioxide	Dark red	Displaced oxygen

Table 16.3 Abnormal breath smell.

POISON	SMELL
Hydrogen cyanide, zinc phosphate, arsenic	Bitter almonds
Phosphorus (elementary)	Smokey/choking

Table 16.4 Abnormal stomach contents.

POISON	COLOUR
Copper sulphate	Green/blue
Chromic compounds	Yellow, orange or green
Acids or alkalis (corrosion of mucosa)	Black

Tables 16.1–16.4 from Bruère AN, Cooper BS, Dillon EA (1990) *Veterinary Clinical Toxicology*. Veterinary Continuing Education, Palmerston North, New Zealand.

COMMON POISONS AND TOXINS

Genus *Rhododendron*

Definition/overview

The genus *Rhododendron* includes rhododendrons (**Fig. 16.2**), azaleas and pieris, all of which are wild or ornamental shrubs found worldwide.

Aetiology

These plants, and others in the Ericaceae family such as laurel, contain the toxic principle grayanotoxin (or andromedotoxin). Ingestion may occur directly from browsing on the shrub itself or from inadvertent access to discarded prunings and clippings. Clinical signs may occur after the ingestion of as little as 0.1% of the goat's body weight in fresh leaves.

Pathophysiology

Grayanotoxin can act directly on the autonomic nervous system, and specifically the vomiting centre in the brain via the vagus nerve.

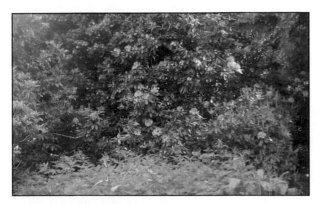

Fig. 16.2 **Rhododendron bushes.**

Clinical presentation

Initial signs include depression, salivation and abdominal pain, with projectile regurgitation (or vomiting) of rumen contents. The consumption of large quantities of plant material may result in rapid deterioration and death. Aspiration of regurgitated contents may lead to pneumonia in recovering goats.

Diagnosis

Clinical signs are characteristic. Leaves or leaf fragments (**Fig. 16.3**) may be present in regurgitated contents or in rumen contents at PME.

Differential diagnosis

Vomiting in goats is unusual, and poisoning with plants from this genus should always be considered first, particularly if they are present in the environment.

Treatment/management/control

If ingestion of a significant amount has occurred, a prompt rumenotomy may be considered (see Chapter 5), removing as much of the leaf debris as possible. Supportive therapy includes oral and/or i/v fluids and an oral activated charcoal suspension, or products such as magnesium hydroxide to reduce rumen toxin absorption. Spasmolytic agents such as butylscopolamine bromide (Buscopan®) may control vomiting. Parenteral antibiotic cover should be given to counteract aspiration pneumonia.

Yew

Definition/overview

Yew (*Taxus* spp.) is found as wild and as ornamental trees worldwide, often growing in churchyards

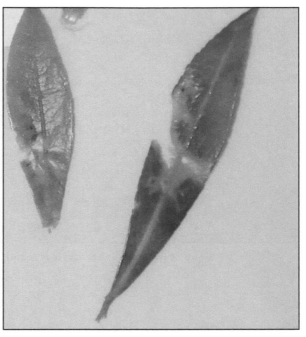

Fig. 16.3 **Rhododendron leaves found in the rumen of a poisoned goat at post-mortem examination.**

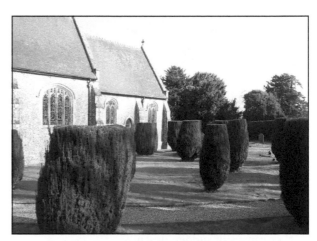

Fig. 16.4 **Yew trees (*Taxus baccata*) in an English churchyard, clipped into ornamental shapes as is common practice. Clippings must be disposed of away from livestock.**

in the UK (**Figs. 16.4, 16.5**). Although it is a common cause of poisoning in other ruminants, it is only occasionally reported in goats.

Aetiology

Most parts of the plant are potentially toxic, containing the cyanogenic glycoside taxine. Goats may eat

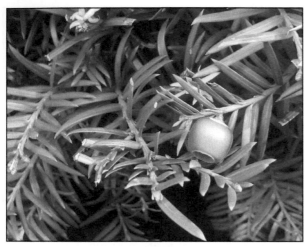

Fig. 16.5 **Close up of yew (*Taxus baccata*) leaves and berry.**

the leaves or branches from the tree, or consume discarded prunings.

Pathophysiology
Taxine is a recognised cardiotoxin, ingestion of a lethal dose causing heart failure and death. Only a very small amount of leaves (about 100) may be required to kill a goat.

Clinical presentation
Affected goats may simply be found dead, often with fragments of yew in their mouth and yew foliage in the vicinity. If still alive, they are profoundly dull with marked cardiac arrhythmia and bradycardia. Yew fragments may be identified in rumen contents.

Differential diagnosis
Other causes of sudden death.

Treatment/management/control
There is no specific antidote. If found alive and poisoning is suspected, a very prompt rumenotomy may be of benefit (see Chapter 5), together with supportive fluid therapy, oral activated charcoal and atropine sulphate for bradycardia.

Other plants, trees and shrubs potentially toxic to goats
See *Table 16.5*.

Oxalate poisoning
Definition/overview
Goats, like other ruminants, are potentially susceptible to poisoning if they eat excessive amounts of oxalate containing plants. Toxicity can also develop following the inadvertent consumption of ethylene glycol.

Aetiology
Oxalate containing plants include sorrel, docks, sugar beet and mangold tops, rhubarb leaves, pigweed, kikuya grass, spinach and chard. Ethylene glycol is a constituent of vehicle antifreeze and degrades to oxalates in the rumen if consumed because of its sweet taste. It appears that goats have an innate ability to degrade and detoxify oxalates in rumen contents compared with other ruminants, therefore typically a large amount needs to be consumed in a short period of time.

Pathophysiology
Oxalates that bypass the rumen and enter the bloodstream combine with calcium ions to produce calcium oxalate, thus resulting in a progressive hypocalcaemia. Calcium oxalate is insoluble, leading to crystal formation mainly in the renal tubules, causing severe renal insufficiency.

Clinical presentation
Generally acute, with the hypocalcaemia resulting in incoordination, muscular trembling and hyperexcitability, followed within hours by profound depression, coma and death if untreated.

Diagnosis
Diagnosis is based on a history of exposure to potentially toxic material, the clinical signs exhibited and laboratory evidence of hypocalcaemia and renal insufficiency in live goats. Crystals may be evident in urine. At PME, plant material may be evident in rumen contents and the kidneys will be enlarged and oedematous with characteristic histopathological changes.

Differential diagnosis
Includes predominantly primary hypocalcaemia, hypomagnesaemia and other causes of a neurological disorder with a sudden onset such as enterotoxaemia, listeriosis, cerebrocortical necrosis, pregnancy toxaemia and hepatic encephalopathy.

Table 16.5 Other plants, trees and shrubs that are potentially toxic to goats.

COMMON NAME	SCIENTIFIC NAME	MAIN PRESENTING SIGNS
Bog asphodel	*Narthecium ossifragum*	Photosensitisation
Castorbean	*Ricinus communis*	Salivation, colic, cardiovascular signs
Foxglove	*Digitalis purpurea*	Sudden death, diarrhoea
Giant hogweed	*Heracleum mantegazzianum*	Stomatitis
Golden chain tree	*Laburnum* spp.	Nervous signs
Hemlock	*Conium maculatum*	Nervous signs, severe dyspnoea, diarrhoea
Houseplants	*Dieffenbachia* spp., Calla lily (*Zantedeschia aethiopica*), *Philodendron* spp.	Stomatitis syndrome
Kale	*Brassica oleracea*	Anaemia, haemoglobinuria, jaundice
Nightshade	*Solanum* spp.	Nervous signs, dyspnoea, bradycardia, gastrointestinal tract irritation
Oleander	*Nerium oleander*	Dyspnoea, cardiac arrhythmia
Ragwort	*Senecio jacobaea* (syn. *Jacobaea vulgaris*)	Liver failure, jaundice
Rape	*Brassica napus*	Anaemia, haemoglobinuria, jaundice
St John's wort	*Hypericum perforatum*	Photosensitisation
Trumpet flower (trumpet)	*Datura* spp.	Nervous signs, dyspnoea, collapse
Water dropwort	*Oenanthe* spp.	Sudden death, nervous signs

Note: Unlike other ruminants, goats appear to have a natural tolerance to oak/acorn (*Quercus* spp.) toxicity.

Treatment/management/control

The prognosis for acute cases is guarded. They must be removed immediately from the likely source, and any hypocalcaemia treated by i/v and s/c calcium borogluconate. Intravenous and/or oral fluid therapy may help to combat the progressive renal damage. Prevention is based on the ability to identify toxic plants and make them inaccessible.

Nitrate poisoning

Definition/overview

Nitrate poisoning occurs worldwide. Goats can develop nitrate poisoning via a number of differing routes and from different sources.

Aetiology

The most common route is ingestion of plants containing high levels of nitrates. Some are cultivated crops such as sugar beet tops, turnip tops, rape, lucerne and maize. Worldwide there are also a number of weeds that can concentrate nitrates, including pigweed, some sorghum grasses and thistles.

Accumulation is promoted by disruption to normal plant growth (e.g. because of overcast or cold weather or drought). Poisoning can also occur from drinking water contaminated with run-off from heavily fertilised fields or by the direct ingestion of nitrogenous fertiliser.

Pathophysiology

Normally nitrates are degraded in the rumen, and the resulting nitrite is converted to ammonia by microbes. Toxicity is associated with excessive intake resulting in nitrite overload. These nitrites are absorbed through the rumen wall, converting haemoglobin to methaemoglobin, thus decreasing oxygen transport. Clinical signs will become evident when 30–40% of the haemoglobin is converted to methaemoglobin. Prognosis deteriorates as conversion continues.

Clinical presentation

Weakness, ataxia, progressive dyspnoea, frothing at the mouth and cyanosis, in addition to diarrhoea and obvious abdominal pain. In severe toxicity goats may simply be found dead.

Diagnosis

Evidence of actual or potential exposure is important. In live goats, or at PME, blood will appear dark brown in colour. It can be sent for laboratory nitrate/ nitrite assay, together with other body fluids such as ocular humour. Sampling and submission arrangements should be discussed with the laboratory as both metabolites may be unstable and degrade rapidly.

Differential diagnosis

Other causes of dyspnoea and cyanosis including anaemia, cardiac abnormalities and choking.

Treatment/management/control

All goats in the group should be immediately removed from any potential source. Rapid treatment is vital to success, using an i/v 1–2% solution of methylene blue at a dose rate of 5–15 mg/kg, repeated after 6–8 hours if necessary.

Copper poisoning

Definition/overview

Both acute and chronic copper poisoning can occur in goats, but they do appear to be inherently more resistant to the effects of increased copper intake than sheep.

Aetiology

Almost all cases encountered will be the result of accidental oversupplementation. These include excessive copper inclusion in rations and *ad-libitum* high copper mineral provision. Accidental drinking of copper sulphate footbaths has been reported.

Pathophysiology

If very high levels are ingested or administered, goats may immediately develop signs of acute toxicity. Chronic daily dietary excess is accumulated in the liver. Levels gradually rise with no clinical signs evident until a critical point is reached. At this point, there is a rapid release of copper from the liver, initiating an acute haemolytic crisis resulting in intravascular haemolysis.

Clinical presentation

Non-specific signs of abdominal pain, mucoid diarrhoea and profound depression are evident in acute toxicity. As haemolysis progresses, affected goats become anaemic, dyspnoeic and jaundiced and the urine is dark brown due to haemoglobinuria.

Diagnosis

Clinical signs should raise suspicion, taking any copper supplementation history into account. Haematology will reveal very low PCV, Hb and erythrocyte counts. Liver enzymes (GLDH, AST, SDH and gGT) will be elevated, as will serum bilirubin levels. Haemoglobin may be demonstrated in urine. At PME, there are widespread signs of jaundice (**Fig. 16.6**), and the liver is invariably pale, soft and yellow in colour. Kidneys are soft, swollen and black in colour (**Fig. 16.7**).

Differential diagnosis

Acute enteritis or abdominal catastrophe for acute toxicity. Other causes of jaundice include brassica (e.g. rape, kale) poisoning and primary liver disease. Other common causes of haemolytic anaemia include blood parasites and clostridial disease.

Treatment/management/control

Any copper source should be removed immediately. Treatment is aimed at removal and clearance

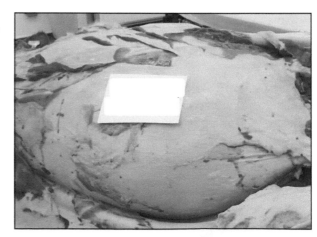

Fig. 16.6 Profound jaundice evident after the carcase is skinned. A confirmed case of copper poisoning in a calf.

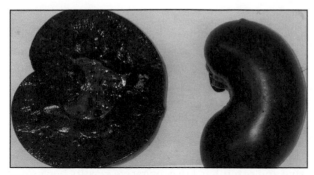

Fig. 16.7 Typical black discolouration of kidneys at post-mortem examination in copper poisoning cases (ovine specimen).

of copper from the blood and body tissues via the use of chelating agents. The most widely used agent is ammonium tetrathiomolybdate at a dose rate of 1.7 mg/kg i/v or 3.4 mg/kg s/c given three times on alternate days. (**Note:** This product is off-licence in many countries.) Control is based on ensuring that there is an actual need for copper supplementation (by liver or blood assay) before the inclusion of copper in the ration or the introduction of other sources of copper.

Urea poisoning
Definition/overview
Urea is used as a feed supplement in high-production dairy goats. Accidental overdosing may occur, causing toxicity.

Aetiology
Poisoning episodes most typically occur after a free access urea-containing product is introduced suddenly or following a period of unavailability, or because of uneven mixing into a ration. Urea is very soluble and can wash out of a ration or feed blocks following heavy rain, and be consumed by goats drinking surface water.

Pathophysiology
Urea is converted in the rumen to ammonia, which, in excess, diffuses out from the rumen into the blood stream. Toxic signs will develop when the liver's ability to cope with these increasing ammonia levels is compromised, resulting in hyperammonaemia.

Clinical presentation
Signs are seen within 90 minutes after ingestion and include abdominal discomfort, rumen atony with or without tympany, muscle and skin tremors, salivation, incoordination, dyspnoea, convulsions and death.

Diagnosis
Diagnosis is based on a known availability or access to urea, often following a period when it has not been available and then reintroduced. Blood ammonia levels can be analysed in live goats, but testing must be undertaken within 30 minutes of sampling (or samples frozen immediately). Serum urea levels will be raised. There are no specific PME findings, although rumen contents pH may become markedly alkaline, exceeding 7.5.

Treatment/management/control
Prognosis is guarded. Treatment options include administration of several litres of ice-cold water via stomach tube into the rumen, together with 0.5–1 litres of vinegar as an acidifying agent – both to slow down ammonia production. Rumenotomy may be indicated in valuable animals. In addition, i/v isotonic saline, together with calcium borogluconate and magnesium sulphate, should be given. Barbiturate or other sedative agents may help against convulsions.

Prevention is by ensuring that any ration containing urea is thoroughly mixed, and that any free access urea source is introduced gradually. Maximum recommended urea inclusion rates are 2–3% of the concentrate portion of a diet, or 1% of the total diet.

Mycotoxins
Overview
Fungal infection of growing plants, or harvested and stored feedstuffs (**Fig. 16.8**), occurs frequently. It can be difficult to pinpoint the specific role or impact of mycotoxins.

Aetiology
Some specific agents, and the disease they cause, are recognised and shown in *Table 16.6*.

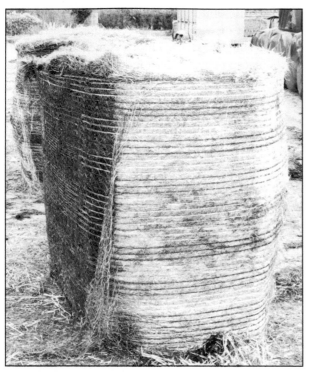

Fig. 16.8 Visibly spoiled hay. Such forages or feedstuffs are not suitable for any type of animal or production group.

Clinical presentation

Signs suggestive of the specific mycotoxins are shown in *Table 16.6*. However, low levels of mycotoxins may result in general suboptimal production.

Diagnosis

Diagnosis is difficult and often circumstantial. Indications that mycotoxins are involved include a large number of animals affected over a short period and no evidence of contagious disease, improvement once feed is withdrawn, mouldy feedstuffs and failure to isolate other pathogens. Mycotoxicosis from pasture typically occurs in the autumn. Fungal isolation from feed is expensive and often has false-negative results because of only localised patches of feed being affected, heat damage having eliminated the fungus but not the toxin, and the causative fungus becoming overgrown by other fungal species.

Differential diagnosis

Contagious or highly infective disease for large number of animals affected in a short time. Other causes of suboptimal performance, in particular nutritional deficiencies, stressors, painful conditions such as lameness. For poor reproductive performance, also abortive and venereal agents.

Treatment/management/control

Remove suspected feed. Clays and other anticaking agents and yeasts have been used as mycotoxin binders (e.g. sodium bentonite: available from mineral suppliers, feed about 20 g per head per day, or 1–2% inclusion in diet; cattle products include Mycosorb®, MTB100®, Nutrasound® and Mycortex®). There is

Table 16.6 **Recognised mycotoxins and their presentation.**

MYCOTOXIN	CROP	DISEASE	GENERAL EFFECT
Aflatoxin B1	Cereals	Aflatoxicosis	Hepatotoxic
Dicoumarol	Sweet clover	Sweet clover poisoning	Coagulopathy
Ergot alkaloids	Cereals, grasses	Ergotism	Diarrhoea, lameness with dry gangrene of extremities
Ergot alkaloids?	*Festuca* spp.	Fescue foot	Necrosis/gangrene lower limb
Lolitrem	Ryegrass	Ryegrass staggers	Incoordination, ataxia
Penitrems	All feeds	N/a	Tremors
Trichothecenes (e.g. *Fusarium* spp.)	Cereals	N/a	Dermonecrotic, coagulopathy
Zearalenone	Cereals	*Fusarium* infertility	Oestrogenic

debate as to whether they really bind the mycotoxins or merely act as rumen buffers, and not all mycotoxins may be bound to the same degree. It is also not established to what degree they bind minerals and vitamins (i.e. whether their feeding can induce imbalances or deficiencies). A response, for example in the form of increased appetite or milk yield, should be seen within about 2 weeks of feeding such binders.

Water source poisons

The quality of the animals' drinking water is often overlooked, and although goats tend to be fairly fastidious and will generally refuse to drink water that is not clean and fresh, its potential role in suspected toxicity cases should be considered.

The most important pollutants are bacteria (especially faecal pathogens), algae (in particular blue-green algae), heavy metals, chemicals and hydrogen sulphide. Excessive levels of magnesium or sulphate may have laxative effects resulting in diarrhoea.

Risk factors for poor water quality include natural water courses, stagnant water in particular when exposed to sunlight (**Fig. 16.9**), lead piping, troughs positioned too low leading to faecal contamination, and poor handling of chemicals on the farm. Troughs and water reservoirs should be emptied and disinfected weekly (e.g. with dilute bleach

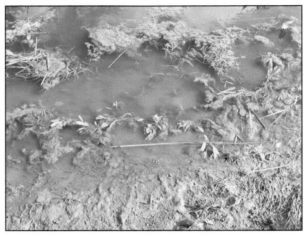

Fig. 16.9 Stagnant pond water with obvious algal overgrowth. Such water sources should be fenced off to avoid toxicity.

[sodium hypochlorite], 30 ml in 1 litre of water, rinsing well after application). Stagnant water should be fenced off and animals provided with mains or well water whenever possible.

Water testing services are readily available. The cost of water analysis is reasonable and a good investment to establish the type and level of any pollutants. The results will also support a more targeted mineral and vitamin supplementation. In dairy herds, ensuring good water quality will support optimum milk production.

EXOTIC AND EMERGING DISEASES

INTRODUCTION

The World Organisation for Animal Health (OIE) has 180 member countries and maintains a list of animal diseases, infections and infestations that it considers of most global importance (currently 117 in total). Each member country undertakes to report the listed animal diseases that it detects in its territory to the OIE, which in turn then disseminates the information to other countries, who can take the necessary preventive action. The organisation provides technical support to member countries for animal disease control and eradication operations. It specifically offers expertise to the poorest countries to assist in the control of animal diseases that cause livestock losses, present a risk to public health or threaten other member countries.

Different countries will implement the OIE list in slightly different ways. In the EU, the diseases relevant to goats and classed as notifiable (i.e. a suspicion of their presence must be reported to the relevant authority) are listed in *Table 17.1*.

Foot and mouth disease (aphthous fever)
Definition/overview

Foot and mouth disease (FMD) is one of the most important and economically devastating infectious diseases, potentially affecting livestock worldwide. All domestic (and many wild) cloven-hoofed species are susceptible including goats, cattle, sheep and pigs. FMD is endemic in parts of Asia, Africa, the Middle East and South America. It is one of the most important entries on the OIE list of scheduled diseases, and there are very strict control measures in place to protect the borders of those countries currently free of infection.

Table 17.1 **Notifiable diseases in goats.**

DISEASE	SPECIES AFFECTED	DESCRIPTION
Anthrax	Most mammals, particularly ruminants and humans	Chapter 17
Aujeszky's disease (pseudorabies)	Mainly pigs – can occasionally infect in-contact goats	Chapter 8
Bovine spongioform encephalopathy	Cattle – very rare confirmation of disease in goats	Chapter 8
Bluetongue	All ruminants	Chapter 17
Bovine tuberculosis	Mainly cattle, but can affect many other domesticated and wild mammal species	Chapter 17
Brucellosis	Goats and sheep, but many mammalian species can be infected	Chapter 2
Contagious agalactia	Goats and sheep	Chapter 12
Contagious caprine pleuropneumonia	Goats are the primary host; in-contact sheep may become infected	Chapter 6
Foot and mouth disease	All cloven hoofed animals	Chapter 17
Goat pox	Goats and sheep	Chapter 11
Peste des petits ruminants	Goats and sheep	Chapter 5
Rabies	All mammals	Chapter 8
Scrapie	Goats and sheep	Chapter 8

The susceptibility of goats to FMD can vary with the breed of animal and the strain of the FMD virus. In the UK outbreak in 2001, for example (caused by serotype O PanAsia strain), clinical disease was rapid in onset and clinically severe in cattle, but lesions were more mild in sheep and goats. FMD was only suspected in one small herd of milking goats after a significant rise in mastitis cases prompted a request for veterinary advice. A number of goats had small 'inconsequential' lesions on the skin of the teats that had become secondarily infected with *Staphylococcus aureus*; no other more typical lesions were evident. FMD seroconversion was widespread, however. Conversely there are strains of serotype O FMD virus circulating in the Middle East where goats and sheep form the majority of the susceptible population. There are many examples where movement of subclinically infected sheep and goats carried FMD into countries previously disease free.

Aetiology

A virus of the family Picornaviridae, genus *Aphthovirus*. There are seven immunologically distinct serotypes: A, O, C, SAT1, SAT2, SAT3 and Asia1, which, significantly, do not confer cross immunity with each other. The virus can be preserved by refrigeration and freezing, but is quickly inactivated by a pH <6.0 or >9.0. This is of real significance as preserved infected meat products have been incriminated as potential sources of disease incursion into countries previously free of infection, such as in the 2001 outbreak in the UK.

Spread of the virus can occur as a result of:

- Direct contact between infected and susceptible animals.
- Direct contact of susceptible animals with contaminated inanimate objects such as hands, footwear, clothing or vehicles.
- Inhalation of infectious aerosols.
- Consumption of untreated contaminated meat products (e.g. swill feeding in pigs).
- Artificial insemination with contaminated semen.
- Airborne spread, especially in temperate zones (up to 60 km overland and 300 km over sea).

- Contact with exposed humans, who can harbour FMD virus in their respiratory tract for 24–48 hours. This is the reason for the common practice of 3–5 days of quarantine (away from susceptible livestock) for personnel exposed in research facilities or while dealing with an outbreak.

Pathophysiology

The incubation period for FMD can vary with the species of animal, the dose of virus, the viral strain and the route of inoculation. In sheep, for example, it is reported to be 1–12 days, with most infections appearing in 2–8 days. Most new infection is contracted by the inhalation route, spreading rapidly within a group of animals before clinical signs become apparent because of the massive viral replication and excretion rates. As a result, many animals may appear to be affected almost simultaneously in a new incident.

Once infected, virus replication leads to an initial pyrexia lasting 2–4 days, during which all secretions are highly infectious. Young kids may die at this stage due to viral myocarditis. Virus then progressively concentrates in the epithelial tissues of the oral cavity and feet, and also occasionally of the teats. Further replication at these sites leads to hydropic degeneration and coalescence of fluid-filled cells to form vesicles. These are thin walled and easily ruptured, leaving raw and very painful areas, leading to the stomatitis and lameness considered to be the characteristic features. These characteristic erosive lesions are much smaller and far less readily observed in goats and sheep compared with cattle, where they may reach 3–4 cm in diameter.

Clinical presentation

FMD in goats can be mild and inapparent, and may only be recognised when other in-contact ruminants (particularly cattle) show more typical signs. In goats that do develop clinical signs, there may be an initial pyrexia (often overlooked) and it is more common for foot lesions than mouth lesions to be identified clinically, in the form of lameness or tenderness on one or more feet. In early cases, vesicles may be found on the coronary band, in the interdigital space (**Fig. 17.1**) and over the soft part of the heels.

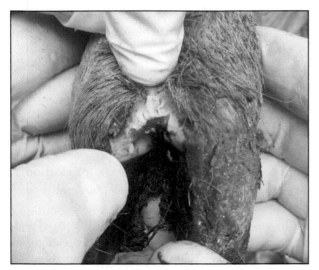

Fig. 17.1 Fresh foot and mouth lesion in the interdigital cleft. (Source: European Commission for the Control of Foot and Mouth Disease; permission granted by the Pirbright Institute.)

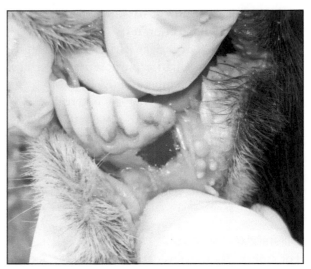

Fig. 17.2 Fresh foot and mouth lesion on the gum. (Source: European Commission for the Control of Foot and Mouth Disease; permission granted by the Pirbright Institute.)

These rupture, exposing raw areas that in turn can become secondarily infected – lameness can be very pronounced, and goats may be reluctant to move or spend more time lying down. Small erosive lesions may develop in the mouth. The common sites are the dental pad and tongue followed by gums, lips, hard palate and cheeks (**Figs. 17.2, 17.3**). They tend to be quite shallow and may heal within 2–3 days. These will lead to saliva drooling, lip smacking and halitosis. Small vesicles may develop on the skin of the udder and teats. These can rupture, become secondarily infected and predispose to mastitis. Indeed, mastitis may be the presenting complaint at the start of an FMD outbreak. It is important that a number of goats within the cohort are examined before FMD can be eliminated clinically, paying particular attention to any in-contact more susceptible species, such as cattle and pigs in which disease is usually more severe and thus more easily recognised. Young kids may be found dead due to viral myocarditis.

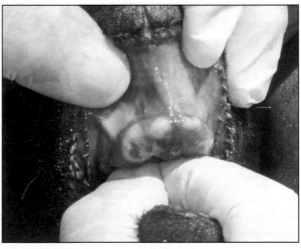

Fig. 17.3 Foot and mouth lesion of 3–5 days' duration on the dental pad. (Source: European Commission for the Control of Foot and Mouth Disease; permission granted by the Pirbright Institute.)

Diagnosis

Unless classical vesicles in the early stages are evident, definitive diagnosis on clinical grounds alone can be problematic, because healing lesions and those that become secondarily infected may not be readily recognisable as FMD lesions. However, suspicion of disease must always be high when a number of goats (or other in-contact susceptible species) show the clinical signs described, particularly if it is known that disease exists in the locality. Most statutory control measures require a suspicion of disease to be reported to the relevant authority, who in turn will instigate a full and rapid investigation including laboratory sampling.

Laboratory testing is based on demonstrating antigen by rapid detection tests such as the reverse transcriptase PCR or antigen ELISA test. Serological screening for surveillance purposes is undertaken using a blocking or competition ELISA test.

Young kids dying during an outbreak can be examined by post-mortem examination (PME). Lesions tend to be confined to the myocardium, in which there may be gross evidence of small, white to grey streaks of necrotic tissue in the myocardial wall, leading to the use of the descriptive term 'tiger heart'.

Differential diagnosis
For mouth lesions, consider orf, bluetongue, feeding trauma, toxic plant or chemical induced stomatitis and, in an individual animal, renal failure and uraemia. For foot lesions consider scald, foot rot, bluetongue and chemical insult.

Treatment/management/control
Treatment is rarely attempted, with control predominantly based on statutory identification of infected premises and slaughter of infected and in-contact animals – a so-called 'stamping out policy'. However, increasingly vaccination programmes are being deployed to support this traditional policy, as vaccines improve in quality and efficacy and tests become available to distinguish between naturally acquired and vaccine acquired antibody.

The overall responsibility for the management and control of any outbreak rests with the animal health policy of each country, underpinned by the global control measures that are in place at the time. The World Reference FMD Laboratory is at the Pirbright Institute in the UK.

Bluetongue
Definition/overview
Bluetongue is an infectious, non-contagious arthropod-borne viral disease of ruminants. Although goats can develop clinical disease, it is not common and usually fairly mild compared with disease in sheep. The causative agent, bluetongue virus (BTV), has a worldwide distribution, including Africa, Asia, Australia, Europe, North America and several islands in the tropics and subtropics, but is confined mainly to the tropical and subtropical regions of each continent, with occasional incursions outside these areas; for example, into northern Europe in the 2006–2008 incident. This resulted in an OIE reclassification of the global susceptibility to between latitudes 53°N to 34°S. This global distribution reflects the distribution of the *Culicoides* spp. vectors that carry and transmit infection between susceptible hosts. Although there are almost 1,500 species of *Culicoides* spp. worldwide, only a very small proportion of around 20 have been identified as potential vectors, and these will vary from region to region.

In any affected country, it is possible to classify the susceptible population into three categories: enzootic (transmission occurs throughout the year), epizootic (mainly in more temperate areas, where transmission is seasonal) and incursive (experience outbreaks when local climatic conditions favour disease transmission by vectors). There is much overlap, however, and local BTV status is also influenced by livestock movements, particularly movement of susceptible animals into infected areas during the midge transmission period.

Bluetongue is a disease listed under the OIE Terrestrial Animal Health Code and must be reported to the World Organisation for Animal Health.

Aetiology
It is caused by an RNA orbivirus in the family Reoviridae. Twenty-four different serotypes have been identified and the ability of each strain to cause disease varies considerably.

Pathophysiology
Worldwide, the disease is most severe in sheep. Infection in goats may be asymptomatic, with goats merely acting as reservoirs of infection. Even when co-located with severely affected sheep, clinical signs may be mild, with lower morbidity and mortality. Available information on the pathogenesis of BTV in goats is minimal and is mainly extrapolated from known information in sheep. Following skin inoculation of infection by biting midges, initial replication occurs in local lymph nodes, resulting in more generalised distribution and viraemia. The virus then appears to

have a predilection for vascular endothelium cells, leading to thrombosis, haemorrhage and oedema in affected tissues, most notably in the mouth, oesophagus, rumen and skin. This in turn results in hyperaemia, erosion and ulcer formation, with clinical signs including stomatitis, glossitis, rhinitis and enteritis.

Clinical presentation

The majority of bluetongue cases in goats tend to be subclinical. Signs described in clinical cases include pyrexia, loss of appetite and milk yield with hyperaemia and mild erosive damage to the oral mucosa. In the occasional more severe case, these oral changes may progress to ulcerative and necrotic changes to the tongue, lips and gums and nostrils (**Fig. 17.4**), resulting in marked salivation. Diarrhoea may also develop. In an outbreak of bluetongue in the Netherlands in 2007, small papular lesions were described on the skin of the udder (**Fig. 17.5**).

Diagnosis

Due to the milder signs exhibited by goats, disease may be overlooked unless more severe signs are evident in other susceptible in-contact species such as sheep. If suspected, antigen detection techniques or serology will confirm infection. Gross pathology is as described above under pathophysiology and clinical signs.

Differential diagnosis

Includes peste des petits ruminants, FMD, contagious pustular dermatitis (orf) and goat pox.

Treatment/management/control

There is no specific treatment. The primary method of control in endemic areas is the use of effective vaccines, administered to give protection during risk periods, which are linked to midge activity. Vaccines used have to reflect the local serotype present or be multivalent, as a single serotype vaccine will give little or no protection against another serotype. Additional control methods are aimed at reducing the exposure to midges, by moving stock indoors when midge activity is high (early evening and dusk, humid still days), providing protective curtains around openings in the buildings, and using insect repellents on the goats and in their environment if approved for use in food producing animals.

In addition, control includes keeping disease out of clean areas by sourcing from known BTV-free areas, and testing and quarantining on arrival.

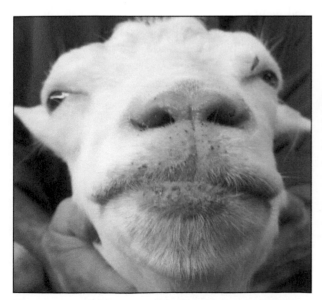

Fig. 17.4 Mild lesions of bluetongue on the muzzle of a goat (Dutch outbreak 2007; courtesy GD Animal Health, Deventer, the Netherlands).

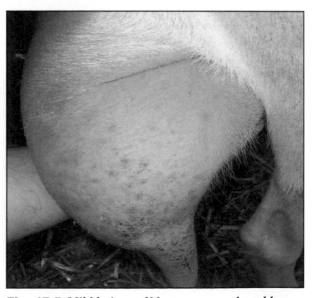

Fig. 17.5 Mild lesions of bluetongue on the udder of a goat (Dutch outbreak 2007; courtesy GD Animal Health, Deventer, the Netherlands).

Tuberculosis

Definition/overview

Although not commonly reported in goats, they are susceptible to infection with bovine, avian and human tuberculosis (TB) infections. They can act as spillover hosts to bovine TB in those areas in which the infection is firmly established in the cattle and associated wildlife populations, such as the UK in which the badger is the main wildlife host. Equally, sporadic cases of avian TB occur when goats are kept in close contact with domesticated or wild birds infected with and excreting the avian TB organisms. There are occasional reports of human TB being passed from an infected owner or keeper to their goat (usually a pet animal). It is an important zoonotic disease when goats and humans are in close contact. TB organisms in milk are inactivated by pasteurisation.

Aetiology

In general mammals are infected with the *Mycobacterium tuberculosis* (MTB) complex, with *Mycobacterium bovis* the type species in cattle, *Mycobacterium avium* in birds and *Mycobacterium tuberculosis* in humans. The causative organisms are referred to as tubercle bacilli, and are very slow growing in the laboratory, requiring specialist media. They show an acid-fast staining characteristic. *M. bovis* has been further divided into a series of spoligotypes – this technique has revolutionised the epidemiological investigations of incidents and breakdowns in the UK.

Pathophysiology

Infection is acquired either orally or by inhalation from other infected animals, birds or contaminated environment. Nursing kids can be infected via contaminated milk or colostrum. *M. bovis* has a predilection for the respiratory tract and *M. avium* for the alimentary tract. *M. bovis* abscesses can develop in the lung parenchyma (**Fig. 17.6**), with more typical TB granuloma formation in lymph nodes (**Fig. 17.7**) and on serosal surfaces such as the pericardial sac and pleura. In advanced cases observed in the UK, other widely distributed visceral lesions were evident (**Fig. 17.8**). Unlike in cattle, the pus is often liquid

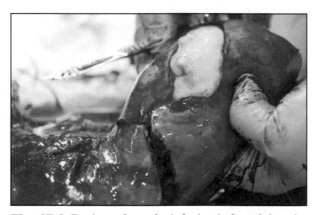

Fig. 17.6 Bovine tuberculosis lesion in lung lobe of a Golden Guernsey goat. Note the liquid pus (rather than caseous as in cattle).

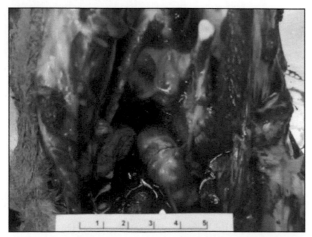

Fig. 17.7 Bovine tuberculosis lesion in retropharyngeal lymph nodes. (© Crown Copyright 2017. Used with kind permission of the Animal and Plant Health Agency.)

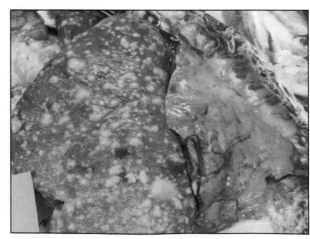

Fig. 17.8 Miliary bovine tuberculosis lesions in liver tissue. (© Crown Copyright 2017. Used with kind permission of the Animal and Plant Health Agency.)

(not caseous) and can erode into airways, resulting in rapid spread among housed goats.

Clinical presentation

In countries where bovine TB occurs, clinical signs reported include weight loss, drop in milk yield, coughing and other non-specific respiratory signs such as lagging behind when driven. However, many infected goats show few clinical signs, with infection only being detected during PME or meat inspection or following surveillance screening. Clinical signs associated with avian TB are more non-specific, with most cases being identified on PME.

Diagnosis

The first cases in an incident are often detected either at meat inspection or PME, with the typical TB granulomata and lung abscesses being identified. Microscopical examination may demonstrate the acid-fast organisms in ZN-stained smears, with confirmation by specialist laboratory cultures. In the live goat, the traditional diagnostic test has been the single intradermal comparative cervical test (SICCT) – or 'TB skin test,' as used in cattle. In the UK, as part of a coordinated effort to control TB, a number of other tests have been applied. These include the gamma-interferon test and, following the genomic sequencing of the *M. bovis* organism, molecular techniques linked to individual and multiple antigen assays are being developed. These latter techniques are showing promising results in infected goat herds. The use of Johne's disease (*M. avium* subsp. *paratuberculosis*) vaccines may complicate the interpretation of some of these tests.

Differential diagnosis

Respiratory presentation needs to be differentiated from lungworm, pasteurellosis and mycoplasma infections. If presented as weight loss without obvious respiratory signs, consider Johne's disease, parasitic gastroenteritis and undernutrition.

Treatment/management/control

TB is an OIE listed disease and is most often controlled by nationally operated coordinated control programmes, which will vary from country to country depending on the level of infection and involvement of wild life reservoirs. Most of these are aimed at controlling disease in cattle, but also include its control in other susceptible species. There are no readily available treatments, and control is most often based on a test and cull policy. Sound biosecurity is important in keeping disease out, and when wildlife sources are an issue, needs to be extensive and well adhered to.

Anthrax

Definition/overview

Anthrax is an overwhelming bacterial infection recognised in many livestock species worldwide. It is endemic in many tropical and subtropical regions of the world, and a sporadic problem in many other countries where it may be notifiable (such as in the UK). It is not a common problem in goats compared with the number of cases reported in other domestic and wild ruminants. Anthrax is also of zoonotic importance.

Aetiology

Caused by *Bacillus anthracis*, a spore-bearing, anaerobic, gram positive, rod-shaped organism. Spores can remain dormant for 50 years or longer.

Pathophysiology

Infection is via the oral route, typically by grazing in areas in which the soil has become contaminated by dormant spores (often brought to the surface by earth movement or flooding and soil erosion). This may be the reason the disease is less commonly reported in goats, which tend to feed above ground level. Once ingested, the endospores germinate at the site of tissue entry and then spread by the circulation to the lymphatics, where the bacteria continue to multiply, producing powerful toxins resulting in an overwhelming septicaemia and toxaemia.

Clinical presentation

The disease is invariably peracute in its course and many affected animals present as sudden death, often with blood exuding from mouth, nostrils or anus. If alive, they are profoundly dull and depressed with severe pyrexia extending over a course of a few hours to a few days.

Diagnosis

If anthrax is suspected, a PME is highly inadvisable, as this would potentially release spores thus further contaminating the environment and acting as a severe zoonotic risk. Smears made from peripheral blood (ear or tail) stained with McFadyens polychromatic methylene blue will show the characteristic pink staining capsules (**Fig. 17.9**).

Differential diagnosis

For sudden death includes enterotoxaemia and other septicaemic conditions such as listeriosis and salmonellosis, clostridial disease, plant and chemical toxicities, bloat or acidosis, hypomagnesaemia and lightning strike.

Treatment/management/control

Treatment is often disappointing because of the rapid course of the disease. High doses of antibiotics such as penicillin or tetracycline may be tried, together with supportive care. In endemic areas, livestock may be vaccinated annually with some success.

The zoonotic potential of the disease cannot be overemphasised. Anyone handling infected carcases, their skins, or fixtures and fittings potentially contaminated with infected blood should wear gloves and a facemask as a minimum protective barrier.

To prevent wider spread within the herd, the carcase should not be moved until anthrax is ruled out, temporarily fencing it off from any herd mates. If confirmed, potentially contaminated soil or bedding is removed and the area disinfected. The water agency and milk buyer may have to be informed.

New and emerging diseases

Worldwide, a number of 'new' or 'emerging' diseases have been described in goats and in other ruminant livestock species. For example, bovine spongiform encephalopathy (BSE) and Schmallenberg virus infection were both newly recognised diseases in the UK and Germany, and then much of Europe, respectively, neither having been reported previously around the world. Locally emerging diseases may be the result of movement of animals, animal (by-)products, personnel or vectors such as midges.

As an example, at the time of publication there is concern in Europe of a possible incursion of Rift Valley fever. Its geographical distribution in 2016 is shown in **Fig. 17.10**, essentially in sub-Saharan Africa. One of the reasons for this concern follows the incursion of BTV by an apparent leap from this same area in Africa to Northern Europe.

Many countries have strict legislation in place to minimise these risks, including restrictions on animal movements and strict policies for visitors at entry points such as airports. The movement of bluetongue infection into northern Europe from its more traditional locations in southern Europe and North Africa was a good example of midge-borne infections which, being airborne, are more difficult to prevent, with emphasis placed more on examination of meteorological and other data to predict incursion of disease.

Underpinning prompt identification of these types of disease is a comprehensive disease surveillance gathering and reporting system, based on clinical observation, routine laboratory testing, border controls and import/export testing, PME and meat inspection.

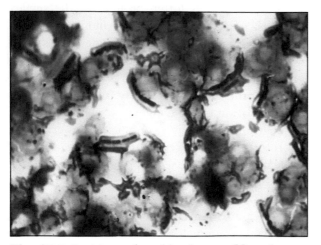

Fig. 17.9 Positive anthrax blood smear. Note the pink capsular stain.

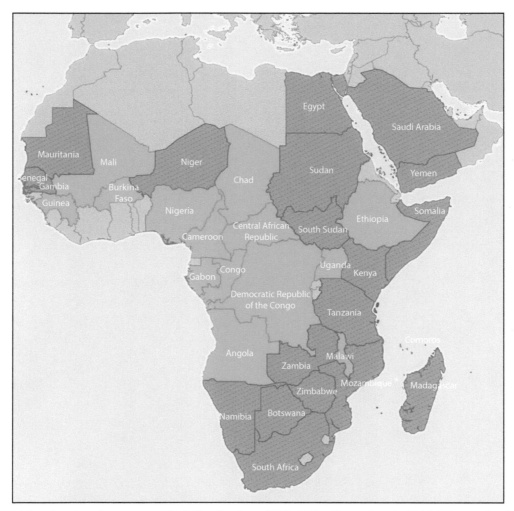

Fig. 17.10 Map showing the geographical distribution of Rift Valley fever virus in 2016. Blue: endemic areas or with substantial outbreaks; green: few cases, periodic virus isolation or serological evidence; brown: status unknown. (Source: Centers for Disease Control and Prevention, Atlanta.)

SEDATION

General principles

For surgical procedures, general anaesthesia (GA) is preferable over sedation, because goats do not tolerate physical restraint under sedation as well as cattle and sheep. In addition, apnoea is relatively common, so it is an advantage having an endotracheal (ET) tube in place. To reduce the risk of aspiration of saliva or regurgitated rumen fluid in a goat under sedation, the animal is positioned with the nose below the level of the throat or upper neck (e.g. by placing a rolled up towel under its neck; **Fig. 18.1**). Starvation, if possible (see General anaesthesia for protocol), is particularly important for procedures

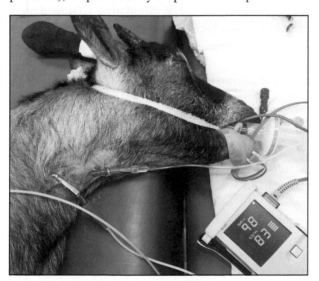

Fig. 18.1 **Some aspects of good anaesthesia practice. The nose is positioned below the larynx in case of regurgitation; an i/v catheter enables fluid therapy and provides immediate venous access if complications arise; the goat is on soft padding; the lowermost eye does not touch the table. Monitoring utilised here includes pulse oximeter (on tongue), oesophageal thermometer (grey tube) and electrocardiogram.**

under sedation, because the airway will not be protected by an ET tube. Blindfolding the animal often prolongs and deepens the level of sedation, and the surroundings should be quiet. The risk of hypothermia must be addressed (see General anaesthesia).

Sedatives

Drug licensing and prescribing restrictions limit the number of available agents for goats in many countries. In the UK, for example, only the first three of the following sedatives can be used under the prescribing cascade at the time of publishing:

- Xylazine hydrochloride: 0.03–0.05 mg/kg i/v or up to 0.1 mg/kg i/m. Ruminants show marked differences in sedative response. Therefore, if a goat is likely to have repeated procedures (e.g. wound dressing), a note of the dose rate used and its effect should be kept on the case file. 'Topping-up' can be difficult with xylazine HCl, with often little noticeable response to additional doses. Especially after i/m administration, sufficient time (minimum 10 minutes) must be allowed for sedation to take effect prior to disturbing the animal, otherwise the full effect may not be achieved. Potential side-effects include bradycardia, hypotension, hypoxaemia and pulmonary oedema. Xylazine HCl should be avoided in cases with urinary obstruction, as it increases urine production. It has oxytocin-like effects, potentially leading to abortion in late pregnancy or retained fetal membranes.
- Detomidine hydrochloride: 0.02–0.04 mg/kg i/v. Potential side-effects are less likely than with xylazine HCl, because of reduced sensitivity to this sedative in ruminants and the lack of oxytocin-like effects at low doses. Medetomidine has been used in goats at

0.01–0.02 mg/kg i/m (or slow i/v to effect), but is off-cascade in the UK.

- Butorphanol: 0.05–0.2 mg/kg i/v or i/m. Potential side-effects are not established in goats.
- Diazepam: 0.2–0.4 mg/kg i/v. This is a useful agent in neonates or compromised patients. In combination with butorphanol, sedation is often deep enough to allow procedures such as radiography. It appears to have an appetite stimulating effect in some goats. Similarly, midazolam is a useful agent, for example for premedication, and may be given i/m as well as i/v, at a dose rate of 0.3–0.6 mg/kg.
- Alfaxalone: 2–3 mg/kg slow i/v to effect.

Reversal

- Atipamezole: 0.02–0.125 mg/kg slow i/v may be given to reverse the alpha-2 agonists (this constitutes off-cascade use in the UK).
- Doxapram hydrochloride also partially reverses the effects of sedatives.

GENERAL ANAESTHESIA

General principles

Regardless of the type of GA, an intravenous catheter should be placed to allow rapid intervention when necessary (**Fig. 18.1**). The jugular, cephalic, saphenous or ear veins are all suitable.

For most surgical procedures, consideration should be given to:

- Preoperative antibiosis (administered at least 30 minutes prior to the start of surgery to ensure tissue perfusion).
- Tetanus cover. Up-to-date vaccination cover (i.e. at least 14 days should have elapsed since full primary course or last booster dose, but not more than 6 months since last booster injection). Alternatively, tetanus antitoxin or an antibiotic with activity against anaerobes may be given at the point of surgery (e.g. procaine penicillin; third-generation cephalosporin is also effective, but subject to responsible use concerns).
- Fly control, depending on time of year. This may be achieved by applying, for example, Battles' Summer Fly Cream to the wound edges and the use of deltamethrin pour-on solutions.

Preoperative starvation

For elective procedures, the goat should be starved prior to GA or sedation. A suitable protocol for morning surgery involves last concentrate meal 24 hours preoperative, forage removed early afternoon, and water removed between 10 pm and midnight. Exceptions to this protocol are neonates and kids up to 3 months of age; they receive their last milk feed at half of normal volume, or are allowed to suckle, 2 hours prior to surgery. This reduces the risk of hypoglycaemia. In peak lactation does, supplementation with an energy precursor such as propylene glycol may be indicated.

Rumen tympany may develop during GA and can be addressed by either passing a stomach tube or, in an emergency, by advancing a 14–16 gauge hypodermic needle into the rumen via the left flank.

Preoperative assessment

Thorough history taking and clinical examination is vital to highlight any particular anaesthetic concerns. The body weight of the patient is determined as accurately as possible. Body condition has an influence on retention of lipophilic drugs and is noted. Where necessary, circulating volume deficits and electrolyte imbalances are corrected as much as possible prior to induction.

Intraoperative support

Attention must be paid to positioning to prevent neuropathies or myopathies. Padding of prominent bony points and supporting legs in their natural posture is advisable. Eyes are protected from trauma, reflux material or surgical scrub by applying a suitable ocular gel and avoiding contact between the lowermost eye and the operating table (**Fig. 18.1**). Placing the head onto a 'doughnut-ring' is useful for this.

Where possible, i/v fluids are administered throughout at a rate of 3–5 ml/kg per hour (unless the goat is hypovolaemic, when a higher dose is required). Hartman's or lactated Ringer's solution is suitable for most patients. In neonates or hypothermic goats, the addition of 1–5% glucose can be beneficial.

Hypothermia

Goats are very prone to hypothermia. For example, rectal temperature may drop to 37.5°C within

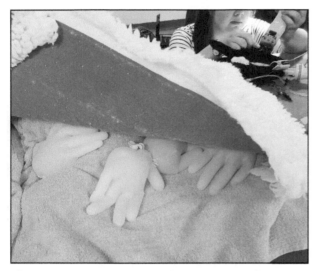

Fig. 18.2 Preventing hypothermia. Use of 'hot hands' (disposable gloves filled with hot water) and a towel placed underneath and around the animal to soak up any fluids (e.g. from scrubbing, lavage).

15 minutes of induction, and may easily fall to 35°C during surgery. Countermeasures include a warm, draught-free operating environment, preventing the animal's coat from becoming soaked with fluids, using warm i/v and lavage fluids, covering as much of the body as possible (e.g. using bubble-wrap or a Baer Hugger™) and using heat pads, hot water bottles or 'hot hands' (**Fig. 18.2**).

Induction

Induction can be achieved by a single drug or a combination of the drugs listed above for sedation. For example, xylazine HCl plus butorphanol as premedication, followed 5–10 minutes later by ketamine at 2–4 mg/kg i/v, given slowly to effect. Additional increments of ketamine may be given if the level of induction is not deep enough to allow intubation. Other induction agents, such as propofol, have been used in goats, but are off-cascade in the UK.

The induction area should be quiet and offer good footing. Premedication is highly recommended. It reduces anxiety in the patient, thereby facilitating catheter placement and induction, can provide analgesia (depending on agent) and typically reduces the required dose of induction and maintenance agents.

Inhalation anaesthesia

An ET tube is placed after induction, and the animal maintained on an isoflurane and oxygen mix (in the UK, currently the prescription cascade can be applied to isoflurane, but not other anaesthetic gases). When using a closed circuit, a flow rate of 2–3 litres is usually sufficient.

A 9–12 mm cuffed ET tube is suitable for adult goats and a 5.5–7 mm tube for young goats up to a few months of age. Placement is easiest with the goat in sternal recumbency, with an assistant fully extending the neck and opening the mouth with the aid of gauze straps. A laryngoscope with an extra long blade is invaluable (**Fig. 18.3**). Lidocaine spray may be applied to the larynx.

Injection anaesthesia

This can be achieved by top-up doses of ketamine using one-third to one-half of the initial induction dose at a time, or by using a ketamine drip (0.2% solution consisting of 200 mg ketamine in 100 ml of physiological saline; dose rate is 1 ml per minute for a 60 kg goat; 50 mg of xylazine HCl can be added to create a double drip). Propofol (5–7 mg/kg i/v)

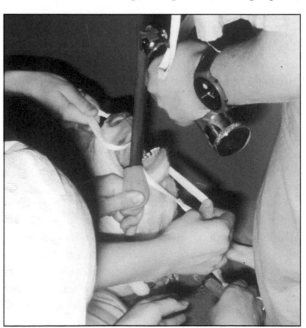

Fig. 18.3 Endotracheal intubation. The goat is in sternal recumbency with its neck and head extended; the mouth is held open with the aid of gauze straps; a laryngoscope with a long blade is used. Note that the assistant is 'topping-up' the i/v induction agent.

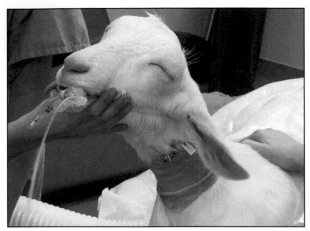

Fig. 18.4 For recovery, the goat is placed into sternal recumbency and the head and neck supported. The goat is extubated once clear signs of chewing and swallowing are present. Note the continued use of a Baer-Hugger™ against hypothermia.

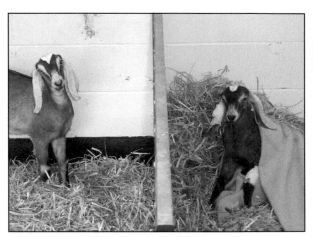

Fig. 18.5 The patient (on the right) is returned into a well-bedded pen and a rug or blanket used as necessary. The i/v catheter (here in the cephalic vein) is retained for several hours in case of late-onset complications during recovery.

is suitable for short procedures and where licensed for use in goats. Injection anaesthesia should only be considered for procedures of up to 1 hour duration. An ET tube should be placed to ensure airway patency and allow rapid intervention if required.

Monitoring

Eyeball position and reflexes give an indication of anaesthetic depth. Circulatory function is monitored through heart rate and rhythm, mucous membrane colour and capillary refill time. Respiratory rate and character and core temperature are monitored (**Fig. 18.1**). Adjunct tools, such as pulse oximetry, capnography and an oesophageal thermometer, and blood gas, glucose and electrolyte analysis are useful where available.

Good communication between the anaesthetist and surgeon is important. Anaesthetic depth can be deepened prior to a particularly painful stimulus, the surgeon asked to temporarily stop if the patient shows a response, and the anaesthetist can take the surgical manipulation into account when interpreting patient parameters (e.g. bradycardia induced by visceral traction).

Recovery

The goat is placed into supported sternal recumbency as soon as possible. Extubation is delayed until obvious signs of chewing are present (**Fig. 18.4**).

If regurgitation occurred during surgery, the ET cuff is left inflated during extubation, otherwise it is withdrawn partially deflated.

Ideally, a narrow gauge tube (e.g. a dog or cat urinary catheter) is available, plus oxygen, to allow intranasal oxygenation if required. A tracheotomy kit should be available for the rare cases that exhibit laryngospasm on extubation.

Hypothermia reducing measures are continued during recovery (**Fig. 18.5**) and the goat's rectal temperature monitored for several hours postoperatively. Offering kids milk or adults food and an electrolyte solution containing sugars as soon as possible after recovery aids thermoregulation.

LOCAL AND REGIONAL BLOCKS

General principles

Local and regional blocks facilitate surgical procedures in the conscious or sedated animal. However, even when surgery is performed under GA, they should be employed whenever possible, both to allow a lighter level of GA, and to aid postoperative analgesia management. Standard aseptic techniques must be used when applying blocks. Prior to injecting the local anaesthetic, one should always aspirate to ascertain that no blood or cerebrospinal fluid (CSF) is present – if present, the needle is redirected. Sufficient time needs to be allowed for a block to take effect.

Drugs

Goats are more sensitive to local anaesthetic agents, therefore a lower maximum dose rate compared with cattle and sheep needs to be observed. Drugs may be diluted between 1:1 to 1:3 drug to sterile saline to increase the volume available for injection (and thereby increase drug distribution across the target tissue or site). Many veterinary preparations of lidocaine HCl and procaine HCl contain adrenaline (syn. epinephrine) – these must not be used for epidural blocks, intravenous regional anaesthesia (IVRA) or distal limb ring blocks. It may be necessary to source a human product that only contains the anaesthetic agent. Anaesthetics that can be used for local or regional blocks include the following:

- Lidocaine hydrochloride 2% (under prescription cascade in the UK): up to 6 mg/kg. As a rule of thumb, a maximum of 0.3 times the animal's body weight can be given in millilitres (e.g. a 75 kg goat can receive 22.5 ml of 2% lidocaine HCl). Onset is within 10–20 minutes and duration about 60–90 minutes (up 120 minutes if the preparation contains adrenaline). Signs of toxicity as a result of overdosing include nystagmus, muscle twitching, convulsions, opisthotonus, hypotension and respiratory arrest. If signs persist for more than 1–2 minutes, diazepam is given at 0.1 mg/kg (off-cascade use in the UK) or thiopental at 5 mg/kg, plus fluid and respiratory support.
- Procaine hydrochloride 5%: no information on maximum dose is available. The authors have used it at up to 15 mg/kg without apparent side-effects (following the same body weight to volume of anaesthetic rule as described above for lidocaine HCl); however, the true safe dose is likely to be much below this level. Procaine HCl has lower tissue distribution, therefore it must be more accurately placed to be effective.
- Bupivicaine (off-cascade use in the UK): up to 2 mg/kg. Onset is within 20 minutes, with a duration of several hours.

Specific blocks

The volumes stated in this section all refer to 2% lidocaine HCl and adult goats. To avoid overdosing in kids, similar volumes, but of 0.7–1% lidocaine HCl, may have to be used. In general, the smallest gauge needle possible should be used.

Paravertebral

A paravertebral block is suitable for laparotomy, offering the advantage over regional infiltration of desensitising the entire flank, including the peritoneum. For an exploratory laparotomy, nerves T13, L1 and L2 are blocked. For a caesarean section, blocking nerve L3 in addition is useful, but may lead to moderate ataxia in the doe. Several techniques may be employed.

The proximal technique is described here. A 5 cm (2 in) long, 18–20 gauge hypodermic needle is placed at the cranial edges of the first to third lumbar vertebrae (plus fourth for nerve L3, if desired), at the mid-point between the spinal column and the tip of each vertebra. The needle is advanced through the interarcuate ligament (syn. ligamentum flavum; located just ventral to the level of the bone), and 4 ml instilled (**Fig. 18.6**). The needle is then withdrawn

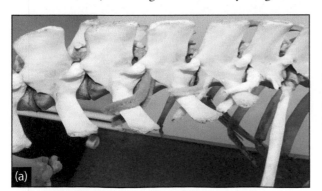
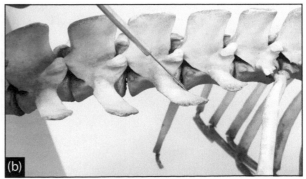

Fig. 18.6 Right lateral view of the lumber spine showing: (a) approximate course of the dorsal and ventral branches of nerves T13 (white), L1 (yellow) and L2 (green); and (b) the position of the needle to anaesthetise the ventral branch of L1.

to above the ligament and 3–4 ml injected while withdrawing the needle further.

Successful blocking of the dorsal branches will lead to loss of skin sensation. Curvature of the spine towards the blocked side (i.e. convex), sweating and rising steam are often observed in a successful block.

Regional flank infiltration

The flank may be desensitised by injecting local anaesthetic subcutaneously and intramuscularly in a linear fashion. A straight-line pattern along the line of incision requires less local anaesthetic (thereby reducing the risk of toxicity), but may interfere with wound healing. An alternative pattern is an inverted L, with the downward arm towards the last rib and the horizontal arm running parallel to the transverse processes. It is important with regional blocks to infiltrate all tissue layers.

Epidural – caudal

A low caudal epidural block is achieved at a dose rate of 0.5 mg/kg, leading to desensitisation of the perineum, tail and usually scrotum. Xylazine HCl at 0.07 mg/kg may be added for prolonged effect. A dose rate of 2–4 mg/kg leads to a high caudal block, desensitising the hind leg, udder, pelvis and caudal abdomen. For the high epidural, the animal's hindquarters may be raised after administration for 5–10 minutes to aid drug distribution. If unilateral tissue desensitisation is required, the desired side is placed lowermost initially until the block has taken effect. With the high block, the animal will become recumbent, requiring assistance to stand during recovery.

For both blocks, the local anaesthetic is administered through the sacrococcygeal (young animals) or first intercoccygeal (mature animals) joint. While moving the tail up and down, the most cranial moving joint is located. A 2.5 cm (1 in), 20 gauge needle is advanced midline, with the hub angled 10–15 degrees caudally. The needle may be advanced to the ventral floor of the spinal canal, then slightly withdrawn and the local anaesthetic injected. There should be no resistance when injecting.

The tail becoming limp indicates a successful block.

Epidural – lumbosacral

This desensitises the flank, pelvis and hind leg. During onset of the block, loss of skin sensation is monitored and, once the most caudal rib region has been reached, the animal's front is elevated to prevent further cranial migration of the block and potential paralysis of the intercostal muscles. The animal will become recumbent, requiring assistance to stand during recovery.

Two to four mg/kg (equivalent to 1 ml/5–10 kg) is injected into the lumbosacral space. The technique is the same as for CSF collection (see Chapter 8); however, the needle is not advanced through the dura mater (i.e. it remains in the epidural space (**Fig. 18.7**). If the subarachnoid space is inadvertently entered, there are two options: (a) the needle is withdrawn into the epidural space and the full

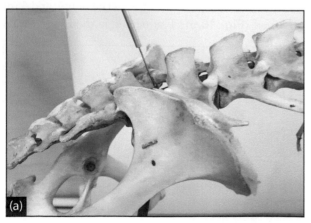
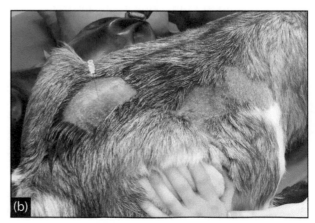

Fig. 18.7 (a) Target area and landmarks for a lumbosacral epidural shown on a skeleton, and (b) needle in position in the patient.

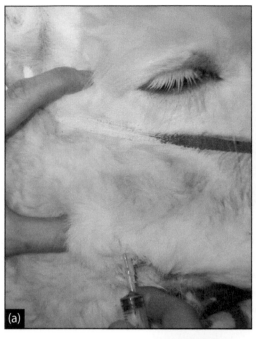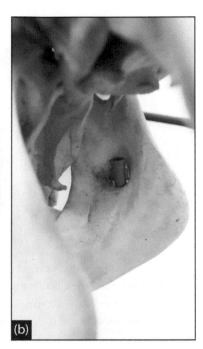

Fig. 18.8 (a) For a mandibular block, a needle is advanced on the medial aspect of the mandible to a point half-way between its ramus and the mandibular joint (indicated by thumb and index finger, respectively, here in an alpaca). (b) Skull with a blue marker inserted into the target area (foramen of the mandibular nerve).

calculated volume administered; or (b) one-third of the calculated volume is administered into the sub-arachnoid space.

Mandibular

This is a useful block for dental work involving the mandibular arcade. It also desensitises the intra- and extraoral soft tissue rostral to the foramen. Three to five ml are injected s/c on the medial aspect of the mandibular ramus, half-way between its ventral border and the mandibular joint (**Fig. 18.8**).

Mental

A mental block desensitises the rostral mandible, including the mandibular symphysis and incisors. It is useful for dental procedures and repair of a fractured symphysis. The mental foramen can be felt on the lateral aspect of the mandible, half-way along the diastema between the incisors and cheek teeth (**Fig. 18.9**). One to two ml is injected over the nerve as it exits the foramen or, for more reliable anaesthesia of the jaw and incisors, 1–3 ml is injected into the canal (with care).

Infraorbital

This block desensitises the upper lip and nose rostral to the foramen, and is useful to deal with traumatic injuries in this area such as dog bites. The landmark is

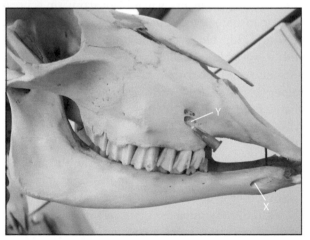

Fig. 18.9 Target positions for a mental nerve block (X) and infraorbital nerve block (Y, with needle inserted), shown on an ovine skull.

1–3 cm above the maxillary premolar teeth and 1–3 cm cranial to the facial tuberosity, usually marked by a palpable depression in the bone (**Fig. 18.9**). One to two ml is injected over the nerve as it exits the foramen. One to three ml injected into the canal (with care) may provide anaesthesia of the first and second premolars.

Auriculopalpebral

An auriculopalpebral block is used to inhibit motor function of the eyelids; for example, to facilitate

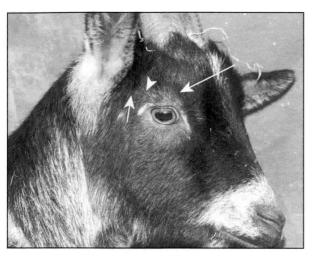

Fig. 18.10 Approximate target points for an auriculopalpebral block (short arrow) and to block the cornual branches of the lacrimal nerve (arrowhead) and infratrochlear nerve (long arrow).

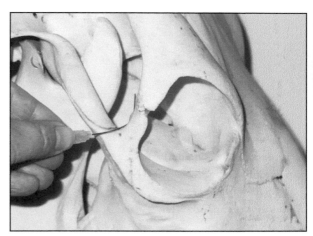

Fig. 18.11 Insertion point and direction of the needle for a Peterson block (shown here on a bovine skull).

examination of the eye when blepharospasm is present or to reduce movement during ocular surgery. (**Note:** This block does not desensitise the eyelids – an additional block such as line infiltration is required.) One to two ml is injected s/c half-way along a line drawn from the lateral canthus to the base of the ear (**Fig. 18.10**).

Peterson

A Peterson block will desensitise the intraorbital soft tissue structures; for example, for enucleation. (**Note:** The eyelids will not be desensitised by this block [i.e. they must be blocked separately]). The risk of injecting local anaesthetic into the optic nerve is probably similar to the retrobulbar block, but needle placement is away from the main ocular structures.

A 5 cm (2 in) hypodermic or spinal needle is shaped into a moderate curve (about 30 degrees) and, with the curvature pointing rostral, is inserted in the corner formed by the zygomatic arch of the temporal bone ventrally and the supraorbital process rostrally (**Fig. 18.11**). The needle is advanced fully to its hub. It may become caught on the coronoid process of the mandible. If this is suspected, the needle is slightly withdrawn and redirected. Five to seven ml are instilled at the depth of the orbit.

Retrobulbar

A retrobulbar block is an alternative to desensitise intraorbital soft tissue structures. Some local anaesthetic may be deposited superficially as the needle is withdrawn, thereby blocking the eyelids.

A 5 cm (2 in) needle is in turn inserted at the 12, 3, 6 and 9 o'clock positions around the orbit, through the eyelid, and advanced to the back of the orbit. Two to three ml are deposited each time.

Cornual

A cornual block may be suitable for disbudding kids (take care not to exceed the toxic dose – see above) or as an adjunct to GA when dehorning adults. The cornual branches of both the lacrimal and infratrochlear nerve must be blocked. One to two ml is injected alongside the temporal ridge, one-third to half-way the distance from the lateral canthus of the eye to the lateral aspect of the horn base. Another 1–2 ml is injected at the dorsomedial aspect of the orbit, close to its margin (**Fig. 18.10**).

Intravenous regional anaesthesia

IVRA is useful for interventions involving the lower limb and foot, including claw amputation or joint lavage. A tourniquet is placed either just below or above the carpus or, in the hind leg, just below or above the tarsus. (**Note:** If above the tarsus, the depression either side of the Achilles tendon must be padded to achieve adequate occlusion.) A short

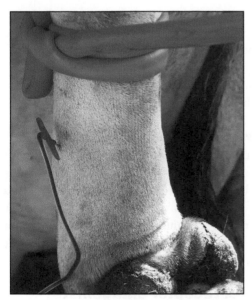

Fig. 18.12 Intravenous regional anaesthesia using a butterfly catheter (shown on a bovine limb).

21–23 gauge needle or, preferably, butterfly catheter is placed into any discernible superficial vein below the tourniquet and 1 ml/15 kg of local anaesthetic injected (**Fig. 18.12**). Care must be taken that the tourniquet remains tightly in place for at least 20 minutes to avoid local anaesthetic entering the general circulation.

Brachial plexus

The distal brachial plexus block desensitises the leg from the elbow distally. From the cranial aspect of the front leg, a needle is inserted horizontally at the medial aspect of the shoulder joint, aiming at the costochondral junction of the first rib. Local anaesthetic is injected as the needle is withdrawn at a dose rate of 2–4 mg/kg lidocaine HCl or 0.5–1 mg/kg bupivacaine.

A proximal block, which desensitises the leg from the mid-humerus distally, is possible, but technically challenging.

Teat blocks

Options to desensitise the teat include: ring block at the base of the teat (avoid adrenaline), IVRA using a household rubber band as a tourniquet around the base of the teat, line block in the shape of an inverted V proximal to a teat wound, and infusion into the teat canal and cistern (to block the mucosal lining).

ANALGESIA

General principles

The value of multimodal analgesia is well recognised. By using different classes of analgesic drugs, which act on different parts of the pain pathway, a complimentary effect is achieved. This produces a better level of analgesia and, potentially, the doses of individual drugs can be kept lower, thereby reducing the risk of side-effects. An example combination is the use of a local block, a NSAID and an opioid. Ideally, analgesia is initiated pre- and perioperatively to limit the amplification of the pain pathway and central sensitisation. Limited information on effective dosing regimes is available in goats, but options that are recognised as useful, either through pharmacological studies or field observations, are listed.

Pain scales remain in their infancy for livestock species and there is no well-validated score for goats. Some aspects of the Glasgow Composite Measure Pain Scale (CMPS) can be extrapolated to judge the likely presence of pain and discomfort. For example, difficulty rising and abnormal gait, response to gentle pressure onto surgical wounds, pain-related vocalisation such as bruxism, restlessness or weight-shifting, or avoidance behaviour.

Opioids

- Butorphanol: 0.1 mg/kg i/v, or 0.1–0.2 mg/kg i/m. Suggested frequency is every 4–6 hours (extrapolated from other species). It is a less potent analgesic than buprenorphine, but can currently be used under the prescription cascade in the UK. Potential side-effects are not known in goats.
- Fentanyl: in other species, the target drug release rate is 1–5 µg/kg/hour (translating to a minimum of 1 × 5 mg patch, which delivers 50 µg/hour for an adult goat). It takes up to 12 hours to reach peak plasma concentrations, with a duration of about 72 hours. Apply to hairless and well-cleansed and dried skin with the aid of a bandage (e.g. axilla, side of neck, lateral or medial antebrachium). Its use is currently off-cascade in the UK. Potential side-effects include bradycardia, respiratory depression, urinary retention and constipation.

- Morphine: 0.05–0.25 mg/kg i/v or i/m, titrated to effect. Analgesic duration is approximately 2–4 hours. Its use is currently off-cascade in the UK. Potential side-effects include (as with most opioids) negative effects on the gastrointestinal tract including ileus; however, the specific risk and its scale in goats is not known.
- Buprenorphine: 0.002–0.01 mg/kg i/v or i/m. It provides the longest duration of the injectable opioids, with a possible duration of 6–8 hours. However, its use is currently off-cascade in the UK. It is also relatively expensive.

Non-steroidal anti-inflammatory drugs

NSAIDs should be used whenever possible. Contraindications include hypovolaemic shock or renal compromise. Ideally, they are given at least 30 minutes prior to surgery. Avoid administration during surgery, as nephrotoxic effects may occur in the sedated or anaesthetised animal because of compromised perfusion. Ketoprofen, flunixin meglumine, carprofen and meloxicam have all been used in goats without apparent side-effects. The recommendations stemming from pharmacological studies of meloxicam in goats are summarised below. For the other NSAIDs, the cattle doses are typically used in the absence of goat-specific information.

- Meloxicam: 0.5 mg/kg i/v. Ideal dosing frequency is unknown, but for analgesia q8–12h may be required. This is based on its rapid distribution and the plasma concentration believed to provide effective analgesia in the horse being maintained in the goat for about 8 hours. No drug was detectable 72 hours after administration in goat studies. Preliminary studies in goat kids (using the i/m route), showed slower clearance compared with adults (i.e. care must be exercised with frequent dosing in young animals).
- Meloxicam: 0.5 mg/kg per os q24h. The drug showed 79% (+/– 19) bioavailability after oral administration. It takes about 15 hours to reach maximum plasma concentration, therefore interim analgesia must be provided. Oral dosing resulted in plasma concentrations that

are regarded as adequate for analgesia in other species. For the use of oral meloxicam, it should be noted that the calibration of the dispensing syringe provided with the product in the UK is 0.1 mg/kg for the dog solution and 0.6 mg/kg for the horse solution.

Corticosteroids

Corticosteroids, via their strong anti-inflammatory action, have some analgesic properties. They must not be used in pregnant does, and other potential side-effects such as immunosuppression must be taken into account. Betamethasone and dexamethasone are suitable for the purpose of analgesia, with an anti-inflammatory effect of 36–72 hours.

NMDA receptor antagonists

Ketamine can be given at subanaesthetic doses as part of a multimodal regime, providing good somatic analgesia. A single dose of 0.1–0.5 mg/kg i/v, i/m or s/c; or i/v infusion at 0.4–1.0 mg/kg/hour, with or without a loading dose of 0.1–0.5 mg/kg.

FLUID THERAPY

Assessing hydration status

Skin tent is a useful measure in the field: when the upper eyelid is pinched, it should return to its normal position within 1–2 seconds. A delayed response of 3–5 seconds indicates about 5–7% dehydration. With 10% dehydration, the skin turgor is typically lost completely (i.e. the skin fold remains).

As dehydration increases, the mucous membranes become drier. From about 8% dehydration, the eyes become sunken; however, the animal's body fat reserves must be taken into account when assessing eye position (with loss of retrobulbar fat in emaciated animals).

Anuria sets in at 10% dehydration and above, and the animal becomes weak and/or recumbent, with a weak pulse. From 12%, the animal becomes moribund.

PCV increases with extracellular fluid (ECF) loss and, after several hours delay, blood loss. Total protein tends to increase with ECF loss, unless there is a protein-losing process present. Lactate can be used to assess hypovolaemia and tissue perfusion.

Fluid rates

The maintenance rate is 2 ml/kg/hour (equivalent to 50 ml/kg/day), translating to 1 drop every 1.5–2 seconds for a 70 kg goat when using a giving set delivering 20 drops per ml. Remember that fluids will be excreted via the kidney. As a rule of thumb, of every litre of i/v crystalloid fluid administered, only a quarter remains in circulation after 1–2 hours. This highlights the need for continued fluid administration until the patient is fully stable.

Goats are relatively susceptible to pulmonary oedema when being overhydrated. Care must be taken with 'shock-doses' of fluids (10–20 ml/kg/hour). Once life-threatening hypovolaemia has been addressed, the remaining fluid deficit is best replaced over 12–36 hours. During surgery, fluid rates may be increased to 5 ml/kg/hour, providing the goat is monitored for overhydration.

Route of administration

If some rumen activity is present, oral fluids may be considered unless the deficit needs to be restored rapidly. They should ideally contain electrolytes. In kids, absence of a suck reflex indicates likely gastro-intestinal tract stasis, and fluid should be administered i/v to ensure absorption.

For the i/v route, placement of an intravenous catheter is highly advisable. For fluid therapy on farm, the catheter may be secured with superglue, thereby enabling the owner to remove it. Suitable veins include the jugular, cephalic, saphenous and ear veins (**Fig. 18.13**).

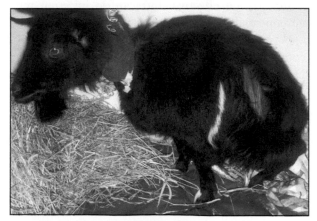

Fig. 18.13 Use of the jugular vein for intravenous fluid therapy, and monitoring urine output, in a Pygmy goat.

Choice of fluids

Crystalloids

Crystalloids are useful to replace ECF losses and as maintenance fluids. Examples and their characteristics are:

- Normal saline (0.9%): isotonic, acidic.
- Hartmann's solution (syn. lactated Ringer's solution): isotonic, alkaline; contains potassium, calcium and bicarbonate or lactate in addition to sodium and chloride.
- Glucose/dextrose solution (5% or 4% plus 0.18% NaCl): slightly hypotonic, acidic. (**Note:** The energy contained in these solutions is negligible in terms of the animal's daily requirements.)
- Hypertonic saline (7.2%): hypertonic, acidic. Main indication is rapid restoration of circulating volume. In large animals, it is widely used because of easier logistics compared with isotonic fluids. However, its effect is short-lived (<2 hours) and isotonic fluids are preferable. Administer at 4 ml/kg over 10–20 minutes. Have clean, warm drinking water within reach of animal during administration. If the animal does not drink voluntarily, administration via stomach tube is required.
- Potassium chloride: add at 10 mEq/litre main fluid where hypokalaemia is present. Adjust fluid rate so that it does not exceed 0.5 mEq/kg/hour.
- Sodium bicarbonate (8.4%): for marked metabolic acidosis. Ideally, the deficit is calculated based on blood gas analysis. The formula using total CO_2 (TCO_2) is:

$$(24 - \text{measured } TCO_2) \times 0.3\text{–}0.5 \text{ body weight}$$
$$(\text{in kg}) = \text{mmol of } NaHCO_3 \text{ required}$$

The 8.4% solution is molar (i.e. 1 ml = 1 mmol)

(**Note:** The true fluid compartment that is affected is 0.6 × body weight; using a factor of 0.3–0.5 provides a safety buffer, but may result in underdosing.)

Colloids

Colloids act as plasma volume expanders and are useful to rapidly expand circulating volume. They may also be considered in animals with hypoproteinaemia (TP <35 g/l) to prevent oedema formation.

Colloids remain in circulation longer than crystalloids. However, they do draw fluids from the interstitial and intracellular compartments and therefore should be combined with isotonic fluids, especially in patients already dehydrated. Products in this group include: 6% hetastarch or pentastarch, Gelofusine®, Haemaccel®, dextran 40 or 70, 7.2% NaCl with starch, and Oxyglobin®. It is important to check the datasheet for potential side-effects (e.g. coagulopathy) or contraindications prior to using these products.

Colloids are given at 5–10 ml/kg and should not be administered at more than 25% of the normal circulating volume of the patient at any one time.

Plasma

The two main indicators for a plasma transfusion are: (1) failure of passive transfer in the neonate; and (2) marked hypoalbuminaemia in mature animals. Goat blood does not separate out readily into solids and plasma, so a centrifuge is required. Despite goats having several blood groups, adverse reactions to plasma transfusion is rare. However, adrenaline and/or dexamethasone should be available in case of a reaction. A blood transfusion set must be used and the flow rate set low for the first 10–20 minutes (1 drop/second) while the goat is observed for adverse reactions.

Blood transfusion

Severe blood loss during surgery may warrant a blood transfusion (as a rough guideline, once >20% of blood has been lost; see Chapter 7).

EUTHANASIA

While being a commonly performed procedure, euthanasia should always be planned carefully. Aspects to consider include:

- Owner's consent and clear, unambiguous instructions that euthanasia is requested.
- Best timing in relation to assistance, disposal, facilities etc. (unless necessitated immediately by the animal's condition).
- Best place, to shield herd mates from procedure, allow easy access to cadaver, avoid undue discomfort by moving diseased animal etc.
- Assistance required and emotional impact on people present.

- Method, including back-up option if first method fails.
- Safety, with potential risks considered from the animal, the environment and the method of euthanasia.
- Disposal of the cadaver.
- Legal aspects (including animal welfare, drug and firearm regulations, environmental protection).

Animal welfare, in particular avoidance of undue stress and discomfort, must be safeguarded during the entire procedure. Signs of death include cessation of heartbeat and respiration, loss of corneal reflex and full dilation of the pupils. Regardless of method used, the animal should be monitored for 15–20 minutes after apparent death.

Sedation may be used where firearms are employed, but should be avoided for lethal injection as drug distribution is often adversely affected by the cardiovascular effects of the sedative.

Lethal injection

An overdose of barbiturates is suitable; for example, pentobarbital sodium (available as a 20–40% solution) at a dose rate of 60–120 mg/kg given as a rapid bolus. The i/v route should be used whenever possible, preferably through an indwelling catheter. In addition to the jugular, cephalic and saphenous veins, the milk vein may be used in lactating does. For injection into the ear vein, the solution should not be stronger than 20% to avoid a burning sensation (dilute with 0.9% NaCl, if necessary). In kids and yearlings, the intraperitoneal route may be effective. Intracardiac injection must never be undertaken in a conscious animal.

A quinalbarbitone sodium/cinchocaine HCl combination is available in the UK (Somulose™, Dechra). The dose rate of approximately 1 ml/10 kg must be given over a defined time of 10–15 seconds to avoid cardiac arrest prior to loss of consciousness.

Free-bullet firearms

Suitable weapons are:

- 0.32 calibre 'humane killer' or 9 mm handgun, used with round nose lead bullets and from a short distance (5–25 cm).
- 0.22 calibre rim-fire rifle, used with round nose lead bullets and from a short distance (5–25 cm).

- Shotgun of 12, 16 or 20 bore used with 4, 5 or 6 birdshot, or 0.410 calibre, held at a short distance (5–25 cm).
- Larger calibre centre-fire rifle, used outdoors from a distance by a trained marksman.

The animal's head must be firmly restrained to ensure accurate placement of the bullet, aided by sedation where required. A free bullet always carries the risk of the bullet exiting the animal's body. The risk of being hit by a ricocheting bullet can be reduced by placing the animal onto soft ground and away from solid walls, avoiding enclosed spaces such as small pens or trailers and limiting the number of people present.

In unhorned goats, the target point is midline just above the eyes in a direction down the line of the spine. In horned goats, if the target point on the forehead is obscured, the animal is shot from behind the poll in a direction towards the angle of the mandible (**Fig. 18.14**). This approach carries a high risk of the bullet leaving the animal. A shotgun is preferable over a pistol or rifle, and the animal must be placed onto soft ground.

When firearms are used, after collapse tonic activity for 10–20 seconds is followed by involuntary kicking. (**Note:** Immediate kicking or paddling indicates an ineffective stun.)

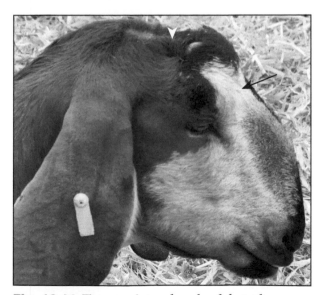

Fig. 18.14 Target point and angle of shot when using a firearm (arrow) and when using a captive bolt or where horns obstruct the normal firearm target (arrowhead).

Captive bolt

A 0.22 calibre trigger-fired penetrating captive bolt is suitable for veterinary euthanasia. Care must be taken to use a cartridge with a suitably high-power charge. In contrast to free-bullet weapons, the captive bolt is placed onto the goat's head prior to discharge. The target point is the same for all goats, regardless of whether horned or not: midline behind the bony mass of the poll, in a direction towards the base of the tongue (**Fig. 18.14**). In neonatal kids, the bolt may be placed on the intersection of two lines drawn between the lateral canthus and the opposite horn bud. Exsanguination or pithing must follow immediately after the stun to ensure outright death.

Conditionally acceptable methods

A non-penetrating captive bolt may be used in animals less than 10 kg bodyweight.

In animals that are unconscious (e.g. under GA or where the initial method of euthanasia did not result in cardiac arrest), the following may be considered:

- Potassium chloride at 1–2 mEq/kg i/v.
- Overdose of magnesium sulphate i/v.
- Exsanguination.
- Combination drug containing tetracaine HCl, mebezonium iodide and embutramid at 4–6 ml/50 kg (T 61™, MSD Animal Health).

Emergency on-farm slaughter of neonatal kids

The UK's Humane Slaughter Association describes the use of external trauma in infant kids – but this procedure must not be used at any other age, and only when veterinary or other skilled intervention is unavailable.

The aim is to humanely kill the kid by delivering a heavy blow to the head. There are two variations of this method:

1. Hold the kid by the back legs and deliver a firm blow to the back of the head with a blunt instrument; for example, an iron bar or hammer.
2. Hold the kid by the back legs and swing it through an arc to hit the back of its head with considerable force against a solid object; for example, a brick wall or metal stanchion.

With both methods, it is essential that the blow is delivered swiftly, firmly and with absolute determination. If there is any doubt that the kid has not been killed effectively, the blow should be immediately repeated.

Death should be ensured by exsanguination, cutting the throat from ear to ear to sever both carotid arteries and both jugular veins. An alternative method is to insert the knife into the ventral base of the neck towards the entrance of the chest to sever all the major blood vessels where they emerge from the heart.

Such a procedure is very much a last resort. Veterinary surgeons developing health plans may include this procedure under emergency slaughter. Under no circumstances should it be used in any other situation.

Unacceptable methods

Methods that must never be used include drowning or smothering, inducing hypothermia, exposure to thermal heat or chemicals, electrocution or use of asphyxiant gases outwith commercial registered units.

CHAPTER 19

POST-MORTEM EXAMINATION AND SAMPLING

INTRODUCTION

Post-mortem examination (PME) is a useful tool when investigating health and welfare issues in goats (**Fig. 19.1**). There are a number of reasons why such an examination may be of value:

- To investigate why a goat has died or been found dead.
- To investigate a problem affecting several animals, when a typical case can be euthanased for examination.
- To investigate a failure in either treatment or preventive medicine protocols, often in collaboration with a pharmaceutical company.
- To investigate welfare infringements instigated by an enforcement authority.
- To target sample viscera for laboratory testing such as liver tissue for copper assay.
- To undertake a specific examination as in the investigation of an abortion outbreak.

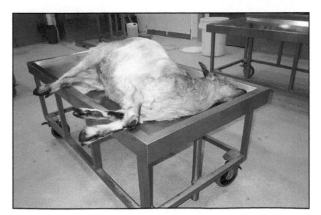

Fig. 19.1 A goat carcase ready for post-mortem examination and sampling.

Case selection is of paramount importance:

- It is important to consider whether a PME is the best approach in investigating the disease outbreak, rather than sampling live goats, which may also be more cost effective. An example is the investigation of a diarrhoea outbreak in young kids in which examination of faeces from a number of live animals may be a better approach.
- The selected case has to be representative of the problem under investigation.
- A goat with residual antibiotic levels following a period of treatment may be useful to investigate the pathology, but be of limited value to identify a possible bacterial cause.
- Severe autolysis can make accurate PME very difficult.

The practitioner's skill as a pathologist may dictate their decision whether to undertake the PME themselves or refer to a specialist laboratory or pathology centre.

HISTORY

A comprehensive history is essential before embarking on any PME, as this will have an influence on the approaches taken, particularly with regard to sampling. Such a history should include as a minimum:

- Age, breed and gender.
- Homebred or purchased (and when).
- Numbers affected, number dead and size of group (morbidity/mortality).
- Clinical signs exhibited prior to death or euthanasia, and any signs of potential relevance in rest of group.

- Treatment history (e.g. anthelmintics, antibiotics).
- Kidding date (if applicable).
- Management – housed/outdoors.
- Management – diet fed, any recent changes.
- Management – vaccination status.
- Management – any recent handling or procedures (e.g. transport, disbudding).

HEALTH AND SAFETY

Anyone undertaking, assisting with or observing a PME should be aware of the health and safety implications. There is a potential risk of cuts or stab wounds, and it is advisable to wear a cut proof glove on the non-cutting hand (under waterproof gloves). Suitable protective overclothing and wellington boots should be worn. These may either be disposable or easily cleaned and disinfected on completion of the PME, and between PMEs to avoid potential cross contamination between carcases. Care should also be taken to avoid injury while lifting heavy carcases.

In addition, there are the risks associated with a number of zoonotic pathogens potentially infecting the carcase or contaminating the environment. In the UK, for example, these are classified by the Advisory Committee on Dangerous Pathogens (ACDP) as:

- Hazard group 2 pathogens. These can cause human disease and may be a hazard to employees, but are unlikely to spread to the community and there is usually effective prophylaxis or treatment available. *Salmonella* spp. and *Cryptosporidium* spp. are examples of hazard group 2 pathogens.
- Hazard group 3 pathogens. These can cause severe human disease and may be a serious hazard to employees. They may also spread to the wider community, but there is usually effective prophylaxis or treatment available. These pathogens include *Coxiella burnetii* (Q fever), *Mycobacterium bovis* (tuberculosis) and *Escherichia coli* O157.

If any of these infectious agents (particularly ACDP Hazard group 3) are suspected, it may be preferable to refer the carcase to a laboratory that can undertake the PME in containment facilities.

PREPARATION

Prior to the PME itself, it is important to have all the instruments and sampling equipment required, including one or more sharp knives or disposable PME scalpels, a hack saw or garden loppers (useful for cutting through ribs), scalpel and forceps for any fine dissection, swabs and sampling pots. These should be readily available with the tops taken off the pots for ease of access, reducing the risk of external contamination of containers. A camera, smartphone or tablet to take images of relevant pathology is useful, and some form of means to record findings, ensuring that notes are made at the time of the examination, and at the end of each carcase if more than one PM is being undertaken (this will ensure that findings are not mixed-up).

POST-MORTEM EXAMINATION APPROACH

It is important to develop a systematic approach to each and every PME undertaken. This will ensure that no organ system is overlooked. There may be a tendency, particularly if the clinical signs suggest (e.g. diarrhoea), to examine the gastrointestinal tract first; this, however, will release gut content thus contaminating the entire carcase and potentially masking other significant pathology.

One author's (DH) approach is as follows:

1. External examination. Entire carcase, then partially skinned to allow access to internal viscera:
   - Note down any identifying ear tag or other identification.
   - Describe the coat covering, including any evidence of ectoparasites.
   - Attribute a body condition to the carcase. Avoid condition scoring a carcase; instead use descriptive terms such as emaciated, thin, moderate, good, overfat condition etc.

- Examine the umbilicus in young kids.
- Examine the udder in females.
- Examine the feet for visible lesions.
- Examine the external mucous membranes for evidence of anaemia.
- For ease of PME activity, cut down through each axilla to lie the front legs flat on the working surface, and cut down and disarticulate through the two hip joints. This should ensure the carcase remains stable and does not move sideways as the examination continues.
- As the carcase is skinned, note any signs of dehydration (subcutaneous tissue has a 'tacky' feel) or jaundice.
- Take a sample of blood (into a plain container; for example a vacutainer) from any free blood flowing from the carcase for possible testing.

2 Open the abdominal cavity – leave viscera in carcase initially:
- Have a superficial look at the intact viscera, but do not open the gut at this stage.
- Note any evidence of spatial displacement, any fluid present (describe nature and quantity).

3 Open the thoracic cavity and examine the contents.
- This can be easily achieved in young kids by cutting along the costochondral junction. In mature animals cut through ribs/sternum using a hacksaw or garden loppers.
- Try not to damage the underlying pericardial sac attached to the sternum.
- Examine initially for excess fluid in the thorax, describe the quantity and consistency, and take a swab or pipette aliquot into a sample container if considered significant.
- By digital palpation, assess whether there are adhesions between the lung and the thoracic wall. Note if fibrinous and easily broken down, or firm and fibrous.
- Remove the complete pluck including the tongue and examine systematically:
  – Examine the lung tissue, initially comparing one lung with the other.

Describe any pathology, and whether bilateral. Examine any focal lesions by excision.
  – Excise into the lumen of the oesophagus and then the larynx and trachea down past the bronchial bifurcation.
  – Examine the bronchomediastinal lymph nodes.
  – Excise the pericardial sac. Describe the quantity and consistency of any fluid present.
  – Examine the heart including each chamber and heart valve.

4 Examine the renal system:
- Remove each kidney. Incise through the capsule, renal medulla and cortex to section the kidney into two halves lengthwise. Can the capsule be easily peeled back? Describe any changes evident (subcapsular haemorrhage, infarct, pale cortex in nephrosis). Repeat with the opposite kidney.
- Examine the ureters, incise into the bladder and examine the penis in males.

5 Examine the reproductive system:
- Pregnant – number of fetuses and stage of pregnancy.
- Recently kidded – any evidence of retained placenta, endometritis.
- Note any kidding injuries to birth canal.
- Examine the testicles – if castrated recently, note any evidence of infection.

6 Examine the remaining abdominal cavity contents systematically:
- Remove the liver and examine grossly. Describe colour, shape, margins and consistency (firm/friable) and incise any superficial lesions.
- Serially section the liver for evidence of deeper lesions.
- Examine the gallbladder. Describe content – note any evidence of liver fluke.
- Examine the caudal vena cava for necrotic change or thrombus formation.
- Examine the intestinal tract grossly. Describe any changes in colour of the serosal surface (e.g. congested).

Palpate between finger and thumb along its length for the subtle thickening often identified in Johne's disease. Incise into the jejunum, ileum and large intestine. Describe any mucosal lesions present. Describe the colour and consistency of the contents, and take a sample if deemed necessary. Strip content into a bowl if parasitic gastroenteritis suspected.

- Take a sample of faeces to test for potential pathogens (e.g. cryptosporidia, coccidia, salmonella, nematode ova).
- Examine associated mesenteric lymph nodes.
- Examine the fore-stomachs – note any evidence of cranial abdominal peritonitis (e.g. reticulitis).
- Examine the abomasal contents – wash into a bowl to examine for nematode infestation, specifically *Haemonchus contortus*, which can often be seen with the naked eye when contents are swirled around the bowl.
- Examine rumen contents. Describe the quantity and consistency (liquid or dry and impacted). Examine specifically for any extraneous material such as leaves of potentially toxic plants (e.g. rhododendron).

7 Examine joints/musculature:
- Excise into joints. Describe the quantity and consistency of synovial fluid, and the joint surface.
- If conditions such as trauma or white muscle disease are suspected, continue to skin the carcase and incise into major muscle masses.

8 Remove the head to examine the oral cavity and brain (if deemed necessary):
- The tongue will have been examined with the pluck.
- Examine the oral cavity for ulceration or diphtheria.
- Examine the dentition, particularly in elderly goats for evidence of tooth loss, overgrowth and gum disease.
- If facilities allow, gain access to the brain either by removing the overlying skull by placing it in a vice and making a diamond-shaped cut (**Fig. 19.2**), or by sagittally sawing the head in half (obtaining two opposing hemi-brain portions). If neuropathological examination is required, place the brain tissue in a container of formol saline intact (i.e. do not section at this stage). Fixation can be achieved by ensuring a minimum 10:1 ratio of fixative to brain tissue.

9 Examine the spinal cord if necessary. Removal of the spinal cord itself can be achieved either by skilfully sawing down the length of the spinal column after all the muscle and viscera have been removed, or by systematic use of bone cutters. This examination may be necessary if swayback is suspected.

10 Finally, give an overall assessment of the carcase quality: fresh or decayed.

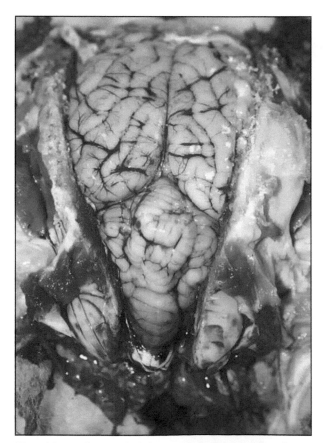

Fig. 19.2 The roof of the cranial cavity removed following diamond-shaped cuts through the skull after skinning. The head must be held firmly for this to be undertaken accurately and safely.

SAMPLING PROTOCOLS

Sample collection will vary depending on the pathology identified or the disease/condition suspected.

Bacteriology

Many organisms are very labile, and may be destroyed by the pH change in tissue as it autolyses in transit to a laboratory. If there is to be a delay in testing samples, then swabs taken aseptically and placed in transport media at the time of the PME or immediately afterwards are far preferable over tissue submission (**Fig. 19.3**). Ideally, samples should only be taken from goats that have not received any antiobiosis prior to death or euthanasia. Once a tissue or specific lesion has been identified for bacteriological sampling, the surface should be seared with a hot spatula (**Fig. 19.4**) and then, using a sterile scalpel, a small nick made in the tissue into which the swab is then inserted (**Fig. 19.5**). Swabs should be clearly labelled.

Histopathology

Any tissue sampled must be fresh to be of any real value: autolysis and freezing/thawing of tissue renders it unsuitable. Sample selection is important. Small cubes of tissue measuring 1–1.5 cm³ should be taken (except brain), including both abnormal and normal tissue for comparison (**Fig. 19.6**). It should

be placed in 10 times its own volume of formol saline fixative. Normal lung tissue will float in fixative. It can be kept below the surface (thus ensuring complete perfusion) by placing a piece of paper towel on top (**Fig. 19.7**).

If fresh gut is available (from very freshly dead or euthanased goats), then 1 cm lengths of gut should be sampled, and opened up such that the mucosa is bathed in fixative (at 10 times the volume of tissue; **Fig. 19.8**). Sample pots should be clearly labelled and allow easy removal of the fixed tissue.

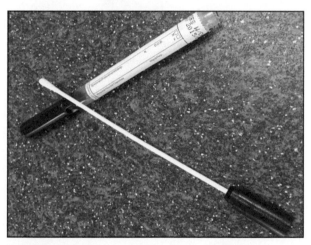

Fig. 19.3 A plain swab placed into a transport medium prior to sending to a laboratory is ideal for ensuring bacterial stability. It should be taken aseptically to avoid contamination.

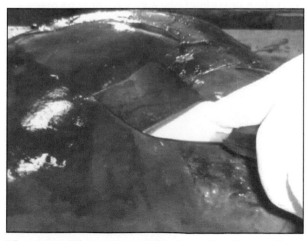

Fig. 19.4 The surface of the tissue (in this case liver) is seared with hot metal (such as a spatula). This will kill off surface contaminants.

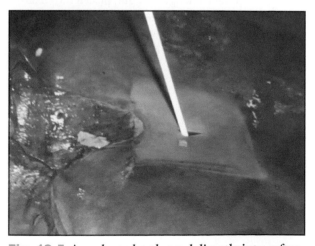

Fig. 19.5 A swab can be plunged directly into softer tissue. This may be facilitated by making a small nick with a sterile scalpel.

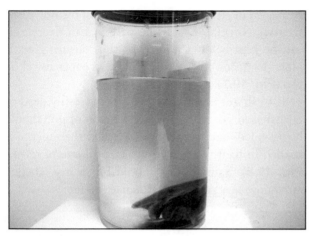

Fig. 19.6 A small portion of tissue placed in 10 times its volume of fixative in a suitable wide-mouthed, leak-proof container.

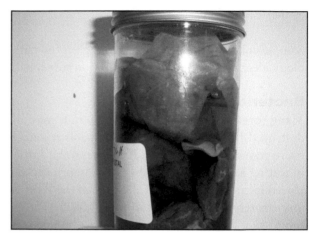

Fig. 19.7 A paper towel has been placed over lung tissue to prevent it from floating, which could result in poor fixation.

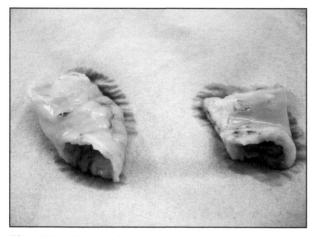

Fig. 19.8 One cm lengths of gut, placed into fixative, ensuring the mucosa surface is in contact with the fixative. This can be achieved by placing the gut over the open ends of a pair of forceps.

Aborted goat kids

Unless the entire kid and placenta can be sent to a diagnostic laboratory for testing, then during a PME:

- With a pipette or syringe, take a sample of any free fluid in either the thoracic or abdominal cavity into a plain vacutainer or other sterile container.
- Take a sample of stomach content aseptically using a vacutainer and needle, or a swab of fluid taken aseptically if minimal amount.
- Take a portion of placenta with at least one cotyledon.

1 LABORATORY REFERENCE INTERVALS

The figures in the tables below are given for guidance only. Laboratories should indicate their own reference intervals with any test results provided. Reference intervals may vary slightly depending on the test procedure, age and type of goat and the geographical location.

Table 1 Red blood cell parameters. (With permission Animal and Plant Health Agency UK)

TEST	UNITS	REFERENCE INTERVAL
Red blood cell count	× 10^{12}/l	10–18
Haemoglobin	g/dl	8–15
Packed cell volume	l/l	0.24–0.39
Mean corpuscular haemoglobin	pg	7–9
Mean corpuscular haemoglobin content	g/dl	31–42
Mean corpuscular volume.	fl	16–34
Platelets	× 10^3/µl (or 10^9/l)	300–600

Table 2 White blood cell parameters. (With permission Animal and Plant Health Agency UK)

TEST	UNITS	REFERENCE INTERVAL	PERCENTAGE OF TOTAL WBCC
White blood cell count (WBCC)	× 10^9/l	6–14	
Neutrophils (mature)	× 10^9/l	1.2–7.2	30–48
Neutrophils (band/immature)	× 10^9/l	Rare	Rare
Lymphocytes	× 10^9/l	2.0–9.0	45–70
Monocytes	× 10^9/l	0–0.5	0–4
Eosinophils	× 10^9/l	0.05–0.5	1–8
Basophils	× 10^9/l	0–0.1	Rare

Table 3 Enzyme assays at 37°C. (With permission Animal and Plant Health Agency UK)

TEST	UNITS	REFERENCE INTERVAL
ALP	IU/l	0–300
AST	IU/l	0–300
CK (CPK)	IU/l	0–100
gGT	IU/l	0–30
GLDH	IU/l	0–10
LDH	IU/l	0–400
Pepsinogen	IU/l	0–1.0
GSH-Px	U/ml RBCs	>60

Table 4 **Other blood biochemistry tests. (With permission Animal and Plant Health Agency UK)**

TEST	UNITS	REFERENCE INTERVAL
Albumin	g/l	29–43
Beta-hydroxybutyrate	mmol/l	0–1.2
Bilirubin – total	µmol/l	0–7
Calcium	mmol/l	2.3–2.9
Chloride	mmol/l	98–110
Copper (plasma)	µmol/l	9–19
Creatinine	µmol/l	54–123
Globulin	g/l	23–46
Glucose	mmol/l	2.4–4.0
Haptoglobin	g/l	<0.1
Magnesium	mmol/l	0.8–1.3
Phosphate	mmol/l	1.0–2.4
Potassium	mmol/l	3.4–6.1
Total protein	g/l	62–79
Sodium	mmol/l	135–156
T4	nmol/l	43–90
Urea	mmol/l	4.0–8.6
Vitamin B12 (cyanocobalamin)	pmol/l	>221
Zinc	µmol/l	>12 adequate <6 deficient

Table 6 **Cerebrospinal fluid.**

TEST	UNITS	REFERENCE INTERVAL
Protein	g/l	<0.4
Nucleated cells	cells/µl	0–8
Red blood cells		Nil
Bacteria		Nil
Beta-hydroxybutyrate	mmol/l	<0.5

Table 7 **Synovial fluid.**

TEST	UNITS	REFERENCE INTERVAL
Protein	g/l	Mean 20
Nucleated cells	cells/µl	Mean 50 (mostly lymphocytes and monocytes)

Table 8 **Peritoneal fluid.**

TEST	UNITS	REFERENCE INTERVAL
Protein	g/l	20–25
Nucleated cells	× 10^9/l	0.2–0.3

Table 5 **Aqueous/vitreous humour.**

TEST	INTERPRETATION
Calcium	<1 mmol/l suggests hypocalcaemia
Magnesium	Aqueous humour <0.33 mmol/l or vitreous humour <0.65 mmol/l suggests hypomagnesaemia
Beta-hydroxybutyrate	>2.5 mmol/l suggests ketosis
Urea	Levels of urea in aqueous humour of >30 mmol/l in ruminants are consistent with significant renal disease, although kidney histopathology is needed for a definitive diagnosis

Table 9 **Urinalysis.**

TEST	UNITS	REFERENCE INTERVAL
pH		7.0–8.0
Specific gravity		1.020–1.040
Osmolarity	mOsm/kg	800–1200
Electrolytes (Na, Cl, P, Ca, Mg)		Low
Protein		Trace
Ketones		Trace (lactating does)
Bacteria	per ml	<10,000 = contamination >100,000 = infection

2 CONVERSION FACTORS

To convert from SI units to old/conventional units, divide by the conversion factor

	SI UNITS	CONVERSION FACTOR	OLD/CONVENTIONAL UNITS
HAEMATOLOGY			
PCV	l/l	0.01	%
RBCs	$\times 10^{12}$/l	1	$\times 10^6$/µl
Erythrocytes	$\times 10^9$/l	1	$\times 10^3$/µl
Nucleated cell count	$\times 10^9$/l	1	$\times 10^3$/µl
Eosinophils	$\times 10^9$/l	1	$\times 10^3$/µl
Fibrinogen	g/l	100	mg/dl
MCV	fl	n/a	fl
MCH	pg	n/a	pg
MCHC	g/l	10	g/dl
BIOCHEMISTRY			
ALP	U/l	1	IU/l
ALT	U/l	1	U/l
ACTH	pmol/ml	0.22	pg/ml
Albumin	g/l	10	g/dl
Ammonia (NH_4)	µmol/l	0.587	µg/dl
Amylase	U/l	1	U/l
AST	U/l	1	U/l
Bilirubin	µmol/l	17.1	mg/dl
Calcium	mmol/l	0.2495	mg/dl
Carbon dioxide	mmol/l	1	mEq/l
Chloride	mmol/l	1	mEq/l
Cholesterol	mmol/l	0.0259	mg/dl
Copper	µmmol/l	0.157	µg/dl
Cortisol	nmol/l	27.59	µg/dl
Creatine kinase (CK)	U/l	1	IU/l
Creatinine	µmol/l	88.4	mg/dl
GGT	U/l	1	U/l
GLDH	U/l	1	U/l
Globulin	g/l	10	g/dl
Glucose	mmol/l	0.0555	mg/dl
Iron, binding	µmol/l	0.179	µg/dl
Iron, total	µmol/l	0.179	µg/dl
Lipase	U/l	1	IU/l
	U/l		Cherry-Crandall U

Continued

	SI UNITS	CONVERSION FACTOR	OLD/CONVENTIONAL UNITS
Magnesium	mmol/l	0.4114	U/l
Osmolality	mmol/l	1	Osm/kg
Phosphorus	mmol/l	0.323	mg/dl
Potassium	mmol/l	1	mEq/l
Protein, total	g/l	10	g/dl
SDH	U/l	1	IU/l
Selenium	µmol/l	0.1266	µg/dl
Sodium	mmol/l	1	mEq/l
Triglycerides	mmol/l	0.0113	mg/dl
Triiodothyronine (T3)	nmol/l	0.0154	µg/dl
Thyroxine (T4)	nmol/l	12.5	µg/dl
Urea nitrogen	mmol/l	0.357	mg/dl
Uric acid	mmol/l	59.48	mg/dl
Vitamin E	µmol/l	2.322	mg/ml

3 FURTHER READING

Textbooks

Cannas A, Pulina G (2007) *Dairy Goats – Feeding and Nutrition*. CABI Publishing, Wallingford.

Clarke KW, Trim CM (2013) *Veterinary Anaesthesia*, 11th edn. Saunders/Elsevier, St. Louis.

Constable P, Hinchcliffe KW, Done SH, Gruenberg W (2016) *Veterinary Medicine: A Textbook of the Diseases of Cattle, Horses, Sheep, Pigs and Goats*, 11th edn. Saunders/Elsevier, St. Louis.

Dugdale A (2010) *Veterinary Anaesthesia – Principles to Practice*. Wiley-Blackwell, Ames.

Fubini SL, Ducharme NG (2016) *Farm Animal Surgery*, 2nd edn. Saunders/Elsevier, St. Louis.

Gordon I (2017) *Reproductive Technologies in Farm Animals*, 2nd edn. CABI Publishing, Wallingford

Harwood DG (2006) *Goat Health and Welfare: A Veterinary Guide*. Crowood Press, Marlborough.

Hendrickson DA, Baird AN (2013) *Turner and McIlwraith's Techniques in Large Animal Surgery*, 4th edn. Wiley-Blackwell, Ames

Matthews JG (2016) *Diseases of the Goat*, 4th edn. Wiley-Blackwell, Chichester.

Mowlem A (2001) *Practical Goat Keeping*. Crowood Press, Marlborough.

Pugh DG, Baird N (2011) *Sheep and Goat Medicine*, 2nd edn. Elsevier Health Sciences, London.

Smith BP (2014) *Large Animal Internal Medicine*, 5th edn. Elsevier, St. Louis.

Smith MC, Sherman DM (2009) *Goat Medicine*. Wiley-Blackwell, Ames.

Solaiman SG (2010) *Goat Science and Production*. Wiley-Blackwell, Ames.

Wolfe DF, Moll HD (1998) *Large Animal Urogenital Surgery*, 2nd edn. Lippincott Williams and Wilkins, Philadelphia.

Review article

Harwood DG (2016) Goat health planning. *In Practice* **38(8):**387–98.

Further information

British Goat Society - https://www.britishgoatsociety.com/

Goat Veterinary Society - http://www.goatvetsoc.co.uk/

National Research Council (2007) *Nutrient Requirements of Small Ruminants: Sheep, Goats, Cervids, and New World Camelids*. The National Academies Press Washington DC. (www.nap.edu), doi.org/10.17226/11654

OIE (World Organisation for Animal Health) (2017) Listed diseases, infections and infestations in force in 2017. http://www.oie.int/en/animal-health-in-the-world/oie-listed-diseases-2017/

Various guides on milk quality, out-of-season breeding and building design available from: The Dairy Practices Council (www.dairypc.org): Small Ruminant Task Force. (Follow link to 'Guidelines', then to 'Small Ruminants')

Note: Page numbers in **bold** refer to figures and in *italics* to tables

abdominal distension 109–10, 129, **129**, **145**
abdominal examination 109–11, **110**
abdominal fluid 111, **111**
abdominal pain 110
abdominal wall, closure 74–5, **75**
abdominocentesis 112, **112**, *354*
abiotrophy 202
abomasum
    bloat (abomasitis) 128–30
    displacement 126–7
    emptying defect 125–6
    examination of contents 350
    nematode parasites 154, **156**
    normal structure and function 125
    ulceration 127–8, **127**
abortion 34–44
    enzootic 36–38
    habitual 44
    infectious causes 35–43
    induced 28, 67
    non-infectious causes 43–4
    sample collection 34–5, 352
accessory sex glands, disorders 52
acetonaemia (lactational ketosis) 303–4
acidosis
    metabolic 245, 302, 304, 343
    neonatal 100
    rumen 122–3, **122**, 186
Actinobacillus lignieresi 126, 169
adenovirus 163
adrenaline 88, 92
agalactia
    contagious 173, 228, 229, 274–5
    post-partum 273
air-hunger signs 165–6, **166**
airways, clearing in newborn 87
Akabane virus 42
albendazole 214
alfaxalone 334
allergic pneumonitis 176–7
alopecia 250–3, 257, 260, 264
Alpine goat **22**
aminoglycosides 82, 245, 247
amitraz solutions 258
ammonium chloride 242
ammonium tetrathiomolybdate (antidote) 319
ampicillin 279
anaemia 155, **155**, **156**, 187–9, 258, 307, 310

anaesthesia *see* general anaesthesia; specific regional blocks
anal/perineal reflex 197
analgesia 341–2
Anaplasma phagocytophilum 42
Anglo-Nubian goat **115**
Angora goats 13, 44
angular limb deformity 217, **218**
anoestrus 22, 23, 24–5
anthelmintic resistance 156–7, 158–9
anthelmintics 157–9
anthrax 329–30, **330**
aphthous fever 323–6, 325
apnoea 333
    primary 87
aqueous humour, analysis 300, *354*
arbovirus infections 42, 330
arterial thrombosis 187
arthritis
    bacterial (joint ill) 227–8
    CAE infection 226, **226**
    Mycoplasma 228–9
arthrocentesis 216, *354*
arthrogryposis 99–100
artificial insemination 26–7, **26**, **27**
artificial rearing 104–6, **104–6**
artificial respiration 87–8
ascites **111**, 179, 184, 308
Aspergillus fumigatus 176
asphyxia, neonate 86–8
aspiration pneumonia 170, 333
ataxia 102, 196, 198, *198*, 202, 210, 211, 303, 307, 317, **320**
    enzootic (swayback) 306–7, **307**
atelectasis 87, **87**
atipamezole 334
atresia ani, recti, coli 96–7, **96**, 129
atrial septal defect 181–2
atropine 88, 290, 293
Aujeszky's disease (pseudorabies) 212–13
aural *see* ear
auriculopalpebral block 339–40, **340**
axillary nerve *205*

babesiosis 193–4
Bacillus anthracis 329
bacteriology 351, **351**
bacteriuria *238*
Bacteroides spp. 82
balanoposthitis 33, **33**, 54–5

base deficit 343
behaviour 4–7
benzimidazoles 157–8, *157*
Besnoitia caprae 260
besnoitiosis 260
17-beta oestradiol 273
beta-hydroxybutyrate (BHB) 302
beta-mannosidosis 101
betamethasone 342
bezoar 126, **126**, 132
biliuria *314*
biochemistry *353–4*
biosecurity 18–20, 227, 275
biparietal diameter (BPD) 62, **63**
birth canal 69, **69**
birth weight 103–4, **104**
blackleg 229
bladder, urinary
   eversion/herniation 84
   rupture 240
   ultrasonography 239, **239**
bleating 6
bleeding diathesis 244
blepharospasm 288, 289, 292, **292**
blindfolding 198
blindness 196, *196*, 198, 203, 210, 214, 295, 302, 303
blood, abnormal colour *314*
blood collection and analysis 180–1, *181*
blood donation 189
blood groups 189
blood parasites 193–4
blood transfusion 189, 344
blood vessel disorders 185–7
blowfly 259–60, **259**
bluetongue 163, 263, 326–7
body condition scoring 8–9, **9**, 47
body reflexes 197
body truss 65, **66**
body weight 14
   at breeding 21
   at weaning 106
   birth 103–4, **104**
Boer goat **5**
bone marrow biopsy 189
bone marrow disease **188**
bone sequestrum 221–3, **222**
borborygmi 110, 132
border disease virus 43
bottle feeding 105, **105**
'bottle jaw' 159
Bovicola limbata 257, **257**
bovine somatotropin 302
bovine spongiform encephalopathy (BSE) 210–11, 330
bovine viral diarrhoea virus 43
brachial plexus block 341
brachygnathia 115
bracken toxicity *237*, *314*
brain
   post-mortem examination 350, **350**
   regions/functions 195, *195*
brain injury, disbudding 201, **202**, 208, **209**
breath, abnormal smell *314*

breeding
   natural service 25–6
   out-of-season 23, 45
   synchronisation 23–4
breeding soundness examination 45–9, *46*
breeds 3, 5
British Goat Society 2
browsing behaviour 7, **7**, 301, 305, 313
Brucella abortus 40
Brucella melitensis 40,50
brucellosis 39–40
buck
   behaviour 25–6, **26**
   body weight 14
   breeding soundness 45–9, **46**
   doe:buck ratio 25
   intersex 24, **24**
   reproductive tract, normal structure and function 45, **45**
   teaser 57
   temporary suppression of fertility 59
bunny hopping gait 195
bunyaviruses 42, 99, 102
bupivacaine 337
buprenorphine 342
burns 253
butorphanol 72, 334, 335, 341
butylscopolamine bromide 71

Cache Valley virus 42
caesarean section 72–5, 337
calciferol 187, 217–8
calcium:phosphorus ratio 242
calcium
   blood and humour levels 299
   deficiency 217, 218, 299–300
   requirements in lactation 300
calcium borogluconate 81, 300, 302
calcium oxalate 316
California mastitis test 277, **277**
campylobacter infection 42–3
   C. fetus fetus 42
   C. jejuni 42
capillary refill time 179
caprine arthritis encephalitis (CAE) 225–7
   mastitis 226, 276, 277
   pneumonitis 176, **176**, 226
caprine arthritis encephalitis virus (CAEV) 225
caprine herpesvirus 1 (CpHV-1) 32–3, 43, 163
capripox viruses 262–3
captive bolt 345
carbetocin 82
carbohydrate overload 113, 122–3, **122–3**, 136, 229–30
carbon dioxide toxicity *314*
carbon monoxide toxicity *314*
cardiac dysrhythmias 180
cardiac murmurs 181, 182
cardiac neoplasia 185
cardiomegaly 184, **185**
cardiomyopathies 184–5, **185**
cardiotoxins 181, 316, *317*
cardiovascular disease 88, 181–5
   signs of 179–80

cardiovascular system, examination 15, 179–81
carprofen 279, 342
cartilage disorders 224–5
caseous lymphadenitis (CLA) 176, **177**, 191–3, **192**
cashmere 3, 14
cast 219, 220, **220**
    hanging pin 220
castration 56–7, **56**, **57**
cats 35, **35**, 36
cefquinome 279
ceftiofur 247
central nervous system (CNS), regions and functions 195, *195*
cephalosporins 82, 278
cerebellar abiotrophy 202
cerebellar hypoplasia 102
cerebellum *195*
cerebral oedema **210**
cerebrocortical necrosis (polioencephalomalacia) 202–4
cerebrospinal fluid (CSF), collection/analysis 199–201,
    200, *354*
cerebrospinal nematodiasis 214
cervix 21, **21**
    dilation failure (ringwomb) 70–1
    laceration 77–8
    prolapse 65–6
cestodes 160–1
Chlamydia abortus (C. psittaci) 37, 50, 293
chlamydiosis 36–8
Chlamydophila pecorum 292
chlorate *314*
choke 121
chorioptic mange 253–5, **254**, **255**
Chorioptes spp. 253–4, **255**
chromosome count 3
circling 203, **203**, 213
claws, lesions 229–35, **230**, **231**, **233**
claws, overgrown 233, **234**
cleft palate (palatoschisis) 97
clenbuterol 71
clinical examination, basic 14–15
colic, signs 110
cloprostenol 67, 71
clostridial metritis 82, 83
clostridial myositis 229
Clostridium perfringens 81, 93, 128, 149–51, *149*, 210
Clostridium septicum 81, 229
Clostridium tetani 209
cloudburst (pseudopregnancy) 63–4, **63**, **64**
coagulopathies *188*
coat 13–14
cobalt deficiency 309–10
    cobalt, dietary levels of 310
coccidiosis 144–6
coenurosis (gid) 213–14
Coenurus cerebralis 213
collagenase inhibitors 290
colloid fluids 343–4
colostrum 90
    CAE transmission 225, **225**, 227
    storage and feeding 91, **91**
colostrum bank 92–3, **93**
complement system 90

computed tomography (CT) 112
congenital disorders 24, 28–9, 85–6, 96, 97–8, 98–100,
    101, 102, 115, 181, 187, 253, 281, 306, 310
conjunctival membranes, colour 155, *156*, **156**, 187, **189**
conjunctival pedicle flap 294
conjunctivitis 162, **162**, **166**, **262**, 274, 293, 295
contagious agalactia 173, 274–5
contagious caprine pleuropneumonia (CCPP) 172–3
contagious ecthyma (orf) 260–1, **261**
contagious ovine digital dermatitis (CODD) 232–3
contagious pustular dermatitis (orf) 260–1, **261**
Cooperia 154
copper analysis, liver biopsy 113
    copper deficiency 102, 306–8
copper, dietary levels of 307
copper, toxicity *314*, 318–19, **318**, **319**
cor pulmonale 185
cornea 285
    damage 286, **286**, **288**, **289**
    oedema 286, 293
    ulceration **286**, 289–90, **289**, **290**, 292
cornual block 340, **340**
corticosteroids
    analgesia 342
    induction of lactation 274
    induction of parturition 67
    necrotic laryngitis 170
    pemphigus foliaceus 250
    peripheral nerve injuries 206
Corynebacterium spp. 50, 54, **177**, 191–3, **192**, 246,
    247, 275, 298
cough 172–3, 175
cowdriosis 181
cows milk **13**
Coxiella burnetti 35, 38, **38**, 348
cranial nerves *286*
cranial nerve reflexes, normal 196
creatine kinase 308
creatinine, peritoneal fluid 240
critical temperature, lower/upper 12
cryptorchidism 51–2, **52**
cryptosporidiosis 142–4, 348
Cryptosporidium parvum 143
crystalloid fluids 343
Culicoides midges 260, 326
cyanide *314*
cyanocobalamin (vitamin B12) 309–10
cyanogenic glycosides 315
cyanosis 179
cypermethrin 258
cystic ovarian disease 25, **25**
cystitis *237*, 245–7, **246**
cystocentesis 241
cystoscopy 239
cystotomy 243–4, **243**, **244**

death, acute/sudden 119, 149, 172, 174, 184, 185, 186, 300,
    308, 316, 317, *317*, 319, 329
death, signs of 344
decoquinate (Deccox) 36
degenerative joint disease (DJD) 224–5
dehorning (adult goat) 267–9, **267–269**

dehydration 342
deltamethrin 258, 259
demodectic mange 256
Demodex caprae 256
dental
    disease 115–18
    formula 114
    radiography 116, **116**, 117
dentition 114
    eruption *114*
dermatitis
    fly bite 259, **259**
    malassezia 264
    mycotic (dermatophilosis) 264
    seborrhoeic 251–2, **252**
    staphylococcal 263–4, **263**
dermatophilosis 264
dermatophytosis (ringworm) 265, **265**
dermatosis, zinc responsive 250–1
detomidine hydrochloride 72, 333–4
developmental abnormalities 85
dexamethasone 67, 206, 274, 342
diabetes 136
diamidine derivatives 194
diazepam 334
Dichelobacter nodosus 231
diclazuril 146
Dicrocoelium dendriticum 160
Dictyocaulus filaria 175, **175**
digestive system
    examination 15
    infectious diseases 142–61
digital dermatitis, contagious ovine 232–3
diminazine 194
dinoprost 67
diphenhydramine 92
disbudding
    complications 201, **202**, 208, **209**, 267
    local anaesthesia 340, **340**
    surgery 267, **267**
disuse atrophy 221
dog tapeworm 213–14
dog-sitting posture 199, 301, **301**, 307
dogs 42
domestication 1
doramectin *157*, 158,
doxapram hydrochloride 87, 334
drenching gun injuries 119–20, **119**
dropped elbow *205*
dropped hock *205*, **205**
dropped stifle 205
drug administration 15–9
dry goat therapy 279
dry matter intake 303–4, **304**
dry period nutrition 300, 303–4
ductus arteriosus 88, 182
'dummy kid' (neonatal malformation syndrome) 102
duodenum 130
dyspnoea 122, 159, 165, 169, 170, 171, 172, 175, 180, 190, 212, 229, 262
dystocia **30**, 68–72, 204
dysuria 29, 52, 240

ear
    clinical examination 295
    haematoma 296–7, **297**
    infectious disease 297–8
    injuries 295–6, **296**
    mange (psoroptic) 257
    tagging 296, **296**
ear tip necrosis 298
Echinococcus granulosus 161
eclampsia 229–300, **299**
Ehmer sling *220*, 223
Eimeria spp. 144–6
Elaphostrongylus cervi 214
electrocardiography (ECG) 180, **180**
electroejaculation (EEJ) 47–8, **48**
electrolytes, fractional excretion 239
electromyography (EMG) 201
embryo transfer 27, **28**
embryonic loss, early 33–4
emerging diseases 330, **331**
encephalitis
    bacterial 208–9
    listerial 206–8
    viral 213
endocarditis 182–3
endometritis 30–1, **30**
endotracheal extubation 336, **336**
endotracheal intubation 335, **335**
energy requirements 8, 301
enilconazole 265
enrofloxacin 247
enteritis, haemorrhagic 145, 147, 149–51, 162, 207, 244
enteritis, parasitic 153–9
enterotoxaemia 149–51, 210, **210**
entropion 287–8, **288**
enucleation 294–5, **294**
environmental enrichment 6, **6**
enzootic ataxia (delayed swayback) 306–7
enzootic calcinosis 218
enzootic haematuria *237*
epididymitis 50–1, **50**
epidural anaesthesia 338–9, **338**
epiphora *166*, 288, **288**, 289, **289**, 293
equine chorionic gonadotropin (eCG) 23
Eric Williams test 110
eructation, failure 121
erythema 252, **252**, 255, 260
erythromycin 132
Escherichia coli 82, 93, 142, 146–7, 208, 227, 246
    mastitis 275, 276
    O157:H7 146, 348
estimated breeding values (EBVs) 4
euthanasia 344–5, **345**
exercise intolerance 175, 179, 181, 183, 329
exophthalmos 291, **291**
exsanguination 346
external coaptation 221
external skeletal fixation 220, **221**
extracellular fluid (ECF), loss 342
eye
    clinical examination 285–7, **285**, **287**
    foreign bodies 287, 288–9, **288**

eye (*continued*)
   infectious disease 291–3
   non-infectious disorders 287–91
   normal structure and function 285
   regional nerve blocks 339–40, **340**
   surgery 290, **290**, 293–5, **294**
   systemic disease affecting 295
   ultrasonography 286–7, **287**
eyelids
   entropion 287–8, **288**
   suturing (tarsorrhaphy) 293
   tears/lacerations 287

facial nerve paralysis 197, **197**, 207
facial sensation 196
faecal egg counts (FECs) 155, **155**, 156, **157**, 187, 189
faecal examination 111
faecal oocyst count 145
failure of passive transfer 91–3
FAMACHA© system 155, *156*, **156**
Farquharson technique 66
Fasciola spp. 159–60
fascioliasis (liver fluke) 159–60, **159**
fat stores 8, **9**
fatty liver necrosis 303–4, **303**
fecundity 22
feed storage 10, **10**
feed supplements 305–6, **305**, **306**
feeding
   dry period 300
   fibre levels 118, 123, **123**
   forage 303–4, **304**
   lactation 303–4, **304**
   prevention of pregnancy toxaemia 302–3
   see also artificial rearing; nutrition
feeding behaviour 7, **7**, 301, 305, 313
female reproductive system 21
   congenital disorders 97–8, **97**
femoral head, erosion **224**
femoral nerve *205*, **205**
fencing 5, **5**, 12
fentanyl 341
fertility
   buck *46*, 47–9
   doe 21
   herd problems 32
   temporary suppression 59
fetal maldisposition 70
fetal membranes, retained 67, 81–2, **81**
fetotomy 75–7, **76**
fetus
   age calculation 62, **63**
   maceration 43
   mummification 35, **36**, 42, 43, 44, **44**
   sexing 62
   signs of distress 70
   signs of life 69–70
fibre, dietary 118, 123, **123**
fibre break 253
fighting 25–6, **26**
figure-of-eight bandage 268–9, **269**

first aid
   fractures 219, 220
   ocular trauma 287
fistula
   discharging 222, **222**
   recto-vaginal 78–9, **78**
   rumen 124, **125**
flank anaesthesia 338
flank incision 72, **73**
flexion tests 216
flies 258–60
floppy kid syndrome 100–1, 304
florfenicol 247
flukicides 160
fluid therapy 342–4
   general anaesthesia 334
   septicaemic kid 94, **94**
flunixin meglumine 27, 94, 279, 342
fluorescein staining 289–90, **290**
fluorogestone acetate 23
fly control 259, 260, 334
fly strike (myiasis) 259, **259**
Foley catheter 243, 244, **244**
follicle stimulating hormone (FSH) 27
follicular cyst 25, **25**
foot abscess 235, **235**
foot disease 229–35
foot examination 13
foot and mouth disease (FMD) 181, 263, 323–6, **325**
foot overgrowth 233
foot trimming 233–4, **234**, **235**
footbaths 232
footrot 230–2
forage 7, **8**, 123
   fungal spoilage 320, **321**
   toxic plants 313, **313**
foramen ovale, closure 88, 182
foreign bodies
   abomasum 126, **126**
   foot 235
   ocular 287, 288–9, **288**
forestomach disorders 121–4
forestomach, normal structure and function 121
fostering 104, **104**
foxes 213
fractures 201, 219–21
fractures, first aid 219, 220
freemartinism 24
frenulum, persistent 52, **53**
fungal pneumonia 176–7
furosemide 245
Fusobacterium spp. 82, 169, 186, 231

gag reflex 196
gait assessment 195–6, 198, 215–6
gallbladder 111, 113, 136
gallbladder, fascioliasis 160, **160**
gamma-glutamyl transferase (gGT) 92
gastroenteritis, parasitic 153–9
general anaesthesia (GA) 334–6
   dehorning 268
   disbudding 267

general anaesthesia (GA) (*continued*)
    exploratory laparotomy 134
    induction 335
    monitoring **333**
    pre- and intraoperative considerations **333**, 334–5
    recovery 336
genetic abnormalities 85, 86, 202, 281, 287–8
genomics 3–4
gestation 61
    see also pregnancy
gestational age 62, **63**
giant cell tumour, oral 118, **118**
giardiasis 163
gid (coenurosis) 213–14
glucose
    intraperitoneal 18, **89**
    intravenous 302
glucose/dextrose solution 343
glutathione peroxidase 308
goat keeping, evolution 1–3
goat meat 3, *4*, **4**
goat plague (peste des petit ruminants) 161–3, 176
goat pox 262–3, **262**
goitre, congenital 101, 310–11
goitre, milk 189–90
goitrogens 310
Golden Guernsey goat **7**
gonadotrophin-releasing hormone (GnRH) 25, 27
goose-stepping *205*
gousiekte 184
grass tetany (grass staggers) 300–1
grazing 7
griseofulvin 265
growth, poor 145, 155, **182**, 187, 310
growth rate, post-weaning 107
gynaecomastia 59

haematocrit *181*, 189
haematology 180–1, *181*, *353*, *355*
haematoma
    aural 296–7, **297**
    penile 53–4
    sporadic 266
    traumatic 219
haematopoiesis 187
haematuria *237*, *238*, *314*
haemoglobinuria *237*, *238*, *314*
haemolysis *188*
Haemonchus contortus 154, 155, 187, 350
haemoptysis 186
haemorrhage *188*
    after castration 57, **57**
    post-parturient 77, **77**
haemothorax 171
hair follicles 13
hair plucks 249, **249**
handling 12–13
hanging pin (transfixation pin) casts 220
'hard udder' 226
Hartmann's solution 343
hay, toxic plants **313**
haylage 7, **8**

head butting 4, **5**
head, regional nerve blocks 339–40, **339**, **340**
head tilt 197, **197**, 298
health plan 18
health and safety, post-mortems 348, 351
heart, examination 179
heart failure 179–80, 183, 184, 185
heart rate 179
heart sounds 179
heart valves 179, 182–3
    see also cardiac valves
heartbeat, absent in newborn 88, **88**
heartwater 181
'heat box' 90, **90**
hepatic *see* liver
hepatic lipidosis 136, 301, 302, 303, **303**
hepatotoxins *314*, *320*
hernia
    inguinal 50, **51**, 132, **132**
    umbilical 137–8, **137**, 140–2
hip dysplasia 224–5, **224**
histopathology 351, **352**
Histophilus somni 183
history taking 14
horns 13
    removal in adult 267–9
housing 11–12, **11**
    and fly worry 259, **260**
    goatlings 107, **107**
    ventilation 11–12, 165, **165**, **166**
human chorionic gonadotropin (hCG) 27
humane killer 344–5, **345**
husbandry systems 2
hydration status, assessment 342
hydrometra 63–4, **63**, **64**
hydronephrosis 240, **241**
hydrops uteri 64–5, **64**
hygiene 19–20
hymen, persistent 28, 29
hyperaesthesia/hypersensitivity 208, 209, 211, 213, 300, 316
hyperkeratosis 251, **251**, **252**
hypermetria *198*, 199, 202
hyphaema 295
hypocalcaemia (milk fever) 299–300, **299**, 302
hypocalcaemia, atypical/secondary 245, 299, 316
hypocupraemia 306–7
hypoglycaemia, neonate 95–6, **95**
hypomagnesaemia (grass tetany) 300–1
hypometria *198*
hypoproteinaemia 181, *181*
hypopyon 295
hypospadias 24, **24**
hypothermia
    general anaesthesia 334–5, **335**, 336, **336**
    neonate 89, **89**
hypotrichosis 253, **253**

identification, individual goats 20
ileal obstruction **111**
ileocolonic junction 130
ileus 132
illness, signs of 6

imidocarb 194
immune response, stimulation 92
immune system 90–5
immunoglobulin (Ig) 90, 91
impetigo, udder 263, **263**
impression smears 249–50
infectious keratoconjunctivitis (pink eye) 291–2
infiltration anaesthesia 336–41
infraorbital block 339, **339**
inguinal hernia 50, **51**, 132, **132**
inhalation anaesthesia 335
injection anaesthesia 335–6
injection site abscesses 266, **266**
injections
    intramuscular 16, **17**
    intraperitoneal 18, **19**
    intravenous 17–18, **18**, 185–6
    needle sizes 18
    subconjunctival 18, **19**, 292
    subcutaneous 16, **17**
injury risks **215**
insect bite reactions 260
insulin 302
intensive dairy farming **2**
intention tremor 202
interdigital dermatitis (scald) 230–2, **231**
intersex 24, **24**
interstitial pneumonitis 226
intestines
    disorders **111**, 128–32, **135**
    normal structure and function 130
    parasites 153–9
    ultrasonography 111, **111**, 131
intramammary tube 279
intramedullary pins 220
intramuscular injection 16–7
intraperitoneal injection 18
intraocular pressure (IOP) 286, **287**
intravenous catheter 17–18, **18**
intravenous fluid therapy 334, 342–4
intravenous injections 17–18, **18**
    venous thrombosis 185–6
intravenous regional anaesthesia (IVRA) 340–1, **341**
intussusception 111, 130, **131**
iodine deficiency 101, 310–11
Ipomoea spp. 202
iris 285, **285**
    adhesions (synechiae) 290, 293, **293**
iritis 293
iron deficiency anaemia *188*
isolation 20, **20**
ivermectin *157*, 214, 298
Ixodes ricinus 42, **258**

jaundice 136, 179, *314*, *317*, 318, **318**
Johne's disease (paratuberculosis) 151–3
joint blocks 216–17
joint fluid 216, **229**, *354*
joint ill (bacterial arthritis) 227–8
joints
    abscess, pedal 235, **235**
    CAE infection 226, **226**

joints (*continued*)
    cartilage disorders 224–5
    congenital contracture 99–100
    dislocation 223
    mycoplasma infection 228–9
    palpation 216
    radiography 216, **217**
jugular veins 179

kale *314, 317*
keratin 251, **252**
keratitis 295
keratoconjunctivitis 262, **262**, 274
keratoconjunctivitis, infectious (pink eye) 291–2
ketamine 335, 342
ketones 301, 302, 303
ketoprofen 342
ketosis 301–4
kidneys 237
    biopsy 239
    lymphosarcoma 245, **245**
    ultrasonography 239, **239**
    see also renal
Klebsiella spp. 246
knuckling reflex 197
kyphosis 218

labour 67–8
lactation 13, 271
    calcium requirements 300
    drying off 272–3, 279
    induction 273–4
    lack of post-partum 273
    in non-bred females 272–3
lactational ketosis 303–4
lambing snare 70, **70**
lameness
    assessment 215–17
    foot **216**, 229–35, **230**, 324–5
laminitis 229–30
lancet fluke 160
laparotomy
    exploratory 134, **135**
    insemination 26–7, **27**
    paravertebral block 337–8, **337**
laryngeal infections 169–70, **169**, **170**
legislation 20
leptospirosis 43
lethal injection 344
leucoencephalomyelitis 226
levamisole 157–8, *157*
libido, deficiency *46*
lice 249, **249**, 257–8, **257**
lidocaine hydrochloride 337
lifespan 14
lighting, artificial 23
limb reflexes 196
limbs
    angular deformity 217, **218**
    nerve blocks 340–1, **341**
    palpation 216
Linognathus spp. 257

Listeria monocytogenes 40, 206, 292, 293
listeriosis 40–1, 206–8
litter size, determination of 62
liver
    abscess 136, **136**
    biopsy 112–13, **113**
    examination 110–11, **112**
    fatty necrosis (hepatic lipidosis) 136, 301, 302, 303, **303**
    metastatic tumours 136, **137**
    normal structure and function 136
    tuberculosis lesions **328**
    white muscle disease, ovine 310
liver fluke 159–60, **159**
local anaesthesia 216–17, 336–41
local anaesthetic agents 337
lochial secretions 83, **83**
locoweeds 202
longevity 14
lordosis 218
louping ill 213
lower motor neurons (LMN) lesions 195
lucerne (alfalfa) **7**, 250
lungs
    abscesses **167**, 176, **177**
    adaptation in newborn 86
    atelectasis 87, **87**
    auscultation 166–7
    consolidation 174, **174**
    premature kid 103
    tuberculosis **328**
lungworm 174–5
luteal cyst 25
lymph nodes 187, *188*
    enlargement 262–3
    neoplasia 190
    tuberculosis lesions **328**
lymphadenitis, caseous (CLA) 176, **177**, 191–3, **192**
lymphoma 190
    ocular 290–1, **291**
    uterine 31
lymphosarcoma 190, **190**, **191**
    kidneys 245, **245**
    oral 118, **118**

maceration 43
macrocyclic lactones *157*, 158, 254–6, 258
    topical 254–5
magnesium
    blood and humour levels 300, *354*
    deficiency 300
    dietary levels 301
magnetic resonance imaging (MRI) 112, **214**
maiden milkers 272–3
Malassezia spp. 264, 298
male reproductive tract 45, **45**
    disorders 52–5
    examination 47–9
malignant oedema 229
mammary gland *see* udder
mandible
    brachygnathia/prognathia 115, **115**
    swelling 117, **117**

mandibular block 339, **339**
mange 253–7, 297–8
Mannheimia haemolytica 174
mannosidosis, acquired 201–2
    beta 101
marching soldier gait 196, 198
mastectomy 283–4
mastitis 275–81
    acute 276, 278
    aetiology 275
    CAE 226, 276, 277
    chronic 276, **276**, 279
    clinical presentation 276, **276**
    control 279–80
    diagnosis 277–8, **277**
    FMD associated 324–5
    gangrenous **271**, **276**, 277, 278–9
    milk appearance **271**
    pathophysiology 275–6
    prevention and control 279–81
    subclinical 277
    treatment 278–9
    tuberculosis associated 275
meat 3, *4*, **4**
meconium retention 96, **96**
medetomidine 333–4
median nerve *205*
mediastinal neoplasia 190
medication 15–9
megaoesophagus 120–1, **120**
megestrol acetate 23
melanoma 266
melatonin 23
meloxicam 279, 342
menace reflex 101, 195, 196
meningeal worm 214
meningitis, bacterial 208–9
mental nerve block 339, **339**
mental state 195, 199
mesenteric torsion 131, **131**
metacestode disease 161
metamizole 71
metatarsal fracture **219**, **220**, **221**
methaemoglobin *314*, 317
methylene blue (antidote) 318
metritis 82–4, **83**
miconazole 264
Microsporum spp. 265
midges 260, 326
milk
    artificial feeding 104–6, **105**
    bulk sample culture 278
    composition 13, *13*
    conductivity testing 278
    in mastitis **271**
    pasteurisation 227
    quality testing 278
    sampling 272
    somatic cell count (SCC) 271, 277, 278
    see also lactation
milk fever (hypocalcaemia) 299–300, **299**
milk goitre 189–90

milking machines 280–1
milking regime 279–80
mineral deficiencies 10, 44, 86, 217, 218, 305–11
mineral supplements 305–6, **306**
misalliance 28
mites
    ears 297–8
    skin (mange) 253–7
modified Ziehl–Neelsen (MZN) smears 37, **38**
mohair 13
monepantel *157*, 158
monorchism 52
Moraxella spp. 292
Morel's disease 265
morphine 342
moxidectin 157–8, *157*
mucous membrane colour 155, *156*, **156**, 179, 187, **189**
Muellerius capillaris 175, **175**
mummification 35, **36**, 42, 43, 44
muscle atrophy 198, 204
muscular dystrophy, nutritional (white muscle
    disease) 308–9
musculocutaneous nerve *205*
musculoskeletal system
    clinical examination 215–17
    infectious disorders 225–9
    non-infectious diseases 217–25, 308–9
Mycobacterium avium 176, 328
Mycobacterium avium subsp. *paratuberculosis* (MAP) 151–3
Mycobacterium bovis 176, 275, 328, 348
Mycoplasma spp.
    arthritis 228–9
    contagious agalactia 274
Mycoplasma agalactiae 228, 274, 292
Mycoplasma arginini 176, 228, 292
Mycoplasma capricolum subsp. *capricolum* 274
Mycoplasma capricolum subsp. *capripneumoniae* 172–3, 228
Mycoplasma conjunctivae 292
Mycoplasma mycoides subsp. *capri* 228
Mycoplasma mycoides subsp. *mycoides 188*, 228, 274
Mycoplasma ovipneumoniae 176
mycotic dermatitis 264
mycotoxins 245, 319–21, *320*
myelography 201, **201**
myiasis
    dermal/skin 258–9
    nasal 169
myoglobinuria *238*, 308
myositis, clostridial 229

nasal cavity, normal structure 165
nasal discharge 162, **162**, 165, **166**, 169
nasal passages, narrowing/obstruction 169
nasolacrimal duct 285, 286
natamycin 265
navel, disinfection 95, **95**
necropsy *see* post-mortem examination
nematodes
    cerebrospinal 214
    intestinal 153–9
    life cycle 154
Nematodirus battus 156

neomycin 245
neonate
    artificial rearing 104–9
    cardiac function 88, **88**
    emergency slaughter 345–6
    hypotrichosis 253, **253**
    immune system 90–5
    metabolic disorders 100–1
    musculoskeletal function 98–100
    neonatal maladjustment syndrome ('dummy kid') 102
    neurological assessment 101–2, 199, **199**
    premature 103, **103**
    respiration 86–8
    rotavirus infection 142
    septicaemia 93–5, **93**, **94**
    thermoregulation 89–90
    urinary function 97–8
    weak 85–6, 306, 310
neoplasia
    heart/cardiac 185
    kidney/renal 245
    liver/hepatic 136
    lung 172
    lymph nodes 190
    male reproductive tract 55, **55**
    ocular 290–1
    oral **118**, 119
    skin/cutaneous 265–6
    udder/mammary gland 272, **273**
    uterine 31–2, **31**, **32**
Neospora caninum 42
neosporosis 42
neovascularisation 286, **286**, **289**
nephrotoxicity 245
nerve blocks 216–17, 337, **337**, 339–41, **339**, **340**, **341**
'nest box' 90, **90**
neurological assessment 101–2, 199, **199**
neurological disease
    infectious 206–8
    neonatal kid 102
    non-infectious 201–6, *317*, *320*
'New Zealand' position 80, **80**
nitrate/nitrate toxicity *314*, 317–18
nitrous fumes 171–2, 313, *314*
'nits' 249, **249**, 257
non-steroidal anti-inflammatory drugs (NSAIDs) 41,
    224, 225, 230, 279, 342
norgestomet 23
notifiable diseases 323, *323*
nutrition 7–10, **11**, 304
    and abortion 44
    calcium/magnesium requirements 300, 301
    dry period 300, 303–4
    trace element deficiencies 250–1, 305–11
    vitamin deficiencies 203, 204, 217–18, 311–12

oak poisoning 245, *314*
obturator nerve *205*
ocular *see* eye
oedema, dependent 151, 155, 179, 184, 191, 244, 260, 310
oesophageal feeder 15, **16**
Oesophagostomum 154

oesophagus
  dilation 120–1, **120**
  obstruction (choke) 121–2
oestrogens 82
oestrus
  behaviour 22–3
  control 23–4
  cycle 22–3, **22**
OIE (World Organisation for Animal Health) 323
omentum 130
omeprazole 128
omphalitis 138, 139
open farms **143**
ophthalmoscopy 286
opioids 341–2
opisthotonus 203, 210, 213
oral cavity, examination 109, **109**, 116–17
oral lesions
  bluetongue 327, **327**
  drenching gun injuries 119–20, **119**
  FMD 325, **325**
  orf 261, **261**
  peste des petits ruminants 162
  tongue 120
  tumours 118–19, **118**
oral medications 15–16, **16**
orchitis 50
orf 260–1, **261**
orogastric tubing 15–6, **16**
osteochondrosis (OC) 224–5
osteodystrophy, mature bone 218–19
osteomalacia 218
osteomyelitis **217, 221**
osteoporosis 218
Ostertagia 154
otitis **197**, 297–8
ovary
  disorders of 24–5, **24**
  normal structure and function 21, **21**
  superovulation programme 27, **28**
over-milking 280
oviduct (fallopian tube), patency test 28, **28**
ovine white liver disease (OWLD) 310
oxalate toxicity 316–17
oxytetracycline 245, 279
oxytocin 82, 278

pain, signs of 6, 110, **110**, 341
palatoschisis (cleft palate) 97
pancreas 136
panniculus reflex 197
pantoprazole 128
paper slide test 197
papillomas (warts) 265–6
paralysis
  flaccid 195, **199**
  spastic 196, 199, 09
paralysis, peripheral nerve 204–6
paraphimosis **54**
parasites
  blood 193–4
  external 253–60

parasites (*continued*)
  gastrointestinal 153–60
  lung 174–5
parasitic gastroenteritis 153–9
paratuberculosis (Johne's disease) 151–3
paravertebral block 337–8, **337**
Parelaphostrongylus tenuis 214
paresis (weakness) 198, 198, 213, 299–300, 301, 306–7, 308
parturient paresis 299–300, **299**
parturition
  correction of fetal maldisposition 70
  dystocia 68–72
  induction 67, 302
  normal 67–8
  post-parturient problems 77–84, 299–301, 303–4
parturition kit 69, **69**
passive transfer 90–1
Pasteurella multocida 174
pasteurellosis 173–4
patellar reflex 196
patent urachus 139, 140–2
pedal joint abscess 235, **235**
pemphigus foliaceus 250
penicillins 31, 82, 209
penis
  deviation 52–3
  examination 45, 47, **48**
  phimosis/paraphimosis 54
  trauma 53–4
pentobarbital sodium 344
pericardial effusion 183–4, **183**
pericardiocentesis 180
pericarditis 183–4
peripheral nerve disorders 204–6, *205*
peritoneal fluid 134, **135**, *354*
peritonitis 78, 79, 109, 112, 124, 127–8, **128**, 134–5
peroneal nerve *205*
peste des petit ruminants (goat plague) 161–3, 176
Peterson block 340, **340**
phenacetin *314*
phenols *314*
phenolsulphonphthalein (PSP) excretion 239
phimosis 54
phlebitis 185, 186
phosphate, serum 240
phosphorus deficiency 217, 218
photosensitisation *237*, 252–3, *317*
phytobezoars 126, **126**
pink eye 291–2
placenta 61, **61**, 62
plants
  causing photosensitisation 252
  containing goitrogens 310
  containing swainsonine 202
  toxic 181, 184, 245, 252, **313, 315, 316**, 314–17, *317*
plasma transfusion 92, **92**, 344
pleural effusion 170–1, 190
pleuritis 171
pleuropneumonia, contagious caprine 172–3
pneumonia
  aspiration 170
  bacterial 173–4, **174**

pneumonia (*continued*)
    fungal 176–7
    parasitic 174–5
pneumonitis
    allergic 176–7
    CAE 176, **176**
pneumothorax 113, 171
poisoning *see* toxicities
polioencephalomalacia (cerebrocortical necrosis) 202–4
polledness 13
population size 1
portosystemic shunts 187
positive pressure ventilation (PPV) 88
post-mortem examination 347–52
    approach 348–50
    case selection 347
    health and safety 348
    history of case 347–8
    sampling 351, **351**, **352**
    value of 347
posture
    abnormalities *198*
    assessment 215–16
potassium, dietary 300
potassium chloride 343
potassium iodide 118, 311
pregnancy
    abdominal contour 109, **110**
    ante-natal preparation 67
    behaviour 6–7
    diagnosis 61–2, **63**
    embryonic loss 33–4
    prepartum problems 63–7, 301–2
    rate 26
pregnancy toxaemia 44, 301–3
prematurity 103, **103**
premedication 335
preoperative preparation 334
prepuce, examination 47, **48**
prion diseases 210–12
procaine hydrochloride 337
procaine penicillin 210, 247
progesterone 23, 273
prognathia 115, **115**
prokinetics 132
prolapse
    rectal 132–4, **133**
    uterine 79–81
    vaginal/cervical 65–6, **65**
propofol 335–6
proprioception, assessment 197
propylene glycol 302
prostaglandin-F2-α (PGF$_{2\alpha}$) 23, 31, 67, 82
prostate gland 47
protein requirements 8
proteinuria *238*
Proteus spp. 246
protozoal infections 142–6, 163
pruritus 212, 251, 254, 255
pseudolactation 272
Pseudomonas spp. 246, 275
pseudopregnancy 63–4, **63**

pseudorabies (Aujeszky's disease) 212–13
Psoroptes cuniculi (*P. caprae*) 257, 298
Psoroptes ovis 297
psoroptic mange 257
puberty 21, 45
pulse 179
punch biopsy 250, **250**
pupillary light reflex (PLR) 196, *196*
pyelonephritis *237*, 245–7
pygmy goat syndrome 251–2, **252**
Pygmy goats 3
pyloric stenosis 125–6
pyometra 30, **64**
pyothorax 171
pyrethroids 258, 259

Q fever 35, 38–9, **38**, 348
quarantine 20, **20**

rabies 212
radial nerve *205*
radioimmune diffusion 92
'rag-doll' neonate 199, **199**
ragwort 252, **313**, *317*
Raillietia caprae 297
rape, oilseed *314*, *317*
rearing, kids 104–7, **105–7**
record keeping 20
rectal prolapse 132–4, **133**
rectal temperature 12
recto-vaginal fistula 78–9, **78**
rectoanal mucosa-associated lymphoid tissue (RAMALT) test 211
recumbency
    hypocalcaemia 299, **299**
    neurological assessment 199
reflexes 195–7
regional anaesthesia 336–41
renal
    artery, embolism *237*
    biopsy 239
    function tests 239
    infarct *237*, 244, **244**
    insufficiency/failure 244–5
reserpine 274
respiratory disease
    infectious 172–5, 226, 328–9
    non-infectious 169–72
    treatment principles 167
respiratory rate 165
respiratory stertor 169
respiratory system
    examination 15, 165–7
    neonate 86–8
    normal structure and function 165
restraint
    CSF collection 199–200, **200**
    dehorning 268
    disbudding 267
    foot trimming **234**
    mastectomy 283
    teat surgery 282

resuscitators 88, **88**
reticuloperitonitis, traumatic 124
retinol 311
retrobulbar block 340
Rhododendron 314–15, **315**
rib fracture, newborn 86, **86**
rickets 217–18
Rift Valley fever 43, 330, **331**
ringwomb 70–1
ringworm 265, **265**
Robert-Jones bandage 220
rock salt **305**
rotavirus 142
routine procedures 18
rubber ring castration 56, **56**
rumen
    acidosis 122–3, **122**, 136, 203
    contractions 119
    examination of contents 350
    fistula 124, **125**
    trocarisation 124
    tympany (bloat) 121–2, 129, 209, 210
rumen fluid 113–14, **114**, 122, 123
rumenitis 122–3, 186, **186**
rumenocentesis 113–14
rumenotomy 124–5

Saanen goat 3, **6**
St John's Wort 252, *317*
saline, hypertonic 343
Salmonella spp. 93, 147, 348
salmonellosis 41, 147–8
salpingitis 82
sample collection
    aborted kid 34–5, 352
    post-mortems 351, **352**
Sarcina spp. 128, **128**, 129
sarcocystosis 120
Sarcoptes scabiei var. *caprae* 255–6
sarcoptic mange 255–6, **256**
scald (interdigital dermatitis) 230–2, **231**
Schirmer tear test 286, **286**
Schmallenberg virus 42, 99, 330
scrapie 210–12
scrotal circumference 47, **48**
seborrhoeic dermatitis (pygmy goat syndrome)
    251–2, **252**
sedation 72, 333–4
    reversal 334
selenium deficiency 184, 308–9
selenium sulphide washes 252, 254, 264
semen
    collection 26, 47–8
    evaluation 47–9
seminal vesiculitis 52
septal defects 181–2, **182**
septic shock 93
septicaemia, neonatal 93–5
sigmoidoscope, human 27, **27**
silage 7, **8**
    listeriosis 40–1, **41**, 206, 208

silage clamp **8**, 313, *314*
sinusitis 169
skin
    examination 249–50
    skin necrosis 252, 253, 262, *320*
    non-infectious disorders 250–3
    parasitic diseases 253–60
skin biopsy 250, **250**
skin innervation, autonomous zones **205**
skin scrape 249, **249**
small ruminant lentivirus (SRLV) 225
smartphone technology **180**
smoke bomb test **166**
smooth muscle relaxants 71, 241
snake bites 172, *188*, 253
sodium bicarbonate 101, 123, 343
sodium iodide 118
somatic cell count (SCC) 271, 277, 278
space requirements 11, 107
sperm
    abnormalities *46*, **47**
    examination 49
spermatic cord, ligation/clamping 56, **57**
spermatogenesis 45, 59
spinal abscess 204, **204**
spinal cord lesions *197*, 201
spleen 187
splinting 219, *220*
squamous cell carcinoma (SCC) 290–1
stance, abnormal **91**, 101, 197, 199, 202, *205*, **205**
staphylococci, coagulase-negative 275
Staphylococcus aureus 258, 263, **263**, 275, 276
Staphylococcus aureus subsp. *anaerobius* 263, 265
Staphylococcus hyicus 263
Staphylococcus intermedius 263
'star-gazing' 203
starvation, pre-operative 334
sticky kid disease 104
stomach contents, abnormal *314*
stomach tube 15–16, **16**, 122
stomatitis *see* oral lesions
strabismus *196*, **196**
straw, feeding **123**
Streptococcus spp. 82, 93, 227, 246
    group D 183
streptothricosis 264
stress 13
Stromal abscess 289–90, **289**
Strongyloides 154
subacute rumen acidosis (SARA) 122–3
subconjunctival injection 18, **19**, 292
suck reflex 196
subcutaneous injection 16
sudden death 119, 149, 172, 174, 184, 185, 186, 300, 308,
    316, 317, *317*, 319, 329
sulphonamides 245
supernumerary teats 281–2, **281**
superovulation programme 27, **28**
suprascapular nerve *205*
surgery, general principles 334–5
swainsonine 202

swayback
    congenital 102, 306–7
    delayed 306, 307, **307**
swelling disease 191, **191**, 312
synechiae 290, 293, **293**
synovial fluid 216, *354*

Taenia multiceps 213
tail flagging 22, **22**
tape strips 249
tapetum lucidum 285
tapeworms 160–1
    carnivore 213–14
tarsorrhaphy 290, 292, 293
taxine 315–16
Taxus baccata 315–6, **315**, **316**
tear apparatus 285
teat biting 272, **272**
teat blocks 341
teat feeders 105, **106**
teat lesions 260–1, 263, **263**, 265, **280**, 325
teats
    fishtail 282
    supernumerary 281–2
    surgery 282–3
    trauma 272, **272**, 280, **280**, **283**
    washing/disinfection 280
Teladorsagia/Ostertagia nematodes 154
tendonectomy 98–9, **99**
tendons
    contracted 98–9, **99**
    injuries 223–4
    laxity 99, 103
terminology 3
testes
    absent/incomplete descent 51–2, **52**
    degeneration/atrophy 49–50, **51**
    examination 47
    hypoplasia 49
    neoplasia 55, **55**
    normal structure and function 45, **45**
    retained 51–2
tetanus 209–10, 334
tethering 12
tetracyclines 31, 38, 82, 229
tetralogy of Fallot 182
thermoregulation 12, 89–90, 103
thiamine (vitamin B1) 203, 204
third eyelid flap 290, **290**, 293
thorax
    auscultation 166–7, 179
    radiography 167, **167**
    tumours 172
thrombosis 185–7
thymus 187
    enlargement 189–90, 266
    neoplasia 172, 190, **191**
thyroid gland 310–11
thyroxine (T4) 310, 311
tibial nerve *205*, **205**
tick-borne diseases 42, 181, 193–4, 213, 258

tick pyaemia 258
ticks 42, 258, **258**
tocopherol 184, 191, 308–9, 312
toclopramide 132
Toggenburg goat **3**
toltrazuril 146
tongue lesions 120
tooth eruption 114–5, *114*
total bacterial count 278
total protein (TP) 91, *181*
toxicities 313–21
    causing abortion 44
    causing nephrosis 245
    causing neurological disease 202
    gases/fumes 171–2, 313
    investigation 313, *314*
    treatment approach 313
    water 321
    see also plants, toxic and specific toxins
Toxoplasma gondii 35, 293
toxoplasmosis 33, 35–6, **35**, **36**
trace element deficiencies 305–11
trachea, narrowing 167, **167**
tracheotomy 167–9, **168**
transcervical intrauterine insemination 27
trauma
    blood vessels 187
    drenching gun 119–20, **119**
    ears 295–7, **296**
    eye 287
    fractures 219–21
    horns 267, **268**
    joint dislocation 223
    tendon 223
    udder/teats 272, **272**, 280, **280**
    uterine tract 29–30, **29**
traumatic reticuloperitonitis 124, 183
treponeme-associated foot disease 232–3, **233**
trichobezoars 126
Trichophyton spp. 265
Trichostrongylus 154
Trichuris 154
trimethoprim/sulphonamides 82, 247
triplets **75**
trough space 7
Truperella pyogenes 82, 119, 169, 170, 183, 186, 227
    mastitis 275, 276
tube cystotomy 243–4, **243**, **244**
tuberculosis 176, **177**, 275, 328–9, **328**
tylosin 229

udder
    atrophy 274
    bluetongue lesions 327, **327**
    enlargement 272, **272**
    examination 271–2
    fibrosis **276**
    impetigo 263, **263**
    induration **271**
    infectious disorders 274–81
    non-infectious diseases 272–4
    surgery 281–4

ulnar nerve *205*
umbilical hernia 137–8, **137**
    repair 140–2
umbilical stump
    bleeding 77, **77**
    care 95, **95**
umbilicus
    infections 138–9, **139**
    normal structure and function 137
    surgery 139–42
underbite 115, **115**
upper motor neuron (UMN) system/lesions 195–7, 198
urachitis 138–9
urachus, patent 139, 140–2
uraemia 98, 240, 244–5
urea:creatinine ratio 239
urea, dietary levels 319
urea poisoning 319
ureters 237
urethra 237
    obstruction 240–1, **240**
urethral process (filiform appendage) 45, **45**, 237
    removal 241
urethrotomy 242–3, **243**
urinalysis 237–8, *238*, **238**, *314*, *354*
urine, abnormal colour *314*
urinary tract
    bladder, calculi 240
    examination 237–9
    neonate 97–8
    normal structure and function 237
urination, frequent 29, 246
urine acidification 242, 247
urine output 94, **94**, 237
urine retention 97–8, **97**
urolithiasis *237*, 240–1, **240**
uroperitoneum, diagnosis 240
uterine artery, thrombus 187
uterus
    acquired disorders 29–30
    amputation 81
    congenital disorders 28–9
    endometritis 30–1, **30**
    neoplasia 31–2, **31**
    normal structure and function 21
    post-partum infection 82–3, **83**
    prolapse 79–81
    rupture 66–7, 79
    torsion 71, **72**
uveitis 290, 293, 295

vagal indigestion 121, 125–6
vagina
    laceration 78
    prolapse 65–6, **65**, 79
vaginal dilation, failure 70

vaginal discharge 30, 43
vaginal speculum **27**
vaginitis, necrotic 84
valethamate bromide 71
vas deferens, ligation 58, **58–9**
vasculitis 187
vasectomy 57–8, **58**, **59**
Velpeau sling *220*, 223
vena cava thrombosis 177, 180, 186–7, **186**
venereal disease 59
venous thrombosis 185–6
ventilation 11–2, **165**, 165, **166**
ventricular dilation 184, **185**
ventricular septal defect (VSD) 181–2, **182**
vestibular syndrome 197, **197**, 198
vitamin A 311
vitamin B group 203, 204, 309–10
vitamin D 187, 217–18
vitamin E 184, 191, 308–9, 312
vitreous humour, analysis 299, 300, *354*
vomiting 315
vulva
    acquired disorders 29, **29**, 30
    congenital disorders 97–8, **97**
    sutures **29**, 80, **80**
vulvoplasty 66
vulvovaginitis 32–3, 43, 54, 59

Walpole's solution 244
warble fly 258
water provision 9, **10**, 251
water quality 305, 321, **321**
wattles 14, 22, **22**
weakness (paresis) 195, 198, *198*, 214, 299–300, 306–7, 308
weaning 106–7
Weingart frame 125
white line disease 234–5
white muscle disease 308–9, **309**
Winkler's cervicoplasty 66
withdrawal reflex 196
world goat population 1–2
World Organisation for Animal Health (OIE) 323
worm burden 187, 189
wounds, non-healing 222, **222**

xylazine hydrochloride 65, 72, 133, 333, 335, 338

yersiniosis 148
yew 315–16, **315**, **316**

zinc deficiency 250–1
zinc sulphate turbidity test 91
zoonotic pathogens 35, 37–40, 43, 142, **143**, 146–8, 161, 163, 191, 212, 255, **261**, 265, 328, 329, 348

T - #0563 - 071024 - C392 - 261/194/17 - PB - 9780367893422 - Gloss Lamination